OFFSPRING

Human Fertility Behavior in Biodemographic Perspective

Panel for the Workshop on the Biodemography of
Fertility and Family Behavior

Kenneth W. Wachter and Rodolfo A. Bulatao, *Editors*

Committee on Population
Division of Behavioral and Social Sciences and Education

NATIONAL RESEARCH COUNCIL
OF THE NATIONAL ACADEMIES

THE NATIONAL ACADEMIES PRESS
Washington, D.C.
www.nap.edu

THE NATIONAL ACADEMIES PRESS • 500 Fifth Street, N.W. • Washington, DC 20001

NOTICE: The project that is the subject of this report was approved by the Governing Board of the National Research Council, whose members are drawn from the councils of the National Academy of Sciences, the National Academy of Engineering, and the Institute of Medicine. The members of the committee responsible for the report were chosen for their special competences and with regard for appropriate balance.

This study was supported by Award No. NO1-OD-4-2139, TO #71 to the National Academies from the National Institute for Child Health and Human Development. Additional funding was provided by the Andrew W. Mellon Foundation. Any opinions, findings, conclusions, or recommendations expressed in this publication are those of the author(s) and do not necessarily reflect the views of the organizations or agencies that provided support for the project.

Library of Congress Cataloging-in-Publication Data

Workshop on the Biodemography of Fertility and Family Behavior.
Offspring : human fertility behavior in biodemographic perspective : proceedings of a workshop / Kenneth W. Wachter, Rodolfo A. Bulatao, editors.
p. cm.
"Panel for the Workshop on the Biodemography of Fertility and Family Behavior."
Includes bibliographical references and index.
ISBN 0-309-08718-X
1. Fertility, Human—Congresses. 2. Demography—Congresses. I. Title: Human fertility behavior in biodemographic perspective. II. Wachter, Kenneth W. III. Bulatao, Rodolfo A., 1944- IV. Title.
QP251.W665 2003
304.6'32—dc21
2003000077

Additional copies of this report are available from the National Academies Press, 500 Fifth Street, N.W., Lockbox 285, Washington, DC 20055; (800) 624-6242 or (202) 334-3313 (in the Washington metropolitan area); Internet, http://www.nap.edu.

Printed in the United States of America.

Suggested citation: National Research Council. (2003). *Offspring: Human Fertility Behavior in Biodemographic Perspective.* Panel for the Workshop on the Biodemography of Fertility and Family Behavior. Kenneth W. Wachter and Rodolfo A. Bulatao, eds. Committeee on Population, Division of Behavioral and Social Sciences and Education. Washington, DC: The National Academies Press.

THE NATIONAL ACADEMIES

Advisers to the Nation on Science, Engineering, and Medicine

The **National Academy of Sciences** is a private, nonprofit, self-perpetuating society of distinguished scholars engaged in scientific and engineering research, dedicated to the furtherance of science and technology and to their use for the general welfare. Upon the authority of the charter granted to it by the Congress in 1863, the Academy has a mandate that requires it to advise the federal government on scientific and technical matters. Dr. Bruce M. Alberts is president of the National Academy of Sciences.

The **National Academy of Engineering** was established in 1964, under the charter of the National Academy of Sciences, as a parallel organization of outstanding engineers. It is autonomous in its administration and in the selection of its members, sharing with the National Academy of Sciences the responsibility for advising the federal government. The National Academy of Engineering also sponsors engineering programs aimed at meeting national needs, encourages education and research, and recognizes the superior achievements of engineers. Dr. Wm. A. Wulf is president of the National Academy of Engineering.

The **Institute of Medicine** was established in 1970 by the National Academy of Sciences to secure the services of eminent members of appropriate professions in the examination of policy matters pertaining to the health of the public. The Institute acts under the responsibility given to the National Academy of Sciences by its congressional charter to be an adviser to the federal government and, upon its own initiative, to identify issues of medical care, research, and education. Dr. Harvey V. Fineberg is president of the Institute of Medicine.

The **National Research Council** was organized by the National Academy of Sciences in 1916 to associate the broad community of science and technology with the Academy's purposes of furthering knowledge and advising the federal government. Functioning in accordance with general policies determined by the Academy, the Council has become the principal operating agency of both the National Academy of Sciences and the National Academy of Engineering in providing services to the government, the public, and the scientific and engineering communities. The Council is administered jointly by both Academies and the Institute of Medicine. Dr. Bruce M. Alberts and Dr. Wm. A. Wulf are chair and vice chair, respectively, of the National Research Council.

www.national-academies.org

PANEL FOR THE WORKSHOP ON THE BIODEMOGRAPHY OF FERTILITY AND FAMILY BEHAVIOR

KENNETH W. WACHTER (*Chair*), Department of Demography, University of California, Berkeley

JOHN N. HOBCRAFT, Population Investigation Committee, London School of Economics

JEROME KAGAN, Department of Psychology, Harvard University

HILLARD S. KAPLAN, Department of Anthropology, University of New Mexico

HANS-PETER KOHLER, Research Group on Social Dynamics and Fertility, Max Planck Institute for Demographic Research, Rostock, Germany

DAVID LAM, Population Studies Center, University of Michigan, Ann Arbor

JANE MENKEN, Institute of Behavioral Sciences, University of Colorado, Boulder

GERALD P. SCHATTEN, Department of Obstetrics, Gynecology and Reproductive Sciences and Department of Cell Biology and Physiology, University of Pittsburgh School of Medicine

RODOLFO A. BULATAO, *Study Director*

ANA-MARIA IGNAT, *Senior Project Assistant*

COMMITTEE ON POPULATION
(June 2000)

JANE MENKEN (*Chair*), Institute of Behavioral Sciences, University of Colorado, Boulder
ELLEN BRENNAN-GALVIN, Woodrow Wilson Center for International Scholars, Washington, DC
JANET CURRIE, Department of Economics, University of California, Los Angeles
JOHN N. HOBCRAFT, Population Investigation Committee, London School of Economics
CHARLES B. KEELY, Institute for the Study of International Migration, Georgetown University
DAVID I. KERTZER, Department of Anthropology, Brown University
DAVID LAM, Population Studies Center, University of Michigan, Ann Arbor
CYNTHIA B. LLOYD, Population Council, New York
W. HENRY MOSLEY, Department of Population and Family Health Sciences, Johns Hopkins University
ALBERTO PALLONI, Center for Demography and Ecology, University of Wisconsin, Madison
JAMES W. VAUPEL, Max Planck Institute for Demographic Research, Rostock, Germany
KENNETH W. WACHTER, Department of Demography, University of California, Berkeley
LINDA J. WAITE, Population Research Center, University of Chicago

BARNEY COHEN, *Director*

Preface

Having children is a biological imperative for the survival of a group, and a wanted child can be a biological coup for a couple, a supreme biological moment—of possible peril and triumph—for a woman. Yet demographic interest in fertility has, for decades, been driven less by such concerns than by the threat of rapid population growth and the issue, for couples and women, of unplanned fertility. This volume seeks to encourage more balance and depth in the treatment of fertility in population studies. It suggests that many fertility behaviors that concern demographers may follow biodemographic templates, are influenced by genetic endowment, are triggered through hormonal pathways, and have been shaped in specific directions in the course of human evolution.

Since the middle of the 20th century, the contrast between small families in developed countries and large families and burgeoning populations in developing countries has fueled concern about deepening poverty, global inequality, and escalating environmental burdens. These concerns have not disappeared, as global population continues to expand. Yet much of the expansion is now effectively a hangover from the high-fertility decades, and many countries, both developed and developing, have entered an era of subreplacement fertility.

The confluence of the largely successful (though still incomplete) worldwide effort to tame high fertility and the emergence of genetic approaches to understanding human behavior provide a stimulus to review the focus of demographic work on fertility, to enlarge its concerns with biological and evolutionary questions. The Committee on Population took on this task with the understanding that researchers in the area were pursuing a variety of independent approaches that required a common, unifying focus. Some work in the area, such as studies of twins and adoptees, has also generated controversy, despite being pursued aggressively. With advice from the Committee on Population, the Board on Life Sciences, and the Institute of Medicine's Board on Neuroscience and Behavioral Health, the National Research Council (NRC) appointed a panel to organize a workshop on the topic. This volume is the result.

The papers contained in this volume were presented at the Workshop on the Biodemography of Fertility and Family Behavior, held at the National Academies in Washington, D.C., in June 2002, building on a preliminary meeting in February 2002 at the Beckman Center in Irvine, California. The workshop in a sense complemented an earlier workshop in April 1996 on biodemographic aspects of longevity (published as *Between Zeus and the Salmon: The Biodemography of Longevity*). Both workshops brought together demographers, evolutionary theorists, geneticists, and biologists to consider questions at the interface between the social sciences and the life sciences.

The papers were subsequently reviewed in draft form by individuals chosen for their diverse perspectives and technical expertise, in accordance with procedures approved by the NRC's Report Review Committee. The purpose of this independent review was to provide candid and critical comments to assist the institution in making the published volume as sound as possible and to ensure that the volume meets institutional standards for objectivity, evidence, and responsiveness to the study charge.

We thank the following individuals for contributing to the review: Nicholas G. Blurton Jones (University of California at Los Angeles), Sue Carter (University of Illinois at Chicago), Peter T. Ellison (Harvard University), John Haaga (Population Reference Bureau), Jennifer Harris (National Institute on Aging), Kristin Hawkes (University of Utah), Jerome Kagan (Harvard University), John J. Lepri (University of North Carolina at Greensboro), Kimber McKay (University of Montana), Monique Borgerhoff Mulder (University of California, Davis), Gerald P. Schatten (University of Pittsburgh School of Medicine), Barbara Smuts (University of Michigan, Ann Arbor), Kim Wallen (Emory University), and Maxine Weinstein (Georgetown University). The review of the entire volume was overseen by Michael Murphy of the London School of Economics. Although these individuals provided constructive comments and suggestions, responsibility for the content of this volume rests entirely with the authors and the institution.

Work on this project was stimulated and encouraged by Christine Bachrach of the National Institute for Child Health and Human Development and was supported under a contract with the institute. We are grateful for her continued attention to the core issues that the volume addresses and to raising many questions that helped shape and enrich the volume. Additional funding was provided by the Andrew W. Mellon Foundation.

We are especially grateful to Kenneth Wachter, who chaired the panel that organized the workshop, providing the spark and vital judgments about appropriate participants. The other members of the panel that organized the workshop each made important contributions in helping delineate relevant topics, identify participants, and critique their contributions, and in some cases writing papers themselves. We also wish to thank Randy Bulatao who, as study director, enriched the workshop with broad perspectives and guided the endeavor through many challenges. Ana-Maria Ignat provided active staff support. Barbara Bodling O'Hare skillfully edited the report and Yvonne Wise guided the manuscript through the publication process.

Jane Menken, *Chair*
Committee on Population

Contents

Tables and Figures

TABLES

FIGURES

OFFSPRING

Human Fertility Behavior in Biodemographic Perspective

1

Biodemography of Fertility and Family Formation

Kenneth W. Wachter

This volume explores the relevance of new developments in biology, genetics, and evolutionary anthropology to our understanding of human fertility behavior and family formation, under the rubric of "biodemography." The biology of fecundity, infecundity, and contraception has long been integral to human population studies. But demographers are only beginning to assimilate findings and approaches from behavioral genetics, molecular genetics, neuro-endocrinology, and cross-species life history analysis and to place them in the context of evolutionary theory. With support from the National Institute of Child Health and Human Development, the National Research Council's Committee on Population has brought together an interdisciplinary group to review this young field of science and reflect on promising opportunities for future research.

"Come, meet our offspring." The parent who says something like that is more likely to be found in a cartoon than in a living room or shopping mall. But the biological term "offspring" summons up a world of interconnections between the having of human children and the deeply scripted life-history dances in which creatures all renew and perpetuate their kind. Conscious choice, conditioned within social and economic systems, is the preoccupation of demographers, along with tabulations of "fertility" in the narrow sense of numbers of children born. But conscious choice colors a few links in a wider loop of impulse and empowerment, in which genes are linked to proteins, proteins to hormones, neurons, and gametes, bodily directives to organized behaviors, bonding, courtship, nurture, and childbearing to the demographic outcome measure, net generational replacement, and finally through the filter of natural selection, back to the evolving genes, bringing the loop full circle. This metaphor, articulated by Randy Bulatao, the director of this National Research Council study, may serve in place of any formal definition to indicate our subject's scope.

In practice, in choosing topics for this volume, the organizing panel began with two areas in which sizable amounts of research familiar to demographers already exist. These areas are twin studies from behavioral genetics and anthropological studies of intergenerational transfers drawing on evolutionary theory. From these two starting points, represented in this volume by Chapters 2 and 7, the panel reached outward, seeking to include a selection of research pertaining to as many as possible of the links in the great loop. Of course, only a sampling is possible. The hope has been to survey and stimulate prospects for new initiatives in boundary-crossing research.

Biology and demography have always been intertwined, even before the days when Darwin was reading Malthus. Demographic studies over recent decades in the area of fertility reinforce the connections. Examples include work on proximate determinants by Kingsley Davis and Judith Blake (1956) and by John Bongaarts and Robert Potter (1983), the fertility exposure analysis of John Hobcraft and Rod Little (1984), the mathematical models of conception and birth of Mindel Sheps and Jane Menken (1973), and the insights into hormonal conditioning of gender roles and demographic outcomes in the 1994 presidential address of Richard Udry to the Population Association of America. (Any selection is necessarily personal.) But the biological and social sciences have both been changing so rapidly that they easily come to seem like strangers, needing fresh introductions to each other.

The most visible interdigitation of the new biology with the new demography, evoked by the name "biodemography" has been in the study of longevity. The Committee on Population published an early overview of that field, *Between Zeus and the Salmon,* in 1997 under the editorship of Wachter and Finch (National Research Council, 1997). The state of play in the areas of fertility and family formation on the occasion of the present volume differs from the state of play in the area of longevity. Students of longevity work with a definitive outcome—death. That contrasts with the many outcome measures and intermediate processes of transition summed up under a general heading like "Fertility Behavior" or "Family Formation." The biodemography of longevity has been channeled in particular directions by a set of initiating discoveries, measurements of hazard curves tapering at extreme ages in Mediterranean fruit flies, Drosophila, and nematode worms. The biodemography of fertility has not gathered force from some canon of particular discoveries but has grown out of overlapping interests. For longevity the biodemographic agenda is closely tied to the practical imperative to forecast the pace of gains against old age mortality in the new century. For fertility the specifically biodemographic agenda does not center on a short list of policy questions but ranges widely across a spectrum of concerns.

Side by side with these differences go a host of commonalities. Most striking are new forms of data presenting opportunities for both areas. These opportunities are described in the Committee on Population's volume *Cells and Surveys* edited by Finch, Vaupel, and Kinsella (National Research Council, 2000). That volume takes up a range of biological indicators—genetic, hormonal, and functional—that will progressively become available in conjunction with detailed survey information on socioeconomic background and demographic choices for population-based samples.

Along with data opportunities, the different branches of biodemography share a reliance on evolutionary theory and on the clues to the human evolutionary environment that anthropology provides. Reproductive fitness in the face of natural selection is measured as a joint function of age-specific rates of survival and fertility. Both figure together in attempts to give mathematical expression to the implications for fitness of age-specific patterns of social support, intergenerational transfers, and constrained resources. Similarly, posited trade-offs between survival and fertility and associated pleiotropic genes (genes with multiple effects) may help explain how demographic schedules come to have the shapes they do.

Biodemography directly encompasses the study of fecundity and the physiology of reproductive success. This field is already vast and active. The Committee on Population decided not to try to cover it, inevitably superficially, in this volume but to concentrate attention on behavior. Here "fertility" denotes the outcome measure of children born, incorporating all the interventions of social and individual choice, while "fecundity" denotes the biological capacity for childbearing. Naturally, no clean separation can be made, but fecundity and infecundity, reproductive disorders, reproductive technology, and the physiology of contraception are kept in the background so as to give space to incipient work on behavioral pathways. Ellison's (2001) *On Fertile Ground* covers aspects related to fecundity that are given less attention here, and Sarah Hrdy's (1999) *Mother Nature* serves as a bridge between these complementary emphases.

RESPONSIBLE RESEARCH

Behaviors relating to fertility and family are central to the creation of life and the well-being of individuals, families, and societies. Understandably, research on these behaviors can be controversial and how societies use scientific knowledge about these behaviors is even more so. Scientists need to be sensitive to the strongly-held and often diverse values that surround fertility and family issues.

Although ethical issues in the responsible conduct of research are not the explicit subject of this volume, they pervade and need to inform all of the topics treated here, and the contributors to this volume held extensive discussions of these issues among themselves. A number of topics specific to genetic studies are treated in Michael Rutter's chapter. Several general principles emerging from the discussions are also worth emphasizing for the sake of productive learning and exchange. It is important for us as scientists to ensure that we represent our science accurately, avoiding the temptation to draw less than fully warranted conclusions that may attract attention but also foster misunderstandings of what we know and what we do not know. It is also important that researchers not leap from scientific findings to policy prescriptions. Science does not tell us what we ought to do. It can inform decisions, but it cannot take the place of social, political, and moral choice.

At the same time, scientists are called on to abandon the arrogant fiction that science can be a "thing apart" from the rest of society. This call involves, on the one hand, recognizing the extent to which our own perspectives and values may influence the science we do and how we interpret it. It involves, on the other hand, recognizing the potential power of scientific "facts" to influence the larger society. It is incumbent on all of us as scientists to do what we can to keep the facts straight, challenging assumptions and methods openly and often, fostering active debate over interpretations of findings and of their implications, and taking these debates outside the boundaries of scientific discussion if necessary to correct misinterpretations.

This volume is organized around contributing disciplines. It moves from work in behavioral genetics to areas of molecular genetics, neuroscience and endocrinology, and comparative integrative biology. These are followed by treatments based on evolutionary theory and anthropology, rounded out by perspectives from economic and social demography.

BEHAVIORAL GENETICS

In Chapter 2, Michael Rutter begins with an overview of what is being learned and what can be learned from behavioral genetics about genetic influences on fertility. It is reasonable to expect some genetic transmission of components of tastes, skills, and impulses that work themselves out in courtship, family planning, and family building. Rutter cites evidence for moderate heritability of traits like social attachment and pair bonding and outcomes like age at first sexual intercourse and marriage dissolution and for number of children. Measures of heritability encapsulate information about genetic influences on differences among people in a population. But Rutter cautions firmly against inferring genetic determinants of differences in levels of traits from group to group and against readily ascribing changes in levels of traits over time to the same factors that modulate individual differences.

The stock in trade of behavioral genetics is the use of twin studies. Rutter spells out the strong assumptions underlying twin study designs and offers caveats, as do Kamin and Goldberger (2002). For demographers interested in courtship, marriage, and family formation, another issue arises, not taken up in Chapter 2, namely, the specialness of identical twins with respect to social experiences where physical appearance matters.

Chapter 3 by Kohler and Rodgers provides an illustrative case study of how current behavioral genetic approaches are being applied in practice to fertility behavior. (A fuller set of examples is found in Rodgers, Rowe, and Miller [2000] and Rodgers and Kohler [2002].) Kohler and Rodgers draw on the Danish twin registry and an associated 1994 survey for fertility and education histories of 2,729 pairs of same-sex twins born over 17 years between 1953 and 1970. They analyze within-pair correlations in numbers of children born to the twins. Their chapter puts on view a whole range of statistical tools employed by practitioners.

Kohler and Rodgers find rapid changes across birth cohorts in correlations for female identical (monozygotic) twins not mirrored by correlations for sororal (dizygotic) twins and show that educational variables partially account for these changes in a statistical sense. Their analysis raises issues discussed further by John Hobcraft in Chapter 12. Kohler and Rodgers interpret their findings as evidence for underlying genetic effects that become visible in family formation choices when given freer rein by social and individual circumstances. In this case, the enabling factor is female education. Measured heritabilities are posited to change rapidly, not because genes change but because conditions change to let the genes have their say.

A debate runs through the chapters of this volume over the prospective uses of heritability estimates and twin-pair correlations from behavioral genetics. It would be eminently desirable if such estimates could aid in picking out traits, variables, and outcome measures most likely to reflect direct and potent genetic propensities. If suitable traits can be singled out and specified, capabilities are in hand to search for "quantitative trait loci," that is, for portions of chromosomes with detectable effects on quantitative traits. Any such guidance would also be welcome for designing studies of gene expression and ultimately for neuro-endocrine analyses.

But it is not clear that heritability estimates can serve these purposes. In Chapter 2, Rutter writes, "within a very broad range, variations among traits in their level of heritability have little or no meaning with respect to theory, policy, or practice." He goes on to say that "evidence that there is a significant heritability for fertility is completely uninformative with respect to causal mechanisms." Rutter sees the search for causal mechanisms as primary and the assessment of genetic influence as secondary, while acknowledging the value of behavioral genetic studies for "a better understanding of the nature-nurture interplay in the development of socially relevant behaviors."

Rutter's chapter can be read as a call for behavioral genetics in a new key. It is possible to go beyond statistical path diagrams and measures of association. Broader opportunities are now opening up for including what Rutter calls "discriminating and sensitive measures of the environment" in behavioral genetic studies. Techniques for direct monitoring of environmental exposures and stimuli for individuals are in rapid development. They dovetail with approaches for making use of biological indicators of hormonal and other physiological responses, as described in the National Research Council's 2000 volume *Cells and Surveys,* already mentioned. Such measures are particularly relevant for studies of fertility behavior, since hormonal signaling must play a role in so many pathways of influence.

The National Longitudinal Study of Adolescent Health ("Add Health"), whose first wave of home interviews were conducted in 1995, is providing researchers with data on familial correlations for a wide range of traits plausibly bearing on fertility. Jacobson and Rowe's (1999) study of depressed moods in adolescents is an example. Where the outcomes of genetic predispositions are likely being modulated by social trends and circumstances, self-selection of individuals into particular niches has to be distinguished from causal influence. Information on school settings and experiences, peer-group composition, and parental treatment, such as Add Health collects, can give a basis for separating out genetic effects from the consequences of self-selection, social homogamy, and friends and family networks. For the topics central to this volume, later waves of the Add Health study should provide more extensive observations of union formation and childbearing as respondents grow toward adulthood.

Conclusions with regard to gene-environment interactions can be particularly convincing when genotypes are measured directly with molecular markers. Rowe at al. (2001) report one example involving numbers of marriages for women. Successes with such approaches are not yet frequent, but technology is improving. Supplementing twin and adoption studies, there are natural experiments taking place willy-nilly all around us which, with ingenuity, can be recognized and analyzed to advantage. The study of change over time stands to benefit from hard thinking about gene-environment correlations and feedbacks. Given such a range of opportunities, it is fair to expect that, for studies of fertility and family formation, the behavioral genetics of the future should bear little resemblance to the behavioral genetics of the past.

NEUROSCIENCE AND ENDOCRINOLOGY

If one said the word "biology" 25 years ago in demography, one would have been talking about the physiology of reproduction and contraception, occupying a couple of weeks in courses on fertility, or perhaps talking about deaths by cause. Since then, biology has spread across the intellectual landscape. This volume is itself an illustration of the phenomenon. Although sensible and cautious writers emphasize the complexity of causal pathways and the intricacy of interactions between genes and environments, the lure of biology is in dreams of explanatory power. Some diseases are present or absent thanks to one mutation in one gene. Hunts for "genes for X" and "genes for Y" sometimes succeed. When they do, they often point forward to the next steps in chains of causation. What can be true for diseases could be true for behaviors.

In Chapter 4, Larry Young describes a genetic discovery that exemplifies the dream. A modest change in one gene appears to be responsible for the presence of pair-bonding behavior in a species of small animals called prairie voles living in the American Midwest. The change is found in males in the regulatory portion of a gene for receptors that respond to the hormone vasopressin. It provides for receptors in an area of the brain associated with rewards. The prairie voles that form pair bonds have occurrences of a particular sequence of 420 base pairs of DNA in their version of the gene, as compared to their neighbors, the montane voles of the Rocky Mountain states, which do not form pair bonds. The full account, involving the hormone oxytocin in females as well as vasopressin in males, reads like a detective story.

What has been found is perhaps something like a switch in a wiring diagram in the middle of a network of interconnected circuitry. A lot of genes in combination make the voles' social attachments possible, but one kind of change in one gene has the eventual effect of turning them on or off. We are not to imagine that enduring love—Petrarch seeing Laura in the church pew—could be nothing other than an extrapotent battery of vasopressin receptors in the poet's brain. But it is clear that some complex behaviors have some clear-cut genetic controls. Triumphs like the one Young describes (only a handful are known so far) encourage us to look for dimensions of human partnering and procreative choice that might be modulated by identifiable genetic variations.

Less widely heralded than genomics but of complementary importance for demographers have been the strides in endocrinology, both in techniques for measuring and monitoring hormone levels and fluctuations and in the unravelling of systems of endocrine signaling. In Chapter 5, Judy Cameron summarizes our present understanding of the hormonal control systems for reproduction in men and women. She emphasizes the directing role of the brain and the complexity of the endocrine "code." The same hormone may stimulate a response at some levels or in some pulsatile patterns and suppress that response at other levels. Many hormonal influences on sexual function are paralleled by influences on sexual desire and behavior.

For the biodemography of fertility, Cameron points to several priorities for interdisciplinary research. One involves effects of extensive artificial exposure to steroids and other endocrinologically active substances now occurring in developed societies through medication, self-medication, and consumer choice. Another follows from experiments documenting the effects of psychosocial stress on hormone secretion, plausibly with implications not only for individual health but also for social gradients. Finally, Cameron directs renewed attention to the question of nutrition and fertility. She notes that biomedical scientists drawing on laboratory data tend to regard energetic stress as "an important regulator of reproductive ecology," posing a contrast, at least in emphasis, to the conclusions of demographers drawing on field data from populations.

In the abstract, one might have imagined that it could be an advantage in evolutionary terms for the reproductive systems of humans and other primates to turn off easily and automatically in the face of hard times. Gains in fitness might be thought to accrue from saving on large physiological and energetic investments in infants when chances for their survival were low and from concentrating resources on procreation when chances for infant survival were high. In fact, however, evolution seems to have honed our reproductive systems to turn on whenever they minimally can. Perhaps evolutionary environments were too unpredictable for automatic regulation to be worthwhile. It is tempting to wonder how different our overpopulated modern world might have been had we come to it endowed with built-in preventive checks on fertility.

INTEGRATIVE BIOLOGY

Happily, both the words "demography" and "population" have grown beyond their etymological roots in words for people and now apply to other species. The mathematical core of demography carries over directly. The species that have figured prominently up to now in the biodemography of longevity, including species of flies and worms, have little in the way of social structure. Now comprehensive demographic data on long-lived species with social structure are beginning to come into being. In Chapter 6, Jeanne Altmann and Susan Alberts treat us to an overview of the remarkable demography of populations of baboons from Amboseli, Kenya, based on observations collected over some 30 years. After setting the life course patterns of humans within the context of other mammals and other primates, they present original data on the pooled age-specific fertility and survival rates of baboon populations and describe the variations of reproduction and survival with abundance of food and dominance status.

The matrilineal dominance hierarchies that Altmann and Alberts describe give a tantalizing analog to the demographer's staple explanatory category, or socioeconomic status. Among the Amboseli baboons, within each group daughters tend to inherit their mother's rank. Rank matters. Low-ranking females have lower fertility. But occasionally, under favorable conditions members split off into a new group, with fewer members to outrank them. Possibly these social arrangements help regulate aggregate group fertility and population growth, with group fission supplying a mechanism for relaxation of constraints.

The account by Altmann and Alberts is a telling example of social behavior altering demographic parameters in another primate. Behavioral flexibility is not unique to humans. Reproductive effort includes both mating and parenting, and both components involve complex social strategizing in other primate species as well as our own. Investment in social relationships has demographic payoffs. It turns out that the patterns of response to food availability in the Amboseli baboons are similar to some of the human patterns described by Carol Worthman in Chapter 10.

Altmann and Alberts calculate quantities called elasticities that describe the sensitivity of population growth to small changes in age-specific rates of fertility and survival and that often serve as measures of susceptibility to forces of natural selection. Growth is much more sensitive to a proportional change in infant or child survival per year than to a proportional change in fertility per year. This finding might be taken to underline the significance of parenting behavior and investment in offspring quality over and above the maximization of offspring ever born. However, overall comparative effects are more complicated to calculate. From a baboon mother's point of view, improving average infant survival by some factor requires improving survival a dozen times over, for a dozen or so infants, whereas raising fertility in a year by the same factor is a one-time investment. Relative returns remain to be assessed. The power of the approach is the ability to perform parallel calculations of demographic trade-offs for humans and other primates, taking advantage of nature's natural experiments.

EVOLUTIONARY ANTHROPOLOGY

The terms of discourse of genetics are particularly attractive for organizing thinking about behaviors because they not only lead forward from genes to physiological mechanisms but also backwards from genes to their evolutionary origins. We ask not only what a gene produces in the body but also where it comes from out of prehistory. For human fertility behavior, we are a long way from carrying out such a program but not so far from understanding how some modern behavior may be rooted in the early exigencies of lineage survival. Such an evolutionary perspective is introduced in Chapter 7 by Hillard Kaplan and Jane Lancaster. Underlying their approach is the idea that natural selection has less to do with specific sequences of behavior and more to do with "norms of reaction," systems for adjustable responses to environmental stimuli. The celebrated diversity of human mating arrangements and reproductive norms and practices may reflect common evolutionary principles working themselves out in highly diverse ecological settings.

Kaplan and Lancaster's chapter is representative of a line of thought in which a kind of economic calculus takes its place alongside the traditional reproductive calculus in the reckoning of long-term fitness in the face of natural selection. This economic calculus involves constraints imposed by feasible age-specific production and consumption, returns to skill, social support, and resource transfers across generations.

In Kaplan and Lancaster's account, the modern concept of a quality-quantity trade-off in the demand for children has an analog for hominid foragers. Compared to chimpanzees, hominids came to concentrate on an ecological food niche, including hunted prey and extracted nutrients, which demanded and rewarded skill and learning. Prolonged juvenile training and dependence, protracted parental investment, larger brains, and longer life spans are seen as coevolving, driven by returns to investment in "embodied capital." In this picture, evolution would have been equipping humans not so much with an instinct toward maximizing total fertility as with instincts for adjusting familial resource transfers in response to the available lifetime returns to such investments.

Elements of this picture are subject to lively debate. An alternative reading of the paleoanthropological data would see the distinctive pacing of human life histories, with extended gestation, juvenile dependence, and training, as tending to precede rather than accompany the evolution of larger and more sophisticated brains. Views differ on how much weight to give to direct provisioning and how much to concomitant gains in status that could enhance mating opportunities. The area is one of active research.

Having outlined their overall perspective, Kaplan and Lancaster proceed in Chapter 7 with a whirlwind tour through human history, from foragers on to horticulturalists, pastoralists, agricultural civilizations, and industrialized societies. They point out along the way relationships between ecological settings and observed outcomes for male-female complementarity in provisioning and parenting, mating and marital systems, and age-specific economic returns. The modern examples are drawn especially from a U.S. perspective. Like the chapters that follow, Chapter 7 provides an entrée to an extensive corpus of existing scientific work.

Steven Gangestad, in Chapter 8, describes how various competing interests of the male and female members of a couple exist alongside their common interest in offspring. He intentionally divides the topic with Kaplan and Lancaster, focusing on conflicting stakes in parenting while they focus on complementarities. Biological processes in which male and female members of a species successively adapt to each other's own gene-promoting stratagems, in a generation-by-generation dance of action and reaction, is called "sexually antagonistic coevolution." Gangestad reports on experiments with *Drosophila*, dung flies, and finches showing such coevolution taking place. He reviews the theoretical implications for humans and describes observations of human behavior under controlled conditions that exemplify the predicted patterns. Among the surprises featured by Gangestad is an increase in a suite of "mate retention tactics" on the part of husbands specifically during the ovulatory phase of their wives' cycles. During the same phase, wives report fantasizing more often about other males. The biological studies provide a context for consideration of contemporary social phenomena in conflicts over parenting effort and marital instability.

Ben Campbell shifts the focus in Chapter 9 to adolescence, specifically reproductive maturation in boys. The topic goes beyond physical sexual maturation to include the endocrinological regulation of emotional and social development. Campbell advances a hypothesis of his own about the possible roles for two adrenal hormones acting progressively over an extended period from just before puberty into early adulthood. Campbell reflects on the evolutionary trade-offs implicated in this part of the human developmental program, on the gap in years between puberty and procreation in many human societies, and on the reversed order of peak growth spurt and menarche for girls compared to puberty and peak growth for boys. He considers refinements of the basic idea that timing of sexual maturation balances the benefits of earlier reproductive opportunities against the costs of risky male-male competition. The availability of biological indicators from populations with differing levels of nutritional advantage and differing norms governing risk taking, competition, violence, affiliation, and mating hold out the promise of testing hypotheses in this area in the coming years.

In Chapter 10, Carol Worthman draws on three approaches—life history theory, reproductive ecology, and developmental psychobiology—and discusses their strengths and limitations and what is to be gained by bringing them together. It is a wide-ranging chapter, taking up a variety of aspects of fertility and family formation not fully treated elsewhere in the volume. Alongside genetic transmission, Worthman stresses the importance of biocultural inheritance. She features the costs of sociality in evolutionary settings, and their implications for established patterns of behavior. She challenges proponents of life history theory to have a more realistic appreciation of the ubiquity of multi-tasking, as it bears on allocations of time and energy between production and parenting. Finally, she describes ideas about genetic plasticity and environmental feedbacks in the shaping of neuronal connections and more generally in physiological and psychological growth after conception that go under the general heading of "developmental Darwinism."

DEMOGRAPHY

The concluding chapters of this volume engage themes of the earlier chapters from demographic perspectives. In Chapter 11, David Lam explores intersections between rational choice models from economic demography and evolutionary approaches to human fertility transitions. Two fertility transitions are at stake—the classic "demographic transition" to near-replacement fertility still under way in many developing countries and the recent transition to below-replacement fertility most visible in a number of European nations. Lam develops the economic formalism for quality-quantity trade-offs and relates it to evolutionary treatments like the one by Kaplan and Lancaster in Chapter 7. For the ultimate goal of predicting fertility levels, quality-quantity frameworks remain in need of a basis for predicting how much child quantity should trade off against how much child quality, which neither approach as yet supplies.

In modern settings, education provides a proxy for child quality. Lam illustrates rational choice theory with empirical results on education, income, women's employment, and fertility in Brazil. It would be interesting, as John Haaga has pointed out in discussing chapters of this volume, to include in such a nexus of variables the gains in status that education may provide to women when entering the marriage market and when negotiating fertility decisions in marriage, as Basu (1999) has described. The human setting is an intriguing parallel to the importance of hierarchical status to evolutionary fitness among some primates illustrated in Chapter 6.

At first encounter, many people expect that evolutionary theory has to have a problem with below-replacement fertility. In principle, it need not. When the environment is transformed, appetites and responses that would once have tended to maximize an individual's descendants may operate instead to reduce them. There are often evolutionary explanations for presently mal-adaptive traits.

Even moderate fertility mediated by quantity-quality trade-offs appears on the face of it mal-adaptive in the Darwinian sense. In Chapter 11, Lam reflects on how odd the demographic dynamics would have to be in the modern world for smaller numbers of high-quality children in one generation to pay off in greater numbers of grandchildren in the next generation.

But it would not be so odd for investments in child quality, status, and command over resources to empower lineages to survive severe rare bouts of hard times and mortality generations apart. In this respect, in the very long run, history and prehistory might not prove so different as they seem.

In Chapter 12, John Hobcraft reviews the prospects for cross-fertilization across the whole range of approaches represented in this volume, from behavioral genetics, experimental biology, endocrinology, evolutionary anthropology, and demography. He underlines the opportunities while recognizing barriers. Returning to the topics with which the volume begins, he scrutinizes problems of analysis that hinder general acceptance of results from the application of behavioral genetics to fertility behavior.

Hobcraft draws attention to the greater readiness of evolutionary anthropologists and behavioral ecologists to incorporate ideas from demography than of demographers to embrace evolutionary perspectives. In his view, "a central challenge facing these approaches . . . is the extent to which they are relevant to our understanding of the demographic transition and of changes in fertility behavior, especially to very low levels of fertility." He expresses a degree of skepticism about the ability of evolutionary theory to make testable predictions. These sections of Chapter 12 provide lively counterpoint to the ideas espoused in Chapters 7, 8, and 9.

Hobcraft goes on in Chapter 12 to describe a framework, developed in association with Kathleen Kiernan, for examining the decision to become a parent, with its long-term implications and uncertainties, in the English and European contemporary settings of low fertility. The biological factors discussed in this volume interact with a broad range of environmental demographic determinants, economic trade-offs, tastes and preferences, gender roles, the calculus of self-interest and joint interest, societal support, and future security. Granting parallels between this framework and behavioral ecology and life history analysis, Hobcraft describes the challenges facing a research agenda for uncovering genetic and neuro-endocrine substructures for fertility behaviors that are now so largely matters of conscious choice.

Is below-replacement fertility a puzzle? Hobcraft balances conflicting views on this central question. Evolution could have arranged for humans to act to maximize the numbers of descendants primarily through our evolved sex drives. In that case, with sexual satisfaction disconnected from the procreation of children by contraception, the lowest of low fertility would be no puzzle. On the other hand, evolution could have emphasized a whole repertoire of innate drives toward pair bonding, nurturing, and parental commitment, originally operating toward assuring the survival of offspring and now constituting instinctive incentives for childbearing. Many of the chapters in this volume present evidence for the salience of such evolved pathways of influence in other species and our own. Are we to regard such inborn impulses as typically being satisfied, in the modern world, with the birth and rearing of a single child? Hobcraft points to changes in mothers' brains during pregnancy and to physiological and psychological reinforcements to nurturing instincts during pregnancy and after birth, which one might interpret as part of an evolved set of mechanisms promoting further births.

Is human nature pro-natal? This term may stand as short-hand for some of the larger issues through which the biodemography of fertility behavior and family formation impinges on the practical demography of policy forecasts. The question makes sense when our evolutionary heritage is viewed not as a built-in program of behavioral directives but as a sounding-board for responses to ever-changing environmental stimuli. For Third World countries, trade-offs between child quantity and quality are seen as propelling transitions away from high fertility. Demographers are struggling to foresee the degree of ease and evenness with which such transitions may proceed across the whole of the globe. Biodemographers are asking about the deep structure of quality-quantity transfers, their evolutionary status and origins, and plausible long-term roles. For the developed world, below-replacement fertility can be seen as a logical concomitant of new gender roles and economic opportunities. Will it be sustained or will it prove a temporary aberration, incompatible in the long term with the instincts with which evolution has endowed us?

DIRECTIONS FOR FUTURE RESEARCH

The biodemography of fertility behavior and family formation is at a stage where lines of communication are being opened up across research domains, ideas are being floated, and groundwork is being laid. The field is not at the point of offering definite competing answers to a handful of sharply-posed questions. It follows that a wide diversity of research directions deserve consideration. Some have been mentioned in earlier sections and are spelled out in a number of the chapters that follow. This volume is not a consensus report, and all that can be offered in this introductory chapter is a personal selection.

Progress depends on data. Exciting opportunities for the future are likely to emerge from the gathering of biological indicators in demographic surveys, a prospect frequently mentioned in this chapter. We may learn whether the conscious reasons offered by individuals for wanting children, or for wanting or not wanting further children, sort themselves out by hormonal levels or other physiological measurements. Linkages between psychosocial stress and reproductive hormones are increasingly well understood from laboratory studies described in Chapter 6. Longitudinal surveys with biological markers are proving their worth in studies of long-term health and successful aging (e.g., National Research Council, 2001) and provide precedents for longitudinal studies of successful marital bonding, family planning, and parenting enriched by coordinated endocrinological and questionnaire-based measurements of stress and resilience.

In the area of behavioral genetics, a need has been described for new starts, moving beyond heritabilities and correlations and emphasizing (to borrow Michael Rutter's phrase) "discriminating and sensitive measures of the environment." Such new approaches might be able to exploit the individual-level time-series measurements of environmental conditions and exposures that are becoming practical. Both evolutionary theory and endocrinological investigations presented, for example, in Chapters 8 and 9 suggest that traits implicated in family formation outcomes, like risk-taking, may be more amenable to genetic analysis than fertility outcomes themselves. Separating genetic influences from self-selection may be aided by accumulating longitudinal data sets like the Add Health Study.

Molecular genetics has its own impetus and will take its own directions. Biodemographers are not for the most part qualified to suggest promising experiments, but they need to be poised to assimilate new molecular discoveries like those presented in Chapter 4. Such discoveries change the conceptual framework for thinking about subconscious sources of decisions and reactions. The suggestions about the kinds of reward circuitry involved in pair-bonding in one other species as described in Chapter 4 might well suggest novel survey designs for demographic fertility surveys. In the wake of advances in endocrinology, as discussed in Chapter 5, studies seem timely to relate psychosocial stress to hormone secretion and to reexamine links between nutrition and fertility.

The ongoing studies of the demography and social interactions of other primates in the wild, illustrated in Chapter 6, are likely to be critically fruitful sources of new ideas and perspectives for biodemography throughout the foreseeable future. In this area, the interests of biologists and the interests of demographers are already well coordinated and mutually reinforcing.

A rich variety of topics from evolutionary anthropology treated in Chapters 7, 8, 9, and 10 holding out promise for future research have been discussed in earlier sections. In the near term, comparative studies of the dynamics of grandparental provisioning and intergenerational support for offspring within an evolutionary framework appear to be at the top of the agenda, bringing together economists, sociologists, mathematical demographers, and anthropologists on common ground.

One gap in coverage in this volume needs to be borne in mind. Despite strenuous efforts, the organizing panel was not successful in recruiting a contribution dealing directly with brain research. Some topics from neuroscience are treated in Chapters 4 and 5, and their relevance is discussed in

Chapter 10, but a comprehensive overview would have been desirable. Rapid advances in brain-imaging techniques are being made. Hamer (2002) cites recent examples in which genetic influence on measured brain activity have proved far stronger than the downstream influences on behavior. Expanding knowledge of the role of the brain and the whole central nervous system in the physiology of sexual response and reproduction is likely to have long-term implications for the understanding of fertility behavior.

A theme that runs through many of the chapters of this volume is the salience of pair-bonding, parent-child bonding, and nurturance as they take their place beside sex and procreation as constituents of fertility behavior. Sexuality research has been a continuing priority within the social science community. Bonding research appears to deserve complementary emphasis. There is much to build on, including the discoveries from molecular genetics reported in Chapter 4, the endocrine pathways described in Chapter 5, the comparative perspective from other primates in Chapter 6, and the evolutionary tradeoffs analyzed in Chapters 7, 8, 9, and 10. As Chapters 11 and 12 make clear, demographers have strong incentives to supplement economic and social theories with an understanding of the biological dimensions of the choices of couples to stop at one child or to go on to further children. Through such pathways, biodemography impinges on the ever-present question of the persistence or transience of below-replacement fertility.

All these research priorities depend on the continuing development of communication and interaction between biological and social scientists. It is interesting to note how some specialists in fields of anthropology, genetics, and integrative biology have adopted ideas and approaches from demography. The mathematical core of demography makes it accessible as well as useful to others, and broader ideas are bound up with the mathematics and may be carried over in the process. Making genetics, neuroendocrinology, integrative biology, and evolutionary perspectives accessible to demographers may be a larger challenge. But the chapters of this volume illustrate the extensive common ground that already exists around the study of fertility behavior and family formation and the promise of future cooperative biodemographic research.

REFERENCES

Basu, A.

1999 Women's education, marriage, and fertility in South Asia: Do men really not matter? Pp. 267-286 in *Critical Perspectives on Schooling and Fertility in the Developing World*. Committee on Population. C. Bledsoe, J. Casterline, J. Johnson-Kuhn, and J. Haaga, eds. Commission on Behavioral and Social Sciences and Eduation. Washington, DC: National Academy Press.

Bongaarts, J., and R.G. Potter
1983 *Fertility, Biology, and Behavior: An Analysis of the Proximate Determinants.* New York: Academic Press.

Davis, K., and J. Blake
1956 An analytical framework. *Economic Development and Cultural Change* 4:211-235.

Ellison, P.T.
2001 *On Fertile Ground.* Cambridge, MA: Harvard University Press.

Hamer, D.
2002 Rethinking Behavior Genetics. *Science* 298:71-72.

Hobcraft, J.N., and R.J.A. Little
1984 Fertility exposure analysis: a new method for assessing the contribution of the proximate determinants to fertility.differentials. *Population Studies* 38:21-45.

Hrdy, S.B.
1999 *Mother Nature: A History of Mothers, Infants, and Natural Selection.* New York: Pantheon.

Jacobson, K.C., and D.C. Rowe
1999 Genetic and environmental influences on the relationships between family connectedness, school connectedness, and adolescent depressed mood: Sex differences. *Developmental Psychology* 35:926-939.

Kamin, L.J., and A.S. Goldberger
2002 Twin studies in behavioral research: A skeptical view. *Theoretical Population Biology* 61:83-95.

National Research Council
1997 *Between Zeus and the Salmon: The Biodemography of Longevity.* Committee on Population. K.W. Wachter and C.E. Finch, eds. Commission on Behavioral and Social Sciences and Eduation. Washington, DC: National Academy Press.
2000 *Cells and Surveys: Should Biological Measures Be Included in Social Science Research?* Committee on Population. C.E. Finch, J.W. Vaupel, and K. Kinsella, eds. Commission on Behavioral and Social Sciences and Eduation. Washington, DC: National Academy Press.
2001 *New Horizons in Health: An Integrative Approach.* Committee on Future Directions for Behavioral and Social Sciences Research at the National Institutes of Health, B.H. Singer and C.D. Ryff, eds., Board on Behavioral, Cognitive, and Sensory Sciences. Division of Behavioral and Social Sciences and Education. Washington, DC: National Academy Press.

Rodgers, J.L., and H.-P. Kohler, eds.
2002 *The Biodemography of Human Reproduction and Fertility.* Boston: Kluwer Academic Publishers.

Rodgers, J.L., D.C. Rowe, and W.B. Miller, eds.
2000 *Genetic Influences on Human Fertility and Sexuality: Theoretical and Empirical Contributions from the Biological and Behavioral Sciences.* Boston: Kluwer Academic Publishers.

Rowe, D.C., C. Stever, D. Chase, S. Sherman, A. Abramowitz, and I.D. Waldman
2001 Two dopamine genes related to reports of childhood retrospective inattention and conduct disorder. *Molecular Psychiatry* 6:429-433.

Sheps, M.C., and J.A. Menken
1973 *Mathematical Models of Conception and Birth.* Chicago: University of Chicago Press.

Udry, J.R.
1994 The nature of gender. *Demography* 31(4):561-573.

2

Genetic Influences on Fertility: Strengths and Limitations of Quantitative Inferences

Michael L. Rutter

There are many different reasons why society should be interested in the number of children being born and the numerous factors that influence this figure.

VARIATIONS IN FERTILITY

First, it is well established that there are strong psychopathological correlates of fertility. Thus, the number of children born to individuals with schizophrenia has tended to be below the general population's average (Jablensky, 2000). To some extent, this is likely to be a function of the social impairments that accompany schizophrenia, but it is also likely to be partly a function of the fact that, at least in the past, many individuals with schizophrenia have spent much of their adult lives in long-term hospital care. In addition, a contributory factor will be the effects on sexual behavior of the drugs used to treat schizophrenia. The situation could well change with the much greater use of so-called atypical drugs that are probably more effective in restoring near-normal social functioning and have lower rates of serious side effects. The expectation is that the use of these drugs will enable more individuals with schizophrenia to live in the community, and this could well have effects on the number of children born to them.

Somewhat similarly, very few individuals with autism have children and very few are born to parents with autism, at least as traditionally diagnosed (Rutter et al., 1997; Rutter, 2000a). For the most part, this is probably a function of the substantial impairment in the ability to develop committed reciprocal social relationships, particularly love relationships. In recent years, genetic findings have made it clear that the liability to autism extends much more broadly than the severely handicapping condition that is traditionally diagnosed. Very little is known about the fertility shown by individuals with this broader phenotype.

Conversely, antisocial behavior is associated with a larger average family size and a considerable tendency to start having children in the teenage years (Rutter et al., 1998; Moffitt and the E-Risk Team, 2002).

Second, there have been major trends in fertility patterns in recent years. The average number of children born to each couple has dropped markedly in most industrialized countries, and in many European countries the number is well below 2—and hence below population replacement rates (Hess, 1995). This has been associated with a parallel marked rise in the average age at which individuals have their first child. It might be expected from these figures that there would have been a very sharp fall in the number of births to teenage parents, but at least in the United States and the United Kingdom, the drop has been quite modest. The implication is that there has probably been a change over time in the *pattern* of births. Another change has been a major increase in the number of multiple births in most industrialized countries, this being a consequence of an increase in the use of various methods of assisted conception (Derom and Bryan, 2000).

Third, in many countries there are marked variations in average completed family size among ethnic groups. For example, in the United Kingdom the average number of children per family is much higher in people of Pakistani or Bangladeshi origin than in "white" families (Modood et al., 1997). There are even more marked differences in the pattern of births. Thus, in the United Kingdom the proportion of children born to one parent of Afro Caribbean origin and one Caucasian parent is very high, whereas the comparable figure is very low for those of Bangladeshi origin (39 versus 1 percent). Similarly, in the United Kingdom there are very marked differences among ethnic groups in the proportion of children reared by a single parent (Modood et al., 1997).

Concerns have been expressed over evidence that in many countries there has been a marked fall in men's sperm counts (Bostofte et al., 1983; Swan et al., 1997). It is not clear whether this has resulted in reduced male fecundity, but there may have been some effects of that kind. Whether there have been parallel changes in female fecundity is not yet known and the fecundity in both sexes needs to be considered in relation to possible effects on number of births (Joffe, 2000).

Finally, there is much evidence of major changes over time in a range of behaviors likely to influence fertility (Rutter and Smith, 1995). For example, there has been a substantial fall in the age at which children first have sexual intercourse, and there has been a marked fall in the proportion of children born within a legal marriage and a corresponding rise in those born to unmarried couples who live together in a committed relationship, with the child's birth being registered in the names of both parents. Divorce rates have risen markedly in most industrialized countries, and there has been a corresponding increase in complex family arrangements involving multiple social parents with children coresiding with a mixture of children born to different pairs of parents (Dunn et al., 1998). Lastly, the ravages of the AIDS (Acquired Immune Deficiency Syndrome) pandemic in many parts of the world, especially southern Africa, are having a devastating effect on family patterns due to the very high death rate among young adults still in their childbearing years.

This brief summary of just a few of the main correlates of variations in fertility serves to emphasize the multiplicity of influences likely to affect people's behavior in relation to mating and childbearing. In addition, of course, the figures on the number of surviving children per couple will be hugely influenced by the rate of infant mortality, which has fallen greatly in the past 100 years (McKeown, 1976). These multiple influences need to be kept in mind when considering possible genetic influences on fertility.

A word about terminology is necessary. "Fecundity" and "fertility" are often used interchangeably (and dictionary definitions encourage this). However, in terms of attempts to understand causal processes, it is helpful to have a means of drawing a distinction between variations in the biological ability to have children and variations in the number of children born to particular groups. Throughout this paper, fecundity will be used to refer to the first (i.e., biological ability to conceive) and fertility to the second (i.e., number of births).

RATIONALE OF QUANTITATIVE GENETIC RESEARCH STRATEGIES

Geneticists have been aware for a long time that similarities between parents and children on some trait or even a familial loading on traits across a broader kinship do not allow an inference about genetic mediation. That is because parents both pass their genes on to their children and shape and select the rearing environments for them. In addition, families will be open to broader societal, environmentally mediated, influences that can create clustering effects. Sophisticated statistical techniques, such as segregation analyses, that can be applied to family data have often been used to infer modes of genetic transmission. However, they are open to numerous methodological hazards and can easily give rise to misleading conclusions. McGuffin and Huckle (1990), with their tongues firmly in their cheeks, illustrated this nicely with their demonstration that attendance at medical school was due to a single recessive gene that was transmitted along Mendelian lines!

Accordingly, reliance has been placed on natural experiments that, in one way or another, can separate genetic and environmental influences. These tend to be thought of in terms of twin and adoptee research strategies. However, both actually involve several different research designs that differ in their patterns of advantages and disadvantages (Rutter et al., 1990, 1999, 2001). Thus, for example, twin strategies include comparisons of separated and nonseparated twins and also studies of the offspring of twins. Similarly, there are several different varieties of adoptee design.

Twin Designs

Equal Environments Assumption

The traditional twin design is predicated on the fact that monozygotic (MZ) pairs share all their segregating genes, whereas dizygotic (DZ) pairs, on average, share just half. The contrast between within-pair correlations or concordances in MZ pairs and DZ pairs can be used to infer the genetic effects on population variance for any particular trait. However, various additional assumptions have to be made. The most important, by far, of these is the equal environments assumption (EEA). This specifies that the environmental variance in MZ pairs is closely similar to that in DZ pairs insofar as the environments are associated with the trait in question. It should be noted that the assumption does *not* require that the environmental variances in the two sorts of the pair are the same but only that, insofar as they are different, they do not relate to the trait being studied. Thus, MZ pairs are much more likely to be dressed alike than are DZ pairs, but this is of no consequence for the vast majority of traits. However, there are some features that, although not directly related to mating behavior or procreation, are likely to influence it. For example, this would be likely to apply to both physical attractiveness and age at puberty. Nevertheless, this is unlikely to violate the EEA because the features are very strongly genetically influenced and therefore would be unlikely to lead to within-pair differences in most circumstances for most traits.

On the other hand, such features may be very informative because they could indicate the route by which genetic effects are mediated. Thus, it is not implausible that part of the genetic effects on population variance in fertility could derive from genetic effects on either physical attractiveness or age at puberty (although it is most unlikely that that is the only mode of genetic mediation). Most reviews by behavior geneticists (e.g., Kendler et al., 1994) have concluded that there is a lack of evidence for violation of the EEA. However, recent evidence has shown that this conclusion is mistaken (Rutter et al., 1999, 2001). It is necessary to note why the conclusion is mistaken as well as its implications for inferences about genetic effects.

Violation of the EEA will come about when two conditions are met. First, there must be a gene-environment correlation. This is necessary because that is the way in which an environmental variance difference between MZ and DZ pairs will arise. In other words, there must be a genetic effect on some environmental feature with the result that the within-pair correlation or concordance for that feature will be greater in MZ pairs than in DZ pairs. Second, the specific environment that has shown evidence of a gene-environment correlation must relate to differences in the trait in MZ pairs. This second condition is necessary because, if it is not, although it may affect influences on other traits, it will not affect the validity of the MZ-DZ comparison in relation to the trait being considered. Evidence for violation of the EEA is available for life events in relation to the liability to depression and the effects of parental negativity, hostility, or criticism on antisocial behavior. That is, parent-child negativity toward each twin is more similar in MZ than DZ pairs, but even in MZ pairs the differences found in negativity are associated with within-pair differences in antisocial behavior. Because MZ twins are genetically identical with respect to the DNA they inherit, the effect of the negativity must reflect some form of environmental mediation. The consequence is that some (but only some) of the MZ-DZ differences will reflect environmental, not just genetic, effects.

Although the conclusion up to now has been resisted by most behavior geneticists, it must be inferred that violation of the EEA is likely to be quite common. That is because gene-environment correlations have been shown to apply to a very broad range of behaviors and are, indeed, likely to be operative with any environment that is susceptible to shaping or selecting as a result of individual behavior. Moreover, there is a good deal of evidence that environments affected by gene-environment correlations are also ones that create an environmentally mediated risk (as demonstrated by genetically sensitive designs; see Rutter, 2000b).

Two further points must be made with respect to possible violation of the EEA. First, some of the differences go in the opposite direction. Thus, the birth-weight differences in MZ pairs tend to be greater than those in DZ pairs. In part, this arises from the transfusion syndrome in which there is a shared circulation between the twins that results in one being "overstuffed" with blood and the other relatively exsanguinated (see Rutter et al., in press). This can only arise in monochorionic MZ pairs and never DZ pairs. Second, there is probably no violation of EEA with respect to those traits in which, although there is multifactorial determination, there is no known specific environmental effect. That would apply, for example, to both schizophrenia and autism. In other words, violation of the EEA must be considered a trait-specific phenomenon and not something that is applicable in all circumstances to all traits.

The question, then, is how much this violation of the EEA is likely to matter with respect to heritability estimates. That is difficult to quantify. What is clear is that, when there is violation of the EEA, part of the effects attributed to genetics will in fact be due to the environment. The net effect is that the estimated heritability will be somewhat too high. That sounds as if it ought to be a major concern, but in practice it probably does not matter as much as one might think. For example, say, an estimated heritability of 40 percent were, in actuality, one of 30 percent, the difference would have no implications for theory, policy, or practice. That is because the level of heritability carries no necessary implications about the ease or difficulty of a change as a result of altered environments. Of course, it would matter if violation of the EEA completely eliminated a genetic effect as previously shown on traditional analyses. Because that has not been put to the test, it is not possible to be definite, but it is quite clear that that is a most implausible consequence.

Where violation of the EEA does matter rather more is in quantification of the effects of specific measured environments. Because they apply to just a portion of the overall environmental effect, they could be influenced to a much greater extent than the overall proportion of the variance attributed to genes or environment. It is necessary, too, to go on to ask whether violation of the EEA is likely to apply to quantitative genetic studies of fertility or, more importantly, to the different traits that together make up the influences on fertility. Because the relevant analyses have not, as yet, been undertaken, it is, once more, not possible to be definite. However, one may infer that some behaviors influencing fertility will be subject to violation of the EEA (that would apply, for example, to antisocial behavior) but it is less likely that it will apply to other features (such as physical attractiveness or age at puberty, neither of which are likely to have much of an effect in MZ pairs). However, with respect to the role of education as an influence on fertility, as discussed in other chapters in this volume, it is quite likely that (although not as yet examined) there may be violation of the EEA. That is because there is good evidence of genetic influences on scholastic achievement (Thompson et al., 1991; Walker et al., 2002) and because environmentally mediated effects of education are probable.

Sampling

As is the case with any research design, the validity of conclusions deriving from twin studies is heavily dependent on the quality of the sampling. Many twin studies have been based on volunteers of one kind or another and, even with samples based on the general population, the final usable sample is necessarily dependent on those who agree to participate. It has been very common for MZ pairs to be overrepresented in twin samples, and, clearly, this constitutes a potential source of bias. There are no good data that would enable an accurate estimate of resulting bias, but, in any case, this will be enormously influenced by the factors associated with willingness or unwillingness to participate in research on twins. Nevertheless, there is reason to be cautious in view of the known possibilities of bias (Berk, 1983; Taylor, 2002).

A second aspect of sampling that matters is the fact that very few studies of twins have included adequate numbers of either ethnic minorities or seriously socially disadvantaged or other high-risk families. This matters because genetic effects may not be equally strong at all points on the distribution of traits. For example, Rowe et al. (1999) found that genetic effects on educational attainment were most marked at the top of the range and least marked at the bottom. Similar effects could well apply to at least some behaviors associated with variations in fertility.

As repeatedly emphasized by behavior geneticists, it is important to appreciate that all estimates of heritability are both population specific and time specific. That is because the statistic is solely concerned with variances in the population studied, and therefore the analyses can only apply to the sample providing the data. If environmental circumstances change, either through the introduction of new environmental influences or because existing ones become more powerful or much weaker, there will be consequent effects on estimates of the strength of genetic influences on population variance. Exactly the same applies, of course, if the changes involve a strengthening or weakening of the pool of susceptibility genes in the population. Heritability is not a measure of the strength of genetic influence at an individual level, it is not a direct function of a particular phenotype, and it is not a reflection of gene frequency or pattern. Accordingly, although heritability is a most useful population statistic, it can (and sometimes does) change rapidly if environmental circumstances or population composition are altered. The rapid change does not mean there has been any change in gene action as it operates within individuals. That is not to say that environmental circumstances cannot influence gene frequencies; both thalassaemia and lactose intolerance provide examples where that seems to have been the case (see Rutter and Silberg, 2002).

With respect to genetic influences on population variance in fertility, there has been emphasis on the ways in which heritability has risen or fallen in an apparently meaningful way in relation to changed environmental circumstances (Kohler et al., 1999). The findings are interesting, but there must be a good deal of skepticism about secular trends in view of the highly conflicting evidence from cohort studies that have examined changes over time in relation to traits for which there have been probably relevant changes in environmental circumstances. For example, Heath et al. (1985) found an increase in the heritability of educational attainment in Norway for males but not females over a time period in which educational opportunities became more widely available. Why should this have applied to one sex and not the other? Conversely, Kendler et al. (2000) found a rise over the 20th century in the heritability of smoking in women but not men. Again, the same question arises. The need in each case is to develop focused hypotheses on why there might be a meaningful sex difference that reflects different patterns of causal processes. The alternative, of course, is that the processes are similar in males and females and that the observed difference reflects only a failure of replication due to chance variation or error. Possible sex differences need to be taken seriously, but they call for rigorous research to test their reality and, if real, their causation (Moffitt et al., 2001; Rutter et al., 2002).

By contrast, Heath et al. (1993) found no difference across cohorts in the heritability of smoking initiation. In a Finnish study, Silventoinen et al. (2000), found a marginal increase over time in the heritability of height (from 76 to 81 percent), but such a small change is not likely to have much theoretical or practical significance. It may be concluded that the research strategy of looking at secular trends is potentially useful, but the results so far have been rather inconclusive. That is probably because so much depends on the specificity of measures and the nature of samples, as well as the fact that the confidence limits for heritability are typically rather wide.

In recent years there has been increasing reliance on statistical modeling in order to provide for more precise estimates of genetic and environmental effects. The basic principle is primarily one of parsimony. In other words, if there is no worsening of a model when one effect is dropped, it may be assumed that the particular effect is not needed. Accordingly, the estimates are recalculated after dropping that variable. In most cases the consequence is an increase in the estimate of genetic effects (although that need not be the case). It sounds like a perfectly reasonable approach, but the problem is that, when confidence limits are very wide (as they often are), an effect may be dropped even though it might actually be quite strong. Also, such modeling procedures can give rise to findings that obviously cannot be valid (see Rutter et al., 1999, for examples). Accordingly, although modeling approaches definitely have their place, they need to be treated with a certain amount of caution. It may often be prudent to rely primarily on the full model in which all the relevant parameters are included.

Gene-Gene Interplay

Typically, traditional genetic analyses assume that all genetic effects are additive. However, it is known that in some circumstances there are synergistic interactions of a nonadditive kind. Sometimes, these involve interactions between different alleles of the same gene (usually referred to as dominance), and in other cases they arise through interactions between different genes (termed epistasis). The most obvious pointer to the likelihood of the operation of such synergistic genetic effects is provided by the finding that the correlation within DZ pairs is well below half of that in MZ pairs. This comes about because, although DZ pairs share, on average, half of their segregating genes, they will share only a quarter of two gene combinations and an eighth of three gene combinations, whereas MZ pairs share all their genes and all their gene combinations. Such effects have been found for both autism (Pickles et al., 1995) and schizophrenia (Moldin and Gottesman, 1997) as well as for some personality traits. Caution is needed in inferring dominance or epistasis because the same divergence between MZ and DZ pairs can arise from contrast effects in ratings of behavior (see Simonoff et al., 1998). Critics of behavior genetics are fond of attacking it on the grounds of the unwarranted presumption of additivity. However, behavior geneticists are well aware of this issue, and it is commonplace nowadays to make explicit tests for dominance or epistatic effects. Moreover, it is perfectly straightforward to include these in any overall model. There is a need to consider such effects, but their likely existence for some traits is not a justifiable reason for doubting behavior genetics.

Gene-Environment Interplay

A somewhat similar issue arises with respect to assortative mating, gene-environment correlations, and gene-environment interactions. Again, old-style traditional genetic analyses have usually made the assumption that none of these are sufficiently operative to warrant being taken into account. It is now clear that for many traits that assumption is unwarranted. Thus, although there is little assortative mating for personality traits, there is substantial assortative mating (in terms of like mating with like) with respect to educational attainment and antisocial behavior (Farrington et al., 1996; Krueger et al., 1998; Plomin et al., 2001), to give two rather different examples. There is also extensive evidence of gene-environment correlations (Plomin, 1994) and growing evidence of gene-environment interaction in relation to emotional and behavioral disturbances (Rutter and Silberg, 2002).

Three points need to be made on this topic. First, unless there is evidence to the contrary, it ought to be assumed that there may be assortative mating, gene-environment correlations, or gene-environment interactions. These should be tested for and, where relevant, included in the analyses. Second, as ordinarily presented, gene-environment correlations and interactions will be included in the estimate for genetic effects, despite the fact that they actually reflect the combination of genetic and environmental influences operating together. On the other hand, it is perfectly possible to disaggregate the genetic term into the portion attributable to baseline genetic effects and the portion reflecting gene-environment interaction (see Silberg et al., 2001). Third, although it has proved problematic up to now to model the effects of gene-environment correlations and gene-environment interactions simultaneously, it now seems that use of Markov chain Monte Carlo techniques provides a way forward (Eaves and Erkanli, in press; Eaves et al., 2002). Accordingly, it should now be possible to determine not only the overall genetic effect but also the extent to which this operates through gene-environment correlations and interactions.

Other Concerns Regarding Behavior Genetics

Over the years, numerous concerns of one sort or another have been expressed in relation to behavior genetics. For the most part, they fall under one of four headings. First, there are the issues that arise out of the biology of twinning. Twins differ from singletons in having a substantially higher rate of obstetric complications at birth and a somewhat higher rate of congenital anomalies (Myrianthopoulos and Melnick, 1977; Rutter et al., 1990). Also, there is the possibility of placentation effects—meaning the effects of the twin pair sharing the same chorion or having two different chorions (Machin and Still, 1995). Evidence on the importance, or otherwise, of such biological differences is fragmentary. They appear to be of negligible importance in relation to language development (Rutter et al., in press), but they might be more important for some kinds of psychopathology (Davis et al., 1995; Prescott et al., 1999).

Second, there is the possibility that the postnatal rearing environment of twins may be somewhat different from that of singletons. The mothers of twins tend to be much more stressed and to have a somewhat higher rate of depression. They also tend to communicate in a somewhat different way because of the different "press" of having two young children at the same developmental level (Thorpe et al., in press). These findings have been shown to be relevant in relation to language development, but it is quite uncertain whether or not they have effects on other behaviors. Certainly, it seems unlikely that the effects will ordinarily be sufficient to invalidate the twin strategy.

Third, there are problems of sampling, which have been raised most forcefully in relation to the two main studies of separated twins (Kamin and Goldberger, 2002). In my view there is some validity to these concerns, and it would be prudent not to place too much weight on separated-twin studies. One of the potential advantages that has been put forward is that they cannot be open to the problem of violation of the EEA because they have been separated and have not had contact with one another. However, this reflects a serious misunderstanding of EEA. Although, of course, separation eliminates the influence of contact, it definitely does not remove the potential effect of gene-environment correlations that could affect environments that matter.

Fourth, concerns have been expressed over the fact that measures of many traits do not show a normal distribution (Capron and Vetta, 2001). This is not a valid criticism because there is no necessary assumption that the "true" distribution is normal and because there are various statistical techniques that can be used to normalize distributions and hence to make them more suitable for the usual genetic analyses. There is no reason to suppose that this creates a significant problem.

Adoptee Studies

At first sight, adoptee designs might seem preferable to twin designs because they provide a cleaner separation of biological heritage and rearing environment. For that reason they have indeed proved very valuable with respect to some phenotypes, most particularly schizophrenia (Kety et al., 1994). However, there are more limitations to adoptee designs than usually appreciated by behavior geneticists. To begin with, social agencies select prospective adoptive parents on the grounds that they will provide a good rearing environment. Of course, they succeed in that goal to only a limited extent, but there is no doubt that extremely adverse environments are greatly underrepresented in samples of adoptive parents (Rutter et al., 2001; Stoolmiller, 1999). Also, adoptive parents tend to be older and better educated than biological parents in the general population. In addition, women who give up their children for adoption are far from a random sample of the general population. With respect to the study of fertility, there is also the obvious problem that, by definition, biological parents cannot include any individuals who have not had children. Finally, in most industrialized countries the number of nonhandicapped children adopted in infancy has dropped greatly. Intercountry adoptions have risen *pari per su* but these involve a much more complicated situation, often including serious early deprivation and adoption after infancy (Selman, 2000).

For all these reasons, it is not likely that adoptee studies will have a major place in the study of fertility, and because, so far as I am aware, there have been no adoptee studies that are relevant, these designs will not be considered further here.

Evolutionary Considerations

If only because the theory of evolution is based on natural selection for reproductive fitness, it is necessary to consider how evolutionary theory might inform the quantitative genetic study of fertility. Indeed, as other chapters in this volume illustrate, it does include most useful pointers as to what might be relevant and also what sorts of mechanisms may need to be considered. Nevertheless, considerable caution is needed in making the leap from evolutionary theory to empirical findings on contemporary human behavior. Thus, as Rodgers et al. (2001) pointed out, Fisher's fundamental theorem of natural selection supposes that, for traits representing reproductive fitness, evolution will result in a progressive reduction of additive genetic variance so that, once evolutionary equilibrium has been reached, there will be no genetic effect on population variance. In fact, the findings show that additive genetic influences account for a substantial proportion of population variance in relation to a range of characteristics that might be thought to be associated with reproductive fitness. That does not necessarily mean that the theorem was wrong, but it definitely does mean that extrapolations need to take account of the numerous features that will lead to results that run counter to the theorem (see also Bock et al., 2000).

Regarding reproductive behavior, it is obvious there are numerous perturbations (such as the availability of contraception and the use of techniques to assist conception) that will alter the situation with respect to fertility. Similar reservations need to be expressed about the concept of sexually antagonistic coevolution as applied to genomic imprinting (see Haig, 2000; also Gangestad, this volume). Mammals are unusual in the way in which embryos are totally dependent on the flow of nutrients from the maternal placenta (Strachan and Read, 1999). Because many imprinted genes are involved in regulating fetal growth, it has been argued that there is a conflict between the parental genomes, with the paternal gains coming from an embryo that aggressively removes nutrients from the mother and the maternal gains from protection of the mother in order to spare resources for future offspring. It is a reasonable notion that this may have played a part in the evolution of imprinting mechanisms, but it is a completely open question whether imprinted genes are particularly important in the regulation of fertility. Of the relatively few imprinted genes in the human that are known at the moment, most concern gross handicapping pathologies (with the specifics of the phenotype being greatly affected by whether the gene comes from the mother or the father), rather than normal behaviors that might influence fertility (see Skuse and Kuntsi, 2002). Of course, that does not mean that imprinted genes are not important in fertility; it simply means that there is a need for more empirical data.

Similarly, the potential evolutionary importance of gene-environment correlations is obvious; Dawkins (1982, 1989) discusses the issue in relation to the concept of "extended phenotypes," and Scarr and McCartney (1983) do so in terms of "niche picking" of environments that are most adaptive for the individual genotype. Clearly, this does and can occur, but niche construction involves a two-way process that fundamentally changes the coevolution dynamics between genetic evolution and cultural change

(Odling-Smee, 1996; see also Rutter and Silberg, 2002). Also, the term niche picking implies an active process that is governed by genes as well as a process that is adaptive. However, the evidence indicates that niche picking is not necessarily socially adaptive and not necessarily primarily driven by genes, although both will be the case in some instances (Rutter and Silberg, 2002).

Implications of Genetic Influences and Behaviors Associated with Variations in Fertility

As the introductory section of this chapter seeks to make clear, fertility is far from a single phenomenon. It represents the effects of a heterogeneous range of behaviors that differ markedly in their origins. Accordingly, little is to be gained by attempting to measure the overall heritability of fertility. Unless further specified with respect to the various routes of genetic mediation, it means little and has no policy or practice implications.

It may be accepted that there are significant genetic effects on a range of traits likely to be influential on fertility, including effects on social attachment (Brussoni et al., 2000), pair bonding (Trumbetta and Gottesman, 2000), age at first sexual intercourse (Dunne et al., 1997), and divorce (Jockin et al., 1996; McGue and Lykken, 1992). Not surprisingly, there is also an overall significant heritability for number of offspring (Rodgers et al., 2001). There are several problems in applying the genetic findings to any of the issues outlined in the first section of this chapter.

First, by their nature, estimates of heritability apply to genetic influences on individual differences within a population. Jensen (1969) famously (or should it be infamously?) tried to use the evidence of genetic influences on a trait (in his case intelligence) within a population to argue that it followed that it was highly likely that, when there were differences in the level of that trait between two populations, the explanation was likely to lie in genetics. Tizard (1975) showed the falsity of that argument by taking the example of human height. Height is a strongly heritable characteristic, but the average height of the population today is much greater than it was 50 or 100 years ago. Tizard analyzed data for London schoolboys over a 50-year span and found a difference of some 12 cm. Other studies have shown much the same thing with respect to adult height in each of the countries in which it has been examined (Kuh et al., 1991; van Wieringen, 1986; Weir, 1952). It is generally assumed, with good reason, that the main explanation for the rise in height is much better nutrition. Certainly, it is most unlikely to be due to a change in the gene pool over this relatively short time span.

Second, there is the somewhat related point that factors that are most influential with respect to individual differences may be rather different from those that are most influential with respect to differences in the *level* of a trait either over time or between different groups. Thus, for example, it is obvious that the features associated with individual differences in unemployment at any one point in time are very different from those that account for the huge rises and falls in unemployment over time in the same country (see Rutter, 1994). Of course, they may be the same or they may overlap greatly, as is probably the case with antisocial behavior (Rutter et al., 1998), but the point is that there is no necessary connection between the two.

Third, within a very broad range, variations among traits in their level of heritability have little or no meaning with respect to theory, policy, or practice. It may be concluded that virtually all human behaviors are genetically influenced to some extent, but the degree to which they are is of little consequence unless the heritability is extremely high. Although there have been no adequate behavior genetic studies of many of the traits that may be important in relation to fertility, it is safe to predict that it is likely they comply with what Bailey (2000) jokingly called his "law"—namely that the heritability will be somewhere in the 20 to 60 percent range and that it does not matter very much exactly where in that range it is.

Finally, there is the crucial point that evidence of a significant heritability for fertility is completely uninformative with respect to causal mechanisms. Of course, the same applies to the parallel evidence that there is an environmental influence. Unless it is known how genetic mediation, or environmental mediation, operates, there are no theoretical or policy implications. Of course, it would be "news" if fertility proved to be the only human trait that involved no genetic component, but that is not what has been found, and it is not the least bit likely that further studies would show that to be the case. In considering how genetic influences might have effects, it is crucial to appreciate that multiple causal routes are likely to be involved and also that indirect chain effects are bound to be involved. For example, the relevant behaviors are likely to include the age of initiation of sexual activity, whether or not contraceptives are used effectively, the extent to which risk-taking behavior incorporates sexual practices that are likely to lead to wanted or unwanted pregnancies, the extent to which the establishment of careers is associated with deliberate postponement of childbearing, the intensity of sexual drive, the degree of affiliative behavior, the age at which cohabitation or marriage is first established, the number of cohabiting or marital partnerships (with the pressure that may be involved in having further children by a new relationship), the willingness to use abortion as a means of fertility control, the strength of desire to have children despite difficulties in conception, the financial resources to make use of expensive methods of assisted conception, and religious attitudes that impinge on any of these behaviors.

This list, although lengthy, is very far from exhaustive and deals only with features likely to operate across the population as a whole. In addition, there are the effects of somatic illness (such as consequences of some sexually transmitted diseases in leading to sterility) and mental disorders, as noted earlier. HIV (human immunodeficiency virus) may bring about early mortality during the childbearing years, and disease or malnutrition will have effects on the number of infants who survive. It is not helpful to jumble all of this together into one overall measure of fecundity or fertility. Rather, the need is to determine how these various behaviors influence fecundity or fertility patterns.

In the first instance, the need is to determine the direct and indirect causal mechanisms in relation to the relevant behaviors. It is only secondarily that it becomes relevant to examine the extent to which such behaviors are genetically influenced. Nevertheless, genetic studies can be very informative in providing a better understanding of nature-nurture interplay in the development of socially relevant behaviors (see Gilger, 2000; Rutter and Plomin, 1997).

In relation to the relative importance of different behaviors, the possibility that the pattern is somewhat different in males and females must be considered and tested for. It is also possible that the pattern of causative influences may not be quite the same in the two sexes (see Rutter et al., 2002, for some of the research implications).

RESEARCH PRIORITIES

It is certainly clear that population variances in childbearing and family building are of considerable public health importance. It is also obvious that an enormous amount remains to be learned about the causal pathways that are most important. In that connection, probably the top priority should be epidemiological/longitudinal studies that span the age period from childhood to midadult life but with the additional requirement that such studies are used in an innovative fashion to test hypotheses about causal processes and, in particular, to use designs of sampling and data analysis that allow one hypothesis to be tested against competing hypotheses. Only in this way is it at all likely that we will learn about the indirect chain effects likely to be crucial. Studies will have to be planned in such a way that they take seriously the possibility of substantial meaningful heterogeneity within populations. These will need to include the possibility of sex differences, ethnic differences, and differences related to geography and social circumstances.

One of the key needs across the whole of behavioral science concerns the separation of genetic mediation from environmental mediation and social selection from social causation. Far too much research is content with the establishment of statistically significant associations without taking seriously the fact that path diagrams, and the like, have little meaning unless these alternatives have been examined, tested, and quantified. Genetically sensitive designs, including the various types of twin and adoptee studies, have a crucially important role to play in that connection. However, it would be a grave error to assume that they provide the only way to test causal hypotheses. There is a rich array of natural experiments of different kinds that can be used for the same purpose (see Rutter et al., 2001). Note, however, that the need here is to use genetically sensitive designs to test for environmental mediation. That constitutes a greatly underused research strategy. Part of the limitation up to now has been the failure of most behavior genetics studies to include discriminating and sensitive measures of the environment.

Third, research strategies need to be developed to test causal hypotheses about both secular trends and between-group differences in patterns of behavior relevant to fertility. There is abundant evidence of major changes in many behaviors of psychosocial importance (Rutter and Smith, 1995), but, although some research has been helpful in ruling out various causal explanations, it has not gotten very far in putting causal hypotheses about possible causal factors to rigorous test. Insofar as secular trends are concerned, it is unlikely that they are due primarily to genetic factors, if only because changes in the gene pool do not develop that quickly in all ordinary circumstances. On the other hand, with respect to the large secular trends in many behaviors, there has been a dilemma because environmental mediation seemed to require a bigger difference in environmental influences than seemed likely. Recently, Dickens and Flynn (2001) have shown that gene-environment correlations could serve as the needed multiplier of environmental effects. They were concerned with the major rise in the mean level of intelligence, but the principle is likely to apply much more widely than that. On the other hand, this remains a suggestion that is still to be tested empirically.

The fourth priority comprises the behavior genetics study of the interconnections among different behaviors that play a part in the causal pathway to fertility patterns. Jockin et al. (1996) found that 30 to 40 percent of the heritability of divorce risk stemmed from genetic factors influencing personality. Similarly, Rodgers et al. (2001) showed that there was a significant shared genetic variance between the number of children born and the age at the first attempt to get pregnant. Potentially, these cross-trait analyses can be very informative about causal mechanisms. For example, is the age of puberty associated with the age of first intercourse because the experience of puberty and the physical changes it entails bring the young person into social situations and styles of heterosexual interaction that make intercourse more likely, or, rather, is it that both share the same genetic liability, with only minor environmentally mediated effects of the experience itself? Similar questions need to be asked with respect to age at first pregnancy and the likelihood of marriage or cohabitation breakdown, risk-taking behavior and promiscuity, and so forth. Relatively few behavior genetics studies have tackled these sorts of issues so far, but there is a considerable potential for such research and it would be of value. It is important to emphasize, however, that it would be unduly narrow to consider such research only in terms of its utility for the understanding of fertility patterns. Rather, it provides a means of understanding the functioning of a wide range of human behaviors that have both adaptive and maladaptive consequences. In that connection, however, there is very little to be said for the value of establishing the heritability of yet another behavior in yet another sample. The time has come to move on to using behavior genetics research to understand causal mechanisms. That is happening already in the field of psychopathology, and it could well serve the same purpose in this field.

Finally, molecular genetics research has a considerable potential both for providing invaluable leads on the possible nature of the neural processes underlying some behaviors and also for elucidation of patterns of nature-nurture interplay (Plomin and Rutter, 1998; Rutter, 2002a, 2002b; Rutter and Plomin, 1997). Although identification of specific individual susceptibility genes for particular behaviors can be expected to open up new avenues of potentially fruitful biological research, the identification of genes, in itself, will not delineate the responsible neural processes. That is to say, finding the genes is just the first step. This has to be followed by research to determine the genes' actions on proteins; this must lead to determination of the effects of these protein products on physiological and biochemical processes in the organism; and then there is the further requirement to determine how these processes lead to the behavior in question (Rutter, 2000a). It will be appreciated that all of this requires a range of rather different sciences, incorporating proteomics, transcriptomics, and integrative physiology and then molecular epidemiology.

Not only does this arduous multistage research route involve many uncertainties, but it will take a very long time. In determining gene actions, animal models have a crucial role to play, but the difficulties and complexities are much increased when dealing with social behaviors likely to be influenced by social contexts that are distinctly human. This determination of what genes do has proved incredibly difficult even with single-gene disorders that require no particular environment for the effects to be evident. It is going to be much more difficult with multifactorial behavioral traits. That is because in most instances it is likely that the genetic effects will derive from normal allelic variations rather than some pathological mutation. Also, it may be expected that none of the genes lead directly to a behavioral trait such as risk taking or novelty seeking or sensation seeking.

Rather, it influences the biological substrate of these traits, but variations in the level of the trait are influenced by environmental, as well as genetic, factors. That raises the crucial parallel issue of the need to determine what environmental influences do to the organism. Are they having effects on the same biological substrate that is influenced by genetic factors or, instead, are they operating in a rather different way? There has been scarcely any research on this issue, and it is much needed.

Potentially, the identification of susceptibility genes will be particularly useful in the study of nature-nurture interplay. The study of gene-environment correlations and interactions has necessarily been a rather uncertain enterprise when it had to rely on "black box" analyses with anonymous genes. This situation will be transformed once it is known which genes these are and what they do. However, if multiple genes are involved (and that will usually be the case), the gains will not be great until most of those genes are identified. Simply finding one gene with very small effects is not likely to be very helpful.

Throughout the whole of this enterprise, it will have to be borne in mind that determination of biological effects will not provide an answer in itself because there will always be further need to determine whether they account for the particular features that have been studied. For example, research has shown that, to a considerable extent, the sex hormone testosterone plays a major role in sex drive in both men and women. However, it has also been shown that testosterone levels are hugely influenced by social experiences. Thus, levels tend to rise in the winner of competitive chess or tennis games and fall in the loser (Booth et al., 1989; Mazur et al., 1992). Also, although it is clear that the surge of testosterone levels at puberty is largely responsible for the rise in libido at that time, it is nowhere near as clear whether individual variations in testosterone level in adult life account for individual differences in sexual activity, let alone with the more indirect connections with fertility. Again, the relevance of testosterone levels for group differences in fertility is even more open to question. Although almost anything is possible in biology, it does not seem plausible that this is responsible for the major ethnic variations in average completed family size or the fall in the same over time in most industrialized countries.

ETHICAL ISSUES

Some critics have raised concerns that the behavior genetics study of social behaviors and evolutionary theory will lead to a highly misleading impression of biological determinism that will bring about a neglect of research into social influences and, even worse, to a failure to act to alleviate or counter adverse social influences (Rose, 1995, 1998; Rose and Rose, 2000). Although a few scientists have made unwarranted claims that could justify that impression, the main messages from genetics and evolutionary theory actually point in the opposite direction. Genetic influences are probabilistic, not determinative, in the case of multifactorial behaviors, and often they act through indirect routes that involve an intrinsic interplay between genes and the environment (Rutter and Silberg, 2002). That consideration makes it crucially important to support research that brings the two together and not separate them.

Evolutionary theory has led to a valuable corpus of knowledge on biological forces that are likely to operate in relation to fertility, and it would be foolish to neglect the insights that it provides. On the other hand, as other chapters in this volume note, it is much more directly helpful for some sorts of questions than it is for others and for some it provides little help. Much the same applies to hormonal effects and to other aspects of biology; they constitute an essential part of the overall understanding, but there are still some puzzles as to how they operate, and they do not give answers to all questions. The first ethical concern, then, is that research could become dominated by a narrow mechanistic deterministic program. Of course, that is a possible danger, but the clear and unambiguous messages from genetic research lead in an entirely different direction. The issue needs to be expressed in an opposite fashion. The topic of human social behavior, including the study of fertility, is of such immense public importance that it would be seriously unethical *not* to investigate its origins and meaning. Genetic research must constitute a crucial part of that research endeavor because it can be so usefully informative on genetic, environmental and developmental mechanisms and especially their interaction (Plomin and Rutter, 1998; Rutter, 2002a, 2002b).

Nevertheless, it is of paramount importance that the research be conducted ethically, as widely recognized in a range of official reports (Medical Research Council, 2000, 2001; Nuffield Council on Bioethics, 1993, 2002b; Royal College of Psychiatrists' Working Party, 2001) as well as papers by individuals (Durfy, 2001; Rutter, 1999). With very few exceptions, the issues related to genetics research into social behaviors are not different from those that apply to any sort of research, and there is no need here to re-review the details. However, a few key points require emphasis.

Most especially the concerns arise from the immense power of modern molecular genetics research and the certainty that, in conjunction with other strategies, it will lead over the next decade or so to a much improved understanding of biological processes. That means that the findings will really matter for society (and bring benefits to it) and, in turn, that it will be open to misuse. The evils of the past, of course, highlight that danger (Devlin et al., 1997), but even if that had not been the case, it is clear that the dangers of misuse are ever present. The challenge is to act in ways that reduce the danger as much as possible and to set in motion procedures to deal with the misuse when it occurs.

Before turning to specific concerns in relation to genetics, some points need to be made with respect to the wide range of community and general population studies that are an essential part of the overall research enterprise as applied to fertility (as discussed in other chapters). Social scientists sometimes wish to argue that when their research involves only observations, interviews, and questionnaires (rather than intrusive medical procedures), there is no need for detailed ethical scrutiny. Obviously, that is a mistaken view not only because of concerns over personal intrusion but also because, if mishandled, even anonymized data can stigmatize groups of individuals. There are also special concerns that apply to research in developing countries, particularly with illiterate individuals (Nuffield Council on Bioethics, 2002a). All human research needs to be subject to independent ethical review. Nevertheless, it needs to be appreciated that those reviewing medical research may well not have the knowledge and experience to assess ethical issues as they apply to social, behavioral, historical, and other nonmedical research. Accordingly, other bodies will need to be established, if they are not already available.

In addition to scrutiny of the research approach itself, attention needs to be paid to the funding source, to the benefits to researchers, and to the appropriateness or otherwise of benefits (or inducements) for participants. Possible conflicts of interest need to be made overt, not only at the point of initial ethical review and at the annual monitoring of research progress but also at the point of publication, as has been increasingly recognized and handled.

With respect to genetic research, several main features warrant attention. First, with any kind of tissue bank in which there is a pooling of tissues for future use by other researchers (whether the banking concerns DNA, umbilical cord blood, placental or other tissues), some modification of the usual approach to informed consent will be needed. That is because neither the precise use of the pooled material nor the researchers using it can be specified in advance (although a range of acceptable research aims can, and should, be specified). The practice that has developed is to require (and specify in the relevant information sheet) that any future use will have to be subject to further independent ethical scrutiny.

Second, genetic information on one family member will inevitably have implications for other family members (who may well not have agreed to participate in the study). The most appropriate guidelines for this issue are still being considered and developed.

Thus, there is the dilemma of when and how to provide feedback to research participants. The usual expectation in the past when dealing with medical research with patients was that participants had the right to expect to be told about test findings that might be relevant to their clinical condition. The situation with respect to large-scale general population studies (whether or not focused on genetics) is quite different in three main respects. First, the clinical implications of many findings (such as allelic variations) will not be known until the research is complete (and maybe not even then). The feedback of findings of unknown meaning is generally considered mischievous and unethical because, if the expert does not know what the findings mean, the feedback cannot be relevant or helpful to the participant. Second, most test measures obtained in large surveys will have been collected by researchers with limited training. The findings should be meaningful at a group difference level but not appropriate for individual diagnosis (and hence not for feedback). Third, some insurance companies are requiring clients to report if they have had a "genetic test," with the anticipation that premiums will be loaded if they have had such a test. They can truthfully answer "no" to that question if there is no feedback and if the research was not focused on the identification of some specific susceptibility gene.

This issue, however, raises two other broader issues. On the one hand, it is already clear that there is no straightforward actuarial calculation that can be based on susceptibility genes that contribute to only part (often a small part) of the risk, that may well be dependent on conjunction with some environmental hazard for their contribution to liability, that may vary in their effects with gender or ethnicity, and that may require interaction with other (not yet identified) background genes. As one or more of these conditions will usually apply, actuarial calculations are bound to be hazardous and potentially profoundly misleading.

On the other hand, the topic raises the fundamental issue of whether society should penalize, sometimes heavily, particular individuals because they have an increased genetic risk. Most societies do not do so in relation to education, which is equally free for the unusually talented, the average, and the handicapped. Why should it be different in relation to genetics?

The final fundamental issue is that of research governance (Royal College of Psychiatrists' Working Party, 2001). Ethical review bodies provide an essential screening or advisory role, but, fundamentally, the ultimate responsibility that research be undertaken ethically, and reported ethically, must be placed on the individual scientist and, through that individual, to the person's employing authority. That is necessary because no set of rules, however exhaustive, can possibly anticipate all new ethical issues. The onus is, and has to be, on each and every researcher.

CONCLUSIONS

It may be concluded that genetic research, both quantitative and molecular, has an important role to play in gaining a better understanding of all that is involved in the processes that lead to variations in fertility. Nevertheless, the extent to which genetic research provides understanding is crucially dependent on the extent to which it leads to good biological studies of a quite different kind. What is more limiting about genetics is that it is primarily concerned with individual differences, rather than population differences in level. It can contribute to the latter but does so more indirectly. Sometimes behavior genetics has been attacked on the grounds of being excessively reductionist in leading to a biological determinism (Rose, 1998). The alternative is often portrayed as a need for a holistic approach. Personally, I do not agree with that way of putting things. In principle, it must surely always be desirable to seek to reduce explanations to some simple underlying principle (see Bock and Goode, 1998). On the other hand, with respect to all forms of social behavior, there will often be a need to undertake research at a systems, as well as an individual, level. That is to say, as May (1998) put it, it may often be necessary to build from physiology to individual behavior to population dynamics to community structure. There are two-way interactions between individuals and their environments, and there is a vital need to examine these with a sensitivity to the fact that many changes take place over lengthy periods of time that cannot easily be reduced to manipulations in a laboratory experiment. That requires an integration across a range of different sciences, and research priorities must reflect that need.

REFERENCES

Bailey, J.M.
2000 How can psychological adaptations be heritable? Pp. 171-180 in *The Nature of Intelligence*. G.R. Bock, J.A. Goode, and K. Webb, eds. (Novartis Foundation Symposium 233.) Chichester: Wiley.

Berk, R.A.
1983 An introduction to sample selection bias in sociological data. *American Sociological Review* 48:386-398.

Bock, G.R., and J.A. Goode, eds.
1998 *The Limits of Reductionism in Biology*. (Novartis Foundation Symposium 213.) Chichester: Wiley.

Bock, G.R., J.A. Goode, and K. Webb, eds.
2000 *The Nature of Intelligence*. Chichester: Wiley.

Booth, A., G. Shelley, A. Mazur, G. Tharp, and R. Kittok
1989 Testosterone, and winning and losing in human competition. *Hormones and Behavior* 23:556-571.

Bostofte, E., J. Serup, and H. Rebbe
1983 Has the fertility of Danish men declined through the years in terms of semen quality? A comparison of semen qualities between 1952 and 1972. *International Journal of Fertility* 28:91-95.

Brussoni, M.J., K.L. Jang, W.J. Livesley, and T.M. Macbeth
2000 Genetic and environmental influences on adult attachment styles. *Personal Relationships* 7:283-289.

Capron, C., and A. Vetta
2001 Comments on "Why have children in the 21st century?" *European Journal of Population* 17:23-30.

Davis, J.O., J.A. Phelps, and H.S. Bracha
1995 Prenatal development of monozygotic twins and concordance for schizophrenia. *Schizophrenia Bulletin* 21:357-366.

Dawkins, R.
1982 *The Extended Phenotype: The Gene as the Unit of Selection.* Oxford: W.H. Freeman.
1989 *The Selfish Gene.* Oxford: Oxford University Press.

Derom, R., and E. Bryan
2000 Improving the treatment of infertility: Towards avoiding high order multiple gestation. *Twin Research* 3:109-112.

Devlin, B., S. Fienberg, D. Resnick, and K. Roeder, eds.
1997 *Intelligence, Genes and Success: Scientists Respond to the Bell Curve.* New York: Copernicus.

Dickens, W.T., and J.R. Flynn
2001 Heritability estimates vs. large environmental effects: The IQ paradox resolved. *Psychological Review* 108:346-369.

Dunn, J., K. Deater-Deckard, K. Pickering, T. O'Connor, J. Golding, and the ALSPAC Study Team
1998 Children's adjustment and prosocial behaviour in step-, single-parent, and nonstep family settings: Findings from a community study. *Journal of Child Psychology and Psychiatry* 39:1083-1095.

Dunne, M.P., N.G. Martin, D.J. Statham, W.S. Slutske, and S.H. Dinwiddie
1997 Genetic and environmental contributions to variance in age at first sexual intercourse. *Psychological Science* 8:11-16.

Durfy, S.J.
2001 Ethical and social issues in incorporating genetic research into survey studies. Pp. 303-328 in *Cells and Surveys: Should Biological Measures Be Included in Social Science Research.* Committee on Population, Commission on Behavioral and Social Sciences and Education, National Research Council. Washington, DC: National Academy Press.

Eaves, L., and A. Erkanli
In press Markov chain Monte Carlo approaches to analysis of genetic and environmental components of human developmental change and GxE interaction. *Behavior Genetics.*

Eaves, L., J. Silberg, and A. Erkanli
2002 Interaction and correlation of genes and life events in the development of depression in adolescent girls. Manuscript submitted for publication.

Farrington, D., G.C. Barnes, and S. Lambert
1996 The concentration of offending in families. *Legal and Criminological Psychology* 1:47-63.

Gilger, J.W.
2000 Contributions and promise of human behavioral genetics. *Human Biology* 72:229-255.
Joffe, M.
2000 Time trends in biological fertility in Britain. *The Lancet* 355:1961-1965.
Haig, D.
2000 Genomic imprinting, sex-biased dispersal, and social behavior. *Annals of the New York Academy of Sciences* 907:149-163.
Heath, A.C., K. Berg, L.J. Eaves, M.H. Solaas, L.A. Corey, J. Sundet, P. Magnus, and W.E. Nance
1985 Education policy and the heritability of educational attainment. *Nature* 314:734-736.
Heath, A.C., R. Cates, N.G. Martin, J. Meyer, J.K. Hewitt, M.C. Neale, and L.J. Eaves
1993 Genetic contribution to risk of smoking initiation: Comparisons across birth cohorts and across cultures. *Journal of Substance Abuse* 5:221-246.
Hess, L.E.
1995 Changing family patterns in Western Europe: Opportunity and risk factors for adolescent development. Pp. 104-193 in *Psychosocial Disorders in Young People: Time Trends and Their Causes.* M. Rutter and D.J. Smith, eds. Chichester, England: Wiley.
Jablensky, A.
2000 Epidemiology of schizophrenia. Pp. 585-298 in *New Oxford Textbook of Psychiatry, Vol. 1.* M.G. Gelder, J.J. López-Ibor, and N. Andreasen, eds. Oxford: Oxford University Press.
Jensen, A.R.
1969 How much can we boost IQ and scholastic achievement? *Harvard Educational Review* 39:1-123.
Jockin, V., M. McGue, and D.T. Lykken
1996 Personality and divorce: A genetic analysis. *Journal of Personality and Social Psychology* 71:288-299.
Kamin, L.J., and A.S. Goldberger
2002 Twin studies in behavioral research: A skeptical view. *Theoretical Population Biology* 61:83-95.
Kendler, K.S., M.C. Neale, R.C. Kessler, A.C. Heath, and L.J. Eaves
1994 Parental treatment and the equal environment assumption in twin studies of psychiatric illness. *Psychological Medicine* 24:579-590.
Kendler, K.S., L.M. Thornton, and N.L. Pedersen
2000 Tobacco consumption in Swedish twins reared apart and reared together. *Archives of General Psychiatry* 57:886-892.
Kety, S.S., P.H. Wender, B. Jacobsen, L.J. Ingraham, L. Jansson, B. Faber, and D.K. Kinney
1994 Mental illness in the biological and adoptive relatives of schizophrenic adoptees. Replication of the Copenhagen study in the rest of Denmark. *Archives of General Psychiatry* 51:442-455.
Kohler, H.-P., J.L. Rodgers, and K. Christensen
1999 Is fertility behaviour in our genes? Findings from a Danish twin study. *Population and Development Review* 25:253-288.
Krueger, R.F., T.E. Moffitt, A. Caspi, and A. Bleske
1998 Assortative mating for antisocial behavior: Developmental and methodological implications. *Behavior Genetics* 28:173-186.
Kuh, D.L., C. Power, and B. Rodgers
1991 Secular trends in social class and sex differences in adult height. *International Journal of Epidemiology* 20:1001-1009.

Machin, G.A., and K. Still
1995 The twin-twin transfusion syndrome: Vascular anatomy of monochorionic placentas and their clinical outcomes. Pp. 367-394 in *Multiple Pregnancy: Epidemiology, Gestation and Perinatal Outcome.* L.G. Keith, E. Papiernik, D.M. Keith, and B. Luke, eds. New York/London: Parthenon Publishing Group.

May, R.
1998 Levels of organization in ecological systems. Pp. 193-202 in *The Limits of Reductionism in Biology.* G.R. Bock and J.A. Goode, eds. (Novartis Foundation Symposium 213.) Chichester, England: Wiley.

Mazur, A., A. Booth, and J.M. Dabbs
1992 Testosterone and chess competition. *Social Psychology Quarterly* 55:70-77.

McGue, M., and D.T. Lykken
1992 Genetic influences on risk of divorce. *Psychological Science* 3:368-373.

McGuffin, P., and P. Huckle
1990 Simulation of Mendelism revisited: The recessive gene for attending medical school. *American Journal of Human Genetics* 46:994-999.

McKeown, T.
1976 *The Role of Medicine: Dream, Mirage or Nemesis?* London: Nuffield Provincial Hospitals Trust.

Medical Research Council
2000 *Personal Information in Medical Research.* London: Medical Research Council.
2001 *Human Tissue and Biological Samples for Use in Research: Operational and Ethical Guidelines.* London: Medical Research Council.

Modood, T., R. Berthoud, J. Lakey, J. Nazroo, P. Smith, S. Virdee, and S. Beishon
1997 *Ethnic Minorities in Britain: Diversity and Disadvantage.* London: Policy Studies Institute.

Moffitt, T.E., and the E-Risk Team (39 authors)
2002 Teen-aged mothers in contemporary Britain. *Journal of Child Psychology and Psychiatry* 43:727-742.

Moffitt, T.E., A. Caspi, M. Rutter, and P.A. Silva
2001 *Sex Differences in Antisocial Behaviour: Conduct Disorder, Delinquency, and Violence in the Dunedin Longitudinal Study.* Cambridge: Cambridge University Press.

Moldin, S.O., and I.I. Gottesman
1997 At issue: Genes, experience, and chance in schizophrenia—positioning for the 21st century. *Schizophrenia Bulletin* 23:547-561.

Myrianthopoulos, N.C., and M. Melnick
1977 Malformations in monozygotic twins: A possible source of environmental influence on the developmental genetic clock. Pp. 206-220 in *Gene-Environment Interactions in Common Diseases.* E. Inouye and H. Nishimusa, eds. Baltimore: University Park Press.

Nuffield Council on Bioethics
1993 *Genetic Screening: Ethical Issues.* London: Nuffield Council on Bioethics.
2002a *The Ethics of Research Related to Healthcare in Developing Countries.* London: Nuffield Council on Bioethics.
2002b *Genetics and Human Behaviour: The Ethical Context.* London: Nuffield Council on Bioethics.

Odling-Smee, F.J.
1996 Niche construction, genetic evolution and cultural change. *Behavioural Processes* 35:195-205.

Pickles, A., P. Bolton, H. Macdonald, A. Bailey, A. Le Couteur, L. Sim, and M. Rutter
1995 Latent-class analysis of recurrence risks for complex phenotypes with selection and measurement error: A twin and family history study of autism. *American Journal of Human Genetics* 57:717-726.

Plomin, R.
1994 *Genetics and Experience: The Interplay Between Nature and Nurture.* Thousand Oaks, CA: Sage.

Plomin, R., and M. Rutter
1998 Child development, molecular genetics, and what to do with genes once they are found. *Child Development* 69:1223-1242.

Plomin, R., J.C. DeFries, G.E. McClearn, and P. McGuffin
2001 *Behavioral Genetics, 4th ed.* New York: Worth.

Prescott, C.A., R.C. Johnson, and J.J. McArdle
1999 Chorion type as a possible influence on the results and interpretation of twin study data. *Twin Research* 2:244-249.

Rodgers, J.L., K. Hughes, H.-P. Kohler, K. Christensen, D. Doughty, D.C. Rowe, and W.B. Miller
2001 Genetic influence helps explain variation in human fertility: Evidence from recent behavioral and molecular genetic studies. *Current Directions in Psychological Science* 10:184-188.

Rose, S.
1995 The rise of neurogenetic determinism. *Nature* 373:380-382.
1998 *Lifelines: Biology, Freedom, Determinism.* Harmondsworth: Penguin.

Rose, H., and S. Rose, eds.
2000 *Alas, Poor Darwin: Arguments Against Evolutionary Psychology.* London: Jonathan Cape.

Rowe, D.C., K.C. Jacobson, and E.J.C.G. van den Oord
1999 Genetic and environmental influences on vocabulary IQ: Parental education level as moderator. *Child Development* 70:1151-1162.

Royal College of Psychiatrists' Working Party
2001 *Guidelines for Researchers and for Research Ethics Committees on Psychiatric Research Involving Human Participants.* London: Gaskell.

Rutter, M.
1994 Concepts of causation, tests of causal mechanisms, and implications for intervention. Pp. 147-171 in *Youth Unemployment and Society.* A.C. Petersen and J.T. Mortimer, eds. New York: Cambridge University Press.
1999 Genes and behaviour: Health potential and ethical concerns. Pp. 66-88 in *Inventing Heaven?: Quakers Confront the Challenges of Genetic Engineering.* A. Carroll and C. Skidmore, eds. Reading: Sowle Press.
2000a Genetic studies of autism: From the 1970s into the millennium. *Journal of Abnormal Child Psychology* 28:3-14.
2000b Psychosocial influences: Critiques, findings, and research needs. *Development and Psychopathology* 12:375-405.
2002a Nature, nurture, and development: From evangelism through science toward policy and practice. *Child Development* 73:1-21.
2002b The interplay of nature, nurture and developmental influences: The challenges ahead for mental health. *Archives of General Psychiatry* 59:996-1000.

Rutter, M., A. Bailey, E. Simonoff, and A. Pickles
1997 Genetic influences and autism. Pp. 370-387 in *Handbook of Autism and Pervasive Developmental Disorders, 2nd ed.* D.J. Cohen and F.R. Volkmar, eds. New York: Wiley.

Rutter, M., P. Bolton, R. Harrington, A. Le Couteur, H. Macdonald, and E. Simonoff
1990 Genetic factors in child psychiatric disorders. I. A review of research strategies. *Journal of Child Psychology and Psychiatry* 31:3-37.

Rutter, M., A. Caspi, and T.E. Moffitt
2002 Making Sense of Sex Differences in Psychopathology: Unifying Issues and Research Strategies. Under editorial review.

Rutter, M., H. Giller, and A. Hagell
1998 *Antisocial Behavior by Young People*. New York: Cambridge University Press.

Rutter, M., A. Pickles, R. Murray, and L. Eaves
2001 Testing hypotheses on specific environmental causal effects on behavior. *Psychological Bulletin* 127:291-324.

Rutter, M., and R. Plomin
1997 Opportunities for psychiatry from genetic findings. *British Journal of Psychiatry* 171:209-219.

Rutter, M., and J. Silberg
2002 Gene-environment interplay in relation to emotional and behavioral disturbance. *Annual Review of Psychology* 53:463-490.

Rutter, M., J. Silberg, T. O'Connor, and E. Simonoff
1999 Genetics and child psychiatry: I. Advances in quantitative and molecular genetics. *Journal of Child Psychology and Psychiatry* 40:3-18.

Rutter, M., and D. Smith, eds.
1995 *Psychosocial Disorders in Young People: Time Trends and Their Causes*. Chichester, England: Wiley.

Rutter, M., K. Thorpe, R. Greenwood, K. Northstone, and J. Golding
In press Twins as a natural experiment to study the causes of mild language delay: 1. Design; twin-singleton differences in language, and obstetric risks. *Journal of Child Psychology and Psychiatry*.

Scarr, S., and K. McCartney
1983 How people make their own environment: A theory of genotype greater than environmental effects. *Child Development* 54:424-435.

Selman, P., ed.
2000 *Inter-Country Adoption: Developments, Trends and Perspectives*. London: British Agencies for Adoption and Fostering.

Silberg, J., M. Rutter, M. Neale, and L. Eaves
2001 Genetic moderation of environmental risk for depression and anxiety in adolescent girls. *British Journal of Psychiatry* 179:116-121.

Silventoinen, K., J. Kaprio, E. Lahelma, and M. Koskenvuo
2000 Relative effect of genetic and environmental factors on body height: Differences across birth cohorts among Finnish men and women. *American Journal of Public Health* 90:627-630.

Simonoff, E., A. Pickles, A. Hervas, J.L. Silberg, M. Rutter, and L. Eaves
1998 Genetic influences on childhood hyperactivity: Contrast effects imply parental rating bias, not sibling interaction. *Psychological Medicine* 28:825-837.

Skuse, D.H., and J. Kuntsi
2002 Molecular genetic and chromosomal anomalies: Cognitive and behavioral consequences. Pp. 205-240 in *Child and Adolescent Psychiatry, 4th ed.* M. Rutter and E. Taylor, eds. Oxford: Blackwell Science.

Stoolmiller, M.
1999 Implications of restricted range of family environments for estimates of heritability and nonshared environment in behavior-genetic adoption studies. *Psychological Bulletin* 125:392-409.

Strachan, T., and A.P. Read
1999 *Human Molecular Genetics, 2nd ed.* Oxford: BIOS Scientific.

Swan, S.H., E.P. Elkin, and L. Fenster
1997 Have sperm densities declined? A reanalysis of global trend data. *Environmental Health Perspectives* 105:1228-1232.

Taylor, A.
2002 The Influence of Non-response on Estimates of Genetic and Environmental Effects in Behavioral-Genetic Models of Twins. Manuscript submitted for publication.

Thompson, L.A., D.K. Detterman, and R. Plomin
1991 Associations between cognitive abilities and scholastic achievement: Genetic overlap but environmental differences. *Psychological Science* 2:158-165.

Thorpe, K., M. Rutter, and R. Greenwood
In press Twins as a natural experiment to study the causes of mild language delay: 2. Family interaction risk factors. *Journal of Child Psychology and Psychiatry.*

Tizard, J.
1975 Race and IQ: The limits of probability. *New Behaviour* 1:6-9.

Trumbetta, S.L., and I.I. Gottesman
2000 Endophenotypes for marital status in the NAS-NRC twin registry. Pp. 253-269 in *Genetic Influences on Human Fertility and Sexuality: Theoretical and Empirical Contributions from the Biological and Behavioral Sciences.* J.L. Rodgers, D.C. Rowe, and W.B. Miller, eds. Boston: Kluwer.

van Wieringen, J.C.
1986 Secular growth changes. Pp. 307-331 in *Human Growth, Vol. 3, Methodology, 2nd ed.* F. Falkner and J.M. Tanner, eds. New York: Plenum Press.

Walker, S.O., S.A. Petrill, F.M. Spinath, and R. Plomin
2002 Nature, Nurture and Academic Achievement: A Twin Study of Teacher Ratings of 7 Year Olds. Manuscript submitted for publication.

Weir, J.B. de V.
1952 The assessment of the growth of schoolchildren with special reference to secular changes. *British Journal of Nutrition* 6:19-33.

3

Education, Fertility, and Heritability: Explaining a Paradox

Hans-Peter Kohler and Joseph L. Rodgers

Wilson (1998:8) promoted the importance of "consilience" in science. Consilience is the "'jumping together' of knowledge by the linking of facts and fact-based theories across disciplines to create a common groundwork of explanation." Such a process—in which disciplinary boundaries break down and then disappear (and then, perhaps, are reconstituted)—is occurring in research on human fertility. Our particular interest is in the interplay between demography and biology, as these two very different disciplines begin to blend in the long-standing effort to develop models and theories to explain human fertility. In fact, in this chapter our focus will be even sharper: We treat the interplay between genetics and fertility.

The signals that such a consilience between geneticists and demographers has been developing can be seen in the work of Adams et al. (1990) and Wood (1994). Udry (1995, 1996) added important impetus. There are two directions in which this disciplinary boundary can be crossed. The early work cited above represented (mostly) research in which demographers crossed the boundary from demography into biology and back again. Udry's (1995) article, "Sociology and biology: What biology do sociologists need to know?," is illustrative. A number of more recent publications show that the boundary is also being crossed in the other direction, as those trained in molecular and behavioral genetics present research using genetic methods but applied to topics in the traditional purview of demographers (e.g., Kohler et al., 1999; MacMurray et al., 2000; Miller et al., 1999, 2000; Rodgers et al., 2001a). Two recent papers in the journal *Demography* apply behavioral genetics methods to human fertility (Rodgers et al., 2001b) and race differences in birth weight (van den Oord and Rowe, 2000).

The controversy that can occur when disciplinary boundaries are crossed in the consilience process is illustrated by the responses to the van den Oord and Rowe paper in a later issue of *Demography* (Frank, 2001; Zuberi, 2001).[1] Similarly, a paper by Morgan and King (2001) that reviews the biological predispositions, social coercion, and individual incentives for having children in contemporary below-replacement fertility contexts resulted in diverging opinions about the usefulness of biodemographic or behavioral genetics approaches in understanding contemporary fertility behavior (Kohler, 2001; Capron and Vetta, 2001).

The idea that the disciplinary boundary can be crossed in either direction suggests two very different questions: What does genetics have to contribute to demographic research on fertility? What can demography contribute to a geneticist's thinking about fertility? These questions cannot easily or naturally be addressed together because the specificity of the models and theories in the two disciplines are at such completely different levels. Further, Wilson (1998:198) implied that an asymmetry exists in how the goals of consilience will be received by the two disciplines. In comparing medical science to social science, he stated, "The crucial difference between the two domains is consilience: The medical sciences have it and the social sciences do not." If he is correct, we can infer that genetics, as emergent from medical science, would be more naturally disposed to such an integrative and cross-disciplinary effort than demography, a social science.

We take the position that consilience is a positive development, that cross-disciplinary research has the potential to generate methods and models that are far beyond the sum of the separate contributions. Those more strongly wedded to a focal disciplinary perspective will undoubtedly be uncomfortable with our specific and also with broader efforts toward consilience. In this paper we are concerned primarily with the issue of how designs and methods that emerge from genetics research (more specifically from behavioral genetics) can contribute to demographic thinking about fertility. In particular, in this specific study we apply behavioral genetics methods to study the relationship of education, fertility, and heritability of fertility.

Before embarking on these specific analyses, we briefly consider the second question: Can demographic methods inform genetics research? In a sense the answer to that question is embedded in population genetics, and that interplay has been occurring for quite some time. Population geneticists are, fundamentally, demographers at heart. Accounting for the distri-

[1] We should note that much of the controversy arising in this exchange was over the use of a race variable rather than behavioral genetics per se.

bution of genes in the population, and studying how gene frequencies change over time through adaptive processes, is similar to the study of various demographic phenomena. The ways that demographers deal with selection (their own type of selection, as opposed to the meaning of the term in genetic/evolutionary contexts) might be one example of a domain in which demography could inform genetics. That consideration, however, is for a different paper at a different time.

How can genetic thinking inform demographic research on fertility? We list several potential answers to this question:

- Behaviors are always constrained by the limits of biological/genetic potential. Humans cannot run at 70 mph, though cheetahs can; each organism's genotype helps define the "reaction norm" involved in performance. In the domain of fertility, humans are limited in the number of offspring they can produce in a given time period (e.g., limited by the menstrual cycle and the gestational period as well as social norms). Those constraints are defined by genetic influences on physiology (which, e.g., limit the human reproductive process to few children at a time) and by genetic influences on behavior (more on that later). Individuals always need to take these restrictions as given in their own decision making and behavior, and even on the population level these biological and genetic limits are fixed within time horizons that may not allow evolutionary adaptation.
- Genes/biology limit not only the theoretical potential at the extremes but also the practical and achievable outcomes. Social behavior has genetic origins. In a distal sense, fertility motivation is influenced genetically (e.g., Miller et al., 2000). Social theories of fertility, which have long ignored the potential for genetic influence, may in fact be much closer to explaining the available variance than is commonly believed (see Rodgers, et al., 2001b). In other words, there may be less social variance available to be modeled than is widely appreciated.
- Genetic influences interact with environmental influences in fascinating and subtle ways. For example, Neiss et al. (2002) showed that, while "education partially mediated the negative association between IQ and age of first birth" in a purely social model, this mediating effect virtually disappeared when genetic influences were entered into the model.
- The assumed existence of preferences that guide behavior is a clear limitation in rational choice or the economic theories often invoked to explain fertility behavior and its change over time. Besides a set of regularity and consistency conditions, however, remarkably little can be said about the preferences for children themselves. Morgan and King (2001), for instance, realized the opportunity that evolutionary theories and behavioral genetics provide for improving our understanding of human preferences for children, and their arguments are closely related to other work that has

tried to interpret the preferences for children and related behaviors, like sexual intercourse, pair bonding, and changing fertility rates in an evolutionary perspective (e.g., Carey and Lopreato, 1995; Foster, 2000; Kaplan et al., 1995; Kohler et al., 1999; Miller and Rodgers, 2001; Potts, 1997; Udry, 1996). Hence, starting from genetic dispositions on the desire to have sex and the "joy" of nurturing, evolutionary reasoning suggests that important aspects of human reproductive behavior are shaped by genetic dispositions (which clearly must be distinguished from genetically "hard-wired" behavior). With proper designs, behavioral genetics models can therefore help to understand human preferences for children and motivations for fertility-related demographic behaviors, such as union formation or parental investments in children, and precursors of fertility such as menarche and sexual initiation.

- Multivariate behavioral genetics modeling has the potential to identify overlapping sources of variance in both genetic and environmental domains. Topics of potential interest to demographers include the following: Are the genetic sources of influence on human fertility of the same nature for early fertility, general fertility, and later fertility? Are genetic influences on fertility similar when considered across generations as those occurring within generations? How do the precursors to fertility—puberty, sexual initiation, marriage, fertility planning—overlap with one another? Further, how do these processes overlap genetically, and environmentally, and how do genetic/environmental processes interact with one another? Rodgers et al. (2001b) and Kirk et al. (2001) illustrate how multivariate analysis can inform our understanding of the overlap between different fertility-related behaviors.

Many of the above issues are of considerable relevance for researchers interested in contemporary patterns of fertility. In the next section we provide an outline of a conceptual framework that facilitates the integration of behavioral genetics modeling and thinking into more standard socioeconomic approaches to fertility and related behaviors. Subsequently, we provide a brief review of the methodology on which behavioral genetics is based. In our empirical analyses, we then apply behavioral genetics design and models to study a question of interest to demographers concerning the role of education in fertility.

INTERPRETING BEHAVIORAL GENETICS IN RESEARCH ON FERTILITY AND RELATED BEHAVIORS

Behavioral genetics is both a way of thinking about causal influence and a set of methods developed to support that thinking. As a way of thinking about causality, it is motivated by the idea that genetic and environmental influences both compete and interact with one another to influence behavior. Gottlieb (2000) criticized the "central dogma" of molecular biology that causality flows in one direction from the genes that activate DNA through proteins that they produce and ultimately to behavior. Rather, he reviewed evidence in support of probabilistic epigenesis, in which the environment also has causal influences on genes and the activation of DNA. Behavioral genetics, however, does *not* have a particular focus on genetic determinism. As Plomin and Rende (1991:162) noted, "The power of behavioral genetics lies in its ability to consider nurture as well as nature—that is, environmental as well as genetic sources of individual differences in behavior." In fact, one of the coauthors of this paper came into the behavioral genetics arena because it provided mechanisms to control for genetic variations in the study of environmental (i.e., social and cultural) influences (e.g., Rodgers, Rowe, and Li, 1994a). For example, Rodgers, Rowe, and May (1994b) showed the influence of taking trips to museums on the mathematical ability in children and the influence of owning books on reading ability in children; each of these influences was a social/environmental influence observed after controlling for genetic processes that make children naturally similar to and dissimilar from one another.

In the application to fertility and related behaviors such as marriage, these interactions of genetic disposition with environmental contexts and individual characteristics can be naturally explored. Traditionally, demographers and related social scientists have emphasized the demand for children as a key factor in explaining contemporary fertility changes. The explanations of a shifting demand for children often focus on changes in education, income, labor market opportunities, female wages, child care arrangements, and so forth, that have been associated with the socioeconomic transformations in developed countries in recent years. These shifts in socioeconomic conditions have also led to changes in many fertility-related behaviors, such as marriage/union formation and female labor force participation, which are also closely related to changing demands for children.

It should be noted that such socioeconomic considerations of fertility change are rarely inconsistent with biological theories. To the contrary, recent evolutionary approaches to demographic change frequently incorporate transformations in the context of fertility decisions through socioeconomic changes or technical innovations. In particular, socioeconomic changes and technological innovations lead to adjustments in the optimal fertility strategies because they alter incentives for allocating scarce resources, such as time and energy, to reproductive efforts, child quality versus quantity, somatic investments, and several other competing uses (e.g., see Hill and Kaplan, 1999; Kaplan et al., 2000; Lam, this volume).

While evolutionary and socioeconomic theories are therefore quite compatible in their general approaches toward explaining levels of fertility, the challenge for incorporating biological dispositions with sociological theories is in the explanation of within-population variations in behavior. In particular, differential biological dispositions of individuals—resulting, for instance, from genetic variations or hormonal influences—can be important determinants of individual behavioral differences in addition to socioeconomic incentives or structural influences. In order to see these potential interactions, we sketch a simplistic, but for our purposes sufficient, framework for fertility decisions in contemporary developed societies (see also Lam, this volume). In particular, the number of children of an individual in these contexts is strongly influenced by the age at marriage/union-formation and the number of reproductive years spent in stable unions, the level of education of the individual and his/her spouse, the abilities for and extent of labor force participation, and similar factors (Becker, 1981; Marini, 1981; Morgan and Rindfuss, 1999; Willis, 1973).

While there is some divergent assessment between economically and sociologically oriented scholars about the extent to which individuals rationally account for the potentially complex interactions between the above behaviors in their life course planning about fertility, it is probably not controversial to assert that individuals conduct conscious life course planning, including plans for marriage and fertility. These life course plans take into account an individual's (potentially incomplete) knowledge about his/her educational opportunities and returns to education, attractiveness in the marriage market (both in terms of physical and socioeconomic characteristics), assessments about opportunities in the labor market, preferences for children, and several other "goods" and/or goals. In addition, these plans are subject to important random elements, for instance, with respect to finding a partner in the marriage market, receiving positive or negative income "shocks" upon entering the labor market, or shocks in the conception and gestation processes leading to the birth of a child.

Individuals are likely to update their life course plans as they learn more about their own relevant characteristics and as they experience different random shocks that affect fertility-related aspects of their life courses. Variations in individuals' life courses—including variations with respect to important fertility outcomes—therefore arise for two reasons: First, individuals' *desired* life courses differ because of different socioeconomic opportunities or constraints and because individuals have different abilities, preferences, physical characteristics, and so forth, that they take into account in making life cycle decisions and plans. Second, the *realized* life courses of individuals differ from their initial plans, as well as among individuals, due to shocks in fertility and fertility-related behaviors/processes, such as an unexpectedly long waiting time to conception or the death of a spouse.

This complex embeddedness of fertility outcome into life course decisions and processes points to a broad framework of genetically mediated influences. In particular, differential genetic dispositions can exert influences on fertility and related behaviors through at least three distinct pathways. On the one hand, biological dispositions affect fertility relatively directly through genetically mediated variations in physiological characteristics affecting fertility outcomes. Genetic influences on fecundity are an obvious example (e.g., see Christensen et al., 2003), but there are also other possibilities, including, for instance, the fact that physical characteristics might render a person especially attractive in the marriage market, which increases the probability of an early marriage because of an unexpected high frequency of attractive marriage offers in early adulthood.

On the other hand, and potentially more interesting in the context of this paper, biological dispositions affect fertility through deliberate fertility decisions and a broad range of fertility-related behaviors that are subject to substantial volitional control. Within this category of influences, we can further distinguish between two different pathways. First, some biological dispositions exert their effect on behavior through conscious decision making and life course planning. Second, biological dispositions may also operate subconsciously on decision processes if individuals are not aware of their background influences on aspects such as emotions, preferences, or cognitive abilities. Examples for the former are individuals' knowledge about their fecundity (e.g., see Rosenzweig and Schultz, 1985) or knowledge about their returns to schooling and delaying fertility (see, for instance, Behrman et al., 1994, 1996). In addition, Halpern et al. (2000) found that "smart teens don't have sex or kiss much either," which is consistent with higher cognitive abilities and an awareness about the high costs of early pregnancies due to foregone opportunities. Further examples of subconscious influences are variations in evolved preferences for nurturing (Foster, 2000; Miller and Rodgers, 2001). Moreover, early sexual activity, which is a predictor of early fertility, has also been related to nonvolitional factors such as hormone levels and body fat (e.g., Halpern et al., 1997, 1999), both of which are subject to strong genetic variations.

In summary, the above interpretations view genetic dispositions as part of individuals' endowments that affect their life course patterns, including those pertaining to fertility and related behaviors, through their effect on (1) conscious decision making and deliberate life cycle planning, (2) nonvolitional processes affecting life course outcomes, and (3) physical characteristics or cognitive abilities that partially determine opportunities in the labor market and marriage market. Instead of focusing on these specific pathways of how genetic dispositions affect fertility outcomes, most current behavioral genetics designs try to identify and estimate the *net* contribution of a broad range of genetically mediated biological factors on the variations in fertility behavior *within* a population or within cohorts.

The advantage of this approach is that it provides an estimate of the overall relevance of genetically mediated biological effects on variations in fertility behavior. This information about the overall relevance of genetically mediated variations is interesting in itself. Moreover, this information will guide future research with respect to the scope of investigating specific mechanisms and pathways of biological influences: If the net overall variation attributed to genetic factors is high, the search for specific pathways (or possibly even specific gene factors) is likely to be more promising compared to a situation in which the overall influence is found to be low. In addition, studies of overall genetic variations in fertility outcomes can suggest specific socioeconomic contexts of cohorts that seem to facilitate genetically-mediated variation in fertility behavior, and these genetic-socioeconomic interactions will provide considerable scope for integrating sociological and biological theories about reproductive behavior.

Although most behavioral genetics work, including that applied to fertility, still focuses on partitioning variances into genetic and environmental components, broader applications are emerging (see Rutter, this volume). On the one hand, more sophisticated modeling and theorizing are supported by an increased availability of data, including large-scale twin and family data that are rich in socioeconomic life course information pertaining to education, marriage/union or labor market history, and genetic relatedness. Such data can be used to estimate multivariate behavioral genetics models that disentangle the pathways of genetic influences, such as the processes affecting marriage/union formation, age at first birth, educational attainment, and so forth. For an example of such an application, see the study by Rodgers et al. (2003), which uses age at first pregnancy attempt as an indicator of (volitional) fertility motivation and lag to pregnancy as a measure of (nonvolitional) fecundity. The study implements a methodology that allows competition between these two domains—the psychological and the biological—in accounting for the genetic variance underlying fertility outcomes.

In addition to suggesting the joint investigation of genetic dispositions and life course processes/decisions, the framework outlined above implies that the relevance of genetic factors for variations in fertility outcomes within cohorts is likely to be strongly conditioned by the socioeconomic context of the cohorts. A possibly surprising—but robust—finding in some of our earlier analyses (Kohler et al., 1999, 2002b), for instance, is a systematic relationship between fertility transitions and patterns in both heritabilities and shared environmental variance in data on female Danish twins: Increased opportunities for education and labor market participation and the emergence of relaxed and flexible reproductive norms in recent decades seem to have strengthened the genetic component in fertility outcomes. Finding these varying influences is consistent with, even predicted by, our understanding of how genetic factors affect fertility decisions that are embedded in broader-context life cycle decision making. For instance, changes in patterns of female labor force participation may heighten the extent to which genetically mediated influences on ability and hence wages affect fertility, or higher mobility may increase the size of the marriage market and therefore strengthen the implications of variation in endowments on the timing and probability of marriage. We have argued (Kohler et al., 1999) that reduced social constraints on fertility and related behaviors, increased opportunities, and more egalitarian societies have increased the relevance of genetically mediated variation in preferences for children on fertility outcomes.

Few of these pathways have been explored in detail, but future studies with twin (or kinship) data that contain extensive socioeconomic information and life course histories can potentially overcome this limitation. Future analyses therefore not only need to estimate sophisticated behavioral genetics models for fertility and related behaviors but also need to allow for interactions between the socioeconomic context, individual characteristics and life histories, and patterns of heritability. In the empirical part of this chapter we apply behavioral genetics designs and models to study one such interaction between genetic dispositions and socioeconomic environments, specifically education, and show how the effect of genetic dispositions on fertility differs between individuals with different education levels. Before we embark on these empirical analyses, we provide a more general introduction to behavioral genetics designs and methods.

BEHAVIORAL GENETICS DESIGNS AND METHODS

The methodology of behavioral genetics begins with research design and then moves to a set of analytic models that can be used to estimate the parameters of the biometrical model. The classic behavioral genetics design is the twin design in which the similarity between identical and fraternal twins is compared on some trait of interest (e.g., completed fertility). Other designs include the family design, the adoption design, and the identical-twins-raised-apart design. As in any research arena, each design has logical weaknesses that leave threats to the validity of conclusions based on those designs. Also, each design rests on a set of assumptions. For example, assumptions of the twin design include no influence of assortative mating and equal environments (e.g., Plomin, 1990).

A complete statement of the behavioral genetics design logic and the basic quantitative genetics model is beyond the scope of this chapter, although we can summarize some of the basic theory and original references. Much of the original design work was done by Fisher (1930). The original and most complete statement of the quantitative genetics model on which behavioral genetics research comes from Falconer (1981). A cogent and comprehensive textbook that reviews the field is that by Plomin et al. (1990), and a more accessible review is contained in Plomin (1990). A common feature of the analytic models used in behavioral genetics work is that the analyses estimate parameters related to genetic variability (usually referred to as heritability, or h^2), shared environmental variability (or c^2), and nonshared environmental variability (or e^2). These parameters represent, respectively, the fraction of variance in a trait or outcome that is due to genetic factors, shared environmental influences like common family backgrounds, and finally individual-specific environmental factors. This interpretation of behavioral genetics results in terms of c^2, h^2 and e^2, however, is correct only in a particular model that specifies how the different factors interact to jointly influence the outcome, quite similar to the fact that the structural interpretation of regression parameters in socioeconomic studies of fertility depends critically on the correctness of the underlying behavioral model and the appropriateness of the estimation strategy. Common—but not necessarily required—assumptions of behavioral genetics models include the additivity of the elements in the model (e.g., additive genetic and environmental influences). In principle, both the design and analytic assumptions are often violated. Extensive study has been given to the nature and effect of violating these assumptions, and these effects are well documented (e.g., Plomin, 1990).

In addition, there have been substantial developments in methods and data innovations that increase the value of twin and family designs. On the one hand, studies of twins are increasingly based on large-scale twin data, sometimes representing the complete population of twins of a country and including longitudinal follow-up (Kyvik et al., 1996, 1995; Pedersen et al., 1991), with low measurement error on key biological and socioeconomic variables and potentially extensive information about nonshared environments in childhood and adulthood. On the other hand, the limitations of the textbook behavioral genetics model are increasingly being overcome, including also in the application of behavioral genetics models to demography. For instance, Kohler and Rodgers (1999) have developed models for binary and ordered models, which are especially suited to the dependent variables such as "having at least one child" or "number of children," and Yashin and Iachine (1997) describe behavioral genetics models suitable for the analysis of mortality or other duration data such as the timing of children. Major advances in disentangling gene-environment interactions are possible with large twin datasets that encompass cohorts that experience substantially different socioeconomic and demographic contexts. For instance, using local regression techniques and cohort interactions, we have shown that genetic influences on fertility have been subject to variations over time (Kohler et al., 1999, 2002b). These local regression techniques therefore account for major gene-environment interactions that occur across cohorts. An alternative possibility is to test gene-environment interactions by incorporating additional socioeconomic conditions and information about the parental household and spouses of the twins. Moreover, these twin models sometimes allow for explicit tests of alternative genetic models, such as dominance effects. An additional development of particular value to demographers is the identification of kinship structure in large national datasets like the National Longitudinal Survey of Youth (NLSY). Using information from the survey, Rodgers et al. (1994) developed an algorithm that specified kinship structure in the children of the NLSY youth data and in another study Rodgers et al. (1999) reported a similar linking algorithm that specified kinship links for the NLSY youth respondents. These links open up the potential to do behavioral genetics analyses on national probability samples (a common criticism of the twins study is its low external validity) using the rich longitudinal and multivariate structure of such data sources.

Behavioral genetics methods have long been criticized by those outside the field (e.g., Lewontin et al., 1984, have defined a popular set of criticisms of the basic behavioral genetics design, including in particular the confounded nature of the genotype of monozygotic twins genotype and similar treatment by their families and peers).[2] Interestingly, the behavioral genetic community itself is filled with internal critics who have carefully scrutinized and criticized these methods, and (arguably) the strongest and most cogent criticisms arise from behavioral geneticists themselves. For example,

[2]In fact, reviewers of the empirical results presented later in this chapter raised the issue of whether the results could have been caused by the greater similarity in appearance/attractiveness of MZ twins compared to dizygotic (DZ) twins. For example, could MZ twin correlations in fertility that are higher than DZ twin correlations in fertility be caused by the greater similarity in appearance/attractiveness for MZ twins? This concern is a form of the well-studied equal environments assumption of behavioral genetics modeling. This assumption has been studied in several ways. "Mislabeling studies" have studied persons (especially twins) misdiagnosed for zygosity; typically, their correlational patterns are similar to their biological zygosity, rather than their presumed (incorrect) zygosity (Scarr and Carter-Saltzman, 1979). Other studies have directly addressed similarity of appearance (e.g., Loehlin and Nichols, 1976). Plomin et al. (1990:319) reviewed these studies and concluded that the data "strongly support the reasonableness of the equal environments assumption." More specifically related to the current research are a number of past studies of fertility based on family designs that come to similar conclusions as our studies of twins (see Rodgers et al., 2001a, for a review). Those family studies include cousins, half siblings, and full siblings (in addition to a few twins). Though siblings are more genetically related than half siblings (for example), they are not likely to be much more similar in appearance or attractiveness. Though the concern over the appearance confound is well founded, evidence has not yet emerged that either behavioral traits in general or fertility in particular are especially influenced by violations of the equal environments assumption. Nevertheless, behavioral genetics texts recommend continued caution.

Turkheimer (1998:782) suggested that "heritability and psychobiological association cannot be the basis for establishing whether behavior is genetic or biological, because to do so leads only to the banal tautology that all behavior is ultimately based in the genotype and brain." Lest one interpret this as dismissive of past behavioral genetics research, Turkheimer (2000) published his "three laws of behavior genetics": (1) All human behavior is heritable; (2) shared environmental influences are typically smaller than genetic influences on behavior; and (3) a great deal of behavioral variability is not based in either genetics or families. In addition, a recent review by Rose (1995:648-649) identified several emerging ideas and enduring issues in behavioral genetics, including a new design based on dividing pairs of MZ twins into those who shared a placenta in utero versus those who did not, and treatment of the question of whether (and how) family environment is relevant to development. Rose concluded: "Few areas of psychology are changing as rapidly as behavior genetics. Few are as filled with excitement and promise. Few are as surrounded by controversy." Wahlsten (1999:599), in his review, described the blending of behavioral genetics and neurogenetics into the field of "neorobehavioral genetics, focusing on single-gene effects," the type of consilience described in the opening sentences of this chapter. Finally, Rutter and Silberg's (2002:465) review of behavioral genetics focused on gene-environment correlations and interactions. They emphasize that "the genes that influence sensitivity to the environment may be quite different from those that bring about main effects."

In summary, therefore, while researchers need to be aware of the specific assumptions underlying behavioral genetics models (see Rutter, this volume), just as they must be aware of the assumptions underlying other domains of empirical work, recent methodological progress provides a powerful set of methods to investigate the relevance of genetic factors also in demography. The broad range of empirical and theoretical possibilities of how these methods can be used and integrated with demography is illustrated in two recent books on genetic influences on fertility and sexuality and the biodemography of fertility (Rodgers et al., 2000; Rodgers and Kohler, 2003).

EDUCATION, FERTILITY TRANSITION, AND FERTILITY OUTCOMES

Our goal in this section is to (begin to) explain a paradox. On the one hand, our previous analyses have shown that genetic factors contribute to variations in fertility outcomes, including the number of children, timing of the first child, and the age at first attempt to become pregnant (e.g., Rodgers et al., 2001a, 2001b). On the other hand, genetic influence related to natural selection changes very slowly; an exception is genetic influence related to mutation that can change abruptly but also idiosyncratically and only in the individual (at least in the short term). But we have also shown that there can be rapid change in both heritabilities (h^2) and coefficients of genetic variation (CVa) across very short periods of time (Kohler et al., 1999). The paradox is that a process, like genetic contributions to variations in fertility, which some would presume to be fixed and virtually immutable, can change rapidly in a short period of time.

Part of the answer to the paradox is that both heritabilities and coefficients of genetic variation are in no sense immutable. On the contrary, the understanding of genetic influences on fertility and related behavior outlined in the previous section suggests transformation in the pattern of how genetic shared environmental and individual-specific environmental factors contribute to variations in fertility outcomes in a population. Nevertheless, our previous research was not able to identify specific socioeconomic changes or characteristics that are the driving forces behind these transformations, and our earlier analyses relied on indirect explanation on the basis of overall socioeconomic and demographic changes across cohorts.

In this study we can overcome this limitation and investigate one particular aspect that is central to socioeconomic and demographic change over time and that is also likely to be an important factor behind the transformation of heritability patterns across cohorts: education.

In the Danish data used by Kohler et al. (1999), the very short periods of time during which heritabilities changed from essentially 0 to .40 and back again corresponded to a demographically important interval: the fertility transition resulting in lower fertility due to the adoption of conscious fertility limitation within marriage. Further, similar to many other European countries, Denmark experienced a second demographic transition staring in the late 1960 and early 1970s (Lesthaeghe and van de Kaa, 1986; van de Kaa, 1987) that was associated with further declines in fertility rates, a rise in cohabiting unions, and ideational changes toward more individualistic values and norms. Despite the somewhat different determinants of fertility change in the first and second demographic transitions the phenomenon of changing heritabilities is replicated, almost exactly, in each fertility transition.

It is worth considering the conceptual role of education in fertility transition in general. Virtually all accounts of fertility transition include education as either the cause or effect (or even both). For example, Cleland (2001:51) noted, "life expectancy and the level of adult education, or literacy, are the strongest predictors of fertility decline." Declining fertility clearly provides opportunity for both women and men to spend the time they previously spent in childbearing and child rearing in other activities. Thus, fertility transition frees up time to support increased educational attainment, especially for women. At the same time, improvements in health care and reductions in mortality (especially maternal and infant mortality) are driven in part by increased technical sophistication—that is, by the education level supporting technological development—inherent in society.

Thus, educational improvements can themselves drive fertility transitions. This causal direction is the one to which Bongaarts and Watkins (1996:639) refer: "As a society develops (modernizes), economic and social changes such as industrialization, urbanization, and increased education first lead to a decline in mortality, and subsequently also to a decline in fertility." Our treatment does not require formal separation of these complex causal interrelationships; in fact, we view both causal directions to be critical features of any complete explanatory system of fertility transition. The variance partitioning methodology that underlies behavioral genetics methods is consistent with the sense derived from the literature on fertility transition that education is embedded in the transitional processes, as both cause and effect.

In this treatment we therefore investigate the relationship between education, heritability, and fertility, with special attention to our earlier finding that heritabilities can change rapidly during periods of rapid fertility change. Education is of particular importance in this context because, as noted above, many accounts and explanations of fertility change refer in some way or another to education. We describe next specific examples of how education can influence family size and vice versa.

Education is considered by some to be the prime cause of fertility transition, acting as the proximal stimulus that improves health care, drives down infant and maternal mortality, contributes to reversals of wealth, increases the ability to "produce" high-quality children in the household, and increases women's opportunities in the labor market. The influence of education continues to be prominent also in posttransitional contexts with low fertility because it is an important determinant of female wages, which determine the opportunity costs of childbearing and shift the relative bargaining of males and females in households with potentially important effects on fertility decisions.

In addition, pursuing education, particularly higher education, is associated with specific social environments that can affect fertility preferences and desires if social interactions affect fertility decisions through social learning or social influence (e.g., Montgomery and Casterline, 1996; Kohler et al., 2002c). Evidence for this important role of education, among many other supportive findings, is the often-cited negative correlation between family size and various indicators related to maternal education (e.g., Higgins et al., 1962; Retherford and Sewell, 1988; Roberts, 1938). Rodgers et al. (2000) additionally asked the question, "Do large families make low-IQ children, or do low-IQ parents make large families?" Based on an analysis of recent national data from the United States, they concluded that the answers are "no" and "yes," respectively.

Both the reasoning and the empirical data reviewed above point to the critical role that maternal education plays in models of fertility transition and posttransitional fertility behavior, and, more specifically, in the role that genetic processes play as influences of fertility during fertility transition. To investigate this role of education from a behavioral genetics perspective, we pursue two different set of analyses. First, we estimate multivariate behavioral genetics models to decompose the variance in fertility into genetic and shared environmental components and to assess the extent to which there are overlapping sources of genetic and shared environmental influences that affect both education and fertility. Second, we extend the results from Kohler et al. (1999) to further consider maternal education as a mediator of the process of how heritabilities change over cohorts and across socioeconomic contexts. In particular, we investigate whether patterns of heritability change across educational categories within cohorts in a similar fashion as across cohorts in our earlier study (Kohler et al., 1999).

DATA

The data for our analyses were obtained from Danish twins born between 1953 and 1970 who participated in the 1994 twin omnibus survey (see Christensen et al., 1998). Included in this survey was information about the level of completed education. The survey data were augmented by a register link (described in more detail below) to include the timing and level of fertility. The analyses are based on same-sex twin pairs with verified zygosity; the sample and cohort sizes are given in Table 3-1. Table 3-2

TABLE 3-1 Number of Twins by Birth Cohort

	Complete Twin Pairs		Complete Twin Pairs (with nonmissing data for fertility and education)	
Cohort	Female	Male	Female	Male
1953-1954	342	418	302	388
1955-1956	400	506	364	488
1957-1958	546	474	508	452
1959-1960	570	594	524	562
1961-1962	648	496	600	442
1963-1964	748	496	678	456
1965-1966	742	586	680	532
1967-1968	712	492	630	422
1969-1970	542	460	504	404
Total	5,250	4,522	4,790	4,146

TABLE 3-2 Completed Education for Females and Males by Birth Cohort

	Cohort			
Completed Education (% within cohorts)	1953-1958	1959-1964	1965-1970	Total
Females				
No education beyond elementary school	12.6	12.7	9.8	11.6
Semiskilled worker	1.5	1.3	1.1	1.3
Standard basic training at apprentice school	2.8	13.2	18.1	12.5
Less than 1 year of higher education	3.3	2.8	1.9	2.6
1 to 3 years of higher education, possibly practical	31.3	28.8	28.1	29.1
3 years of higher education (e.g., technician, pedagogue)	24.2	18.4	10.4	16.8
More than 3 years of academic higher education	15.4	12.4	7.7	11.4
Still in the process of training	5.7	7.8	20.8	12.2
Males				
No education beyond elementary school	9.7	9.8	8.8	9.5
Semiskilled worker	7.1	7.4	4.2	6.3
Standard basic training at apprentice school	3.9	9.0	13.0	8.7
Less than 1 year of higher education	1.7	2.3	0.6	1.6
1 to 3 years of higher education, possibly practical	24.4	24.8	27.9	25.7
3 years of higher education (e.g., technician, pedagogue)	20.8	18.4	13.0	17.4
More than 3 years of academic higher education	21.9	19.0	9.3	16.8
Still in the process of training	4.4	5.6	20.0	9.9

summarizes the completed education for males and females in the different cohorts in our study.

Education levels in Denmark are relatively high for all cohorts, with more than 60 percent of individuals pursuing some kind of tertiary education. The most important change in female education has been the decline of women with no education beyond elementary education and an increase in women with training at apprentice school. A surprising finding in Table 3-2, however, is the absence of an increase in higher education across cohorts, while in younger cohorts the proportion of individuals with more than 3 years of education has diminished due to an increasing number of individuals still in the process of training.[3]

The most important aspect for our analysis has been the changes in the number with primary and secondary education, while changes in the level of higher education, or tertiary education, seem to have little potential to be related to heritability patterns. Table 3-3 therefore reports the mean and standard deviation of years in primary and secondary education, which are the most important education measures in our subsequent analyses (the questionnaire asked "How many years did you go to school? (Elementary school, high school, higher preparatory school)").

In contrast to the proportion of each cohort obtaining various forms of tertiary education, there is a clear cohort trend for both males and females toward prolonged education. The number of years in primary and secondary education increased almost monotonically for females from about 10.5 years (cohort 1953-1954) to 11.9 years (cohort 1969-1970) and for males from about 10.1 years (cohort 1953-1954) to 11.2 years (cohort 1969-1970).

The 1994 twin omnibus survey also contains information about fertility of twins. In addition, we have obtained the fertility histories of participating twins from a link with the civil registration system (see Kohler et al., 2002a, for a description). This link has the advantage that it covers the period up to the end of 1998 (instead of up to 1994 as reported in the survey), and it also contains information about the timing of births and sex of the children. Moreover, these register data are free of potential recall errors.

Our analyses are thus based on the fertility information obtained from the register link that covers all births until the end of 1998. The average numbers of children born by birth cohort are given in Table 3-4. Female cohort fertility has been relatively constant across the cohorts born in the early 1960s (see also Knudsen, 1993) and then declines. This decline is partly due to the fact that women in these younger cohorts had not completed their childbearing by the end of 1998, which is the last year for which births to twins were obtained from the register. Male fertility follows a similar trend, with the primary difference that the decline of fertility

---

[3]The youngest cohorts in Table 3-2 were only 24 years old at the time of the survey in 1994 and therefore had not completed tertiary education. In the 1965-1970 cohorts 20 percent of the male [and 20.8 percent of the female] respondents were still in training. Since this training primarily pertains to the highest education categories in the table, it can be expected that the 1965-1970 cohort attained the highest education levels in the table. Updated information about this completed education will be available soon from new survey data collected in 2002.

TABLE 3-3 Years of Primary and Secondary Schooling

Cohort	Females Mean	Females Standard Deviation	Males Mean	Males Standard Deviation
1953-1954	10.52	1.87	10.05	2.10
1955-1956	11.07	1.92	10.47	1.84
1957-1958	11.12	1.69	10.53	1.74
1959-1960	11.10	1.48	10.77	1.99
1961-1962	11.24	1.68	10.70	1.97
1963-1964	11.45	1.64	10.73	1.87
1965-1966	11.52	1.79	10.95	1.95
1967-1968	11.71	1.81	11.23	2.05
1969-1970	11.86	1.74	11.16	2.02

TABLE 3-4 Number of Children Born Until End of 1998

Cohort	Females Mean	Females Standard Deviation	Males Mean	Males Standard Deviation
1955-1956	1.68	1.01	1.71	1.18
1957-1958	1.65	1.15	1.74	1.14
1959-1960	1.80	1.05	1.59	1.22
1961-1962	1.76	1.06	1.44	1.07
1963-1964	1.64	1.10	1.39	1.12
1965-1966	1.43	1.03	1.05	1.05
1967-1968	1.11	0.98	0.75	0.90
1969-1970	0.78	0.89	0.47	0.72

across cohorts began earlier—starting for cohorts born in the late 1950s—and is more pronounced. This difference is likely to be caused by the somewhat later age pattern of childbearing and the age difference between mothers and fathers.

A potential criticism of a study of the fertility of twins is that twins are not a random draw of all children. Twins are more likely to be born prematurely and to have lower birth weights than nontwins. In this survey DZ twins were born more frequently to older mothers for the birth years covered. A close congruence between the fertility patterns of twins and those of the general population is therefore an essential precondition in order to generalize the results of twin-based investigations into biosocial determinants of fertility to the general population. In Kohler et al. (2002a) we estimated the fertility of the general Danish population at ages 34, 35, and 40 and combined different fertility indices (number of children, parity progression measures, age at first birth) with corresponding measures for the twins population (combined and separately by zygosity). The comparison was restricted to 14,600 twins in complete same-sex pairs born in 1945-1965, including the twins pairs from the present study. The comparison in Kohler et al. (2002c) found a very close correspondence between the fertility level and its change across cohorts in both the twins and the general population. There exist only a few statistically significant differences; the primary difference pertained to the fact that female twins seem to have a slightly later onset of childbearing, which may be due to sibling influences because twins always have at least one sibling (e.g., see Murphy and Knudsen, 2002). There are virtually no relevant differences between the fertility patterns of MZ and DZ twins.

MULTIVARIATE BEHAVIORAL GENETICS MODELS FOR EDUCATION AND FERTILITY

Our first set of analyses considers jointly the genetic and shared environmental variance components in completed education and fertility. We restrict these analyses to cohorts born prior to 1963—that is, the subset of cohorts at least 35 years old in 1998 when our fertility data were censored. For these cohorts we can therefore investigate completed or almost-completed fertility. We then analyze the number of children born to twins, together with a measure of completed education that was obtained by converting the education categories in Table 3-2 into years of tertiary education.[4]

The data include 539 female MZ, 844 female DZ, 524 male MZ, and 822 male DZ twin pairs with nonmissing information on education and fertility. The correlations for within-twin pairs obtained for our measure of completed education (years of tertiary schooling) are 0.37 for DZ males, 0.49 for MZ males, 0.34 for DZ females, and 0.50 for MZ females and for fertility 0.17 for DZ males, 0.30 for MZ males, 0.16 for DZ females, and 0.38 for MZ females. These within-variable patterns clearly suggest the presence of genetic components because the MZ twin correlations are nota-

[4]In particular, the categories were scaled as follows: (a) no education beyond elementary school, semiskilled workers, and standard basic training at apprentice school: zero years of tertiary education; (b) less than 1 year of education: 0.5 years; (c) 1 to 3 years of education, possibly practical: 2 years; (d) 3 years of education (e.g., technician, pedagogue): 3 years; (e) academic education of more than 3 years: 5 years; (d) still in education: 2 years or number of years corresponding to already completed education (if more than 2). For cohorts born prior to 1963, only 7 percent of females and 5 percent of males were still in training.

bly higher than the DZ twin correlations. Also, for females the within-MZ twin-pair correlation for fertility is more than twice as large as the corresponding correlation for DZ twins. This pattern is suggestive of the possibility of nonlinear genetic influences such as dominance or epistasis. Detailed analysis of these effects, however, is beyond the scope of this chapter.

The starting point for most biometrical analyses using behavioral genetics designs is the ACE model, in which A refers to a latent genetic influence, C to a latent common (or shared) environmental influence, and E to a combination of measurement error and nonshared environmental influence. The relative importance of these influences is usually expressed in terms of heritability, h^2, which is equal to the proportion of total phenotypic variance attributable to (additive) genetic variance, and the coefficient of shared environmental influences, c^2, which is equal to the proportion of the total variance related to differences in shared-environmental conditions, such as parental background, and socialization. Estimates for heritability and shared environmental influence are conditional on a specific behavioral genetics model and are typically obtained by either structural equations modeling (SEM) or a regression method called DeFries-Fulker (or DF) analysis (DeFries and Fulker, 1985). SEM approaches use maximum likelihood as the fitting criterion and require both a structural model explaining the relationship between the constructs of the model and a measurement model explaining the relationship between the constructs and the variables used to measure the constructs. Mx (Neale et al., 1999) is a statistical software package that implements SEM methodology specifically to estimate behavioral genetics models.

Once the basic ACE model is fit to a particular dependent variable (often called the "phenotype" in the literature), additional adjustments can be made in the models to help understand the processes that generated the data. For example, fitting dominance models instead of additive models is possible (e.g., an ADE model). Dropping parts of the model with statistically meaningless parameter values results in fitting AE or CE models.

In the context of this chapter, the most interesting and valuable extension of the basic ACE model is the bivariate or multivariate model, in which overlapping sources of variance are evaluated. We estimate this model in Mx using the Cholesky decomposition model shown in Figure 3-1 for females and Figure 3-2 for males.[5,6] Because completed education is

---

[5]To save space, we have only represented the model for one member of the kin pair; the other twin's model is identical, and the two are linked with bidirectional paths between the A and C components.

[6]In a related application (Rodgers et al., 2003), we fit similar bivariate behavioral genetics models to evaluate whether there was overlapping variance between the number of children and age at first pregnancy attempt.

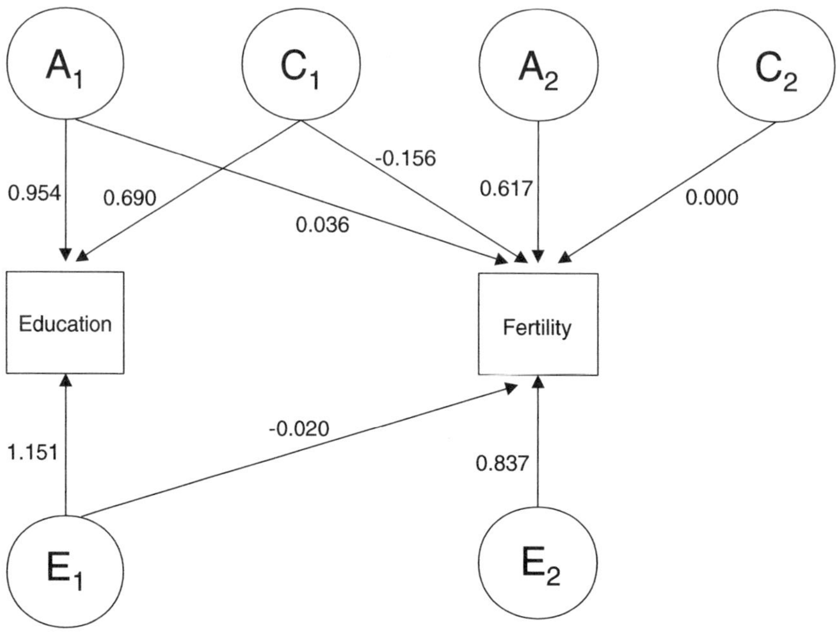

FIGURE 3-1 Bivariate behavioral genetics model for education and fertility, females.

entered first, this bivariate behavioral genetics model provides information regarding the degree to which the same set of genetic and environmental factors influence variations in education and fertility. In addition, the model provides estimates of residual amounts of genetic and environmental variance that affect fertility independent of variations associated with education.

For females the results of the bivariate behavioral genetics model shown in Figure 3-1 imply a heritability of our education measure (years of tertiary education) of $h^2 = 0.33$ (95 percent CI: 0.17 to 0.48) and a coefficient of shared environmental influences of $c^2 = 0.18$ (95 percent CI: 0.06 to 0.30). For fertility the coefficients of heritability and shared environmental influences are equal to $h^2 = 0.35$ (95 percent CI: 0.23 to 0.42) and $c^2 = 0.02$ (95 percent CI: 0.0 to 0.1). The model therefore suggests that about 33 percent of the variance in our education measure and 35 percent of the variance in fertility are related to genetic factors, while 18 percent and 2 percent, respectively, are related to shared environmental influences.[7] The model

[7] The coefficient h^2 (or c^2) is calculated by dividing the sum of squared coefficients on the A paths (or C paths) leading to education (or fertility) by the total trait variance obtained as the

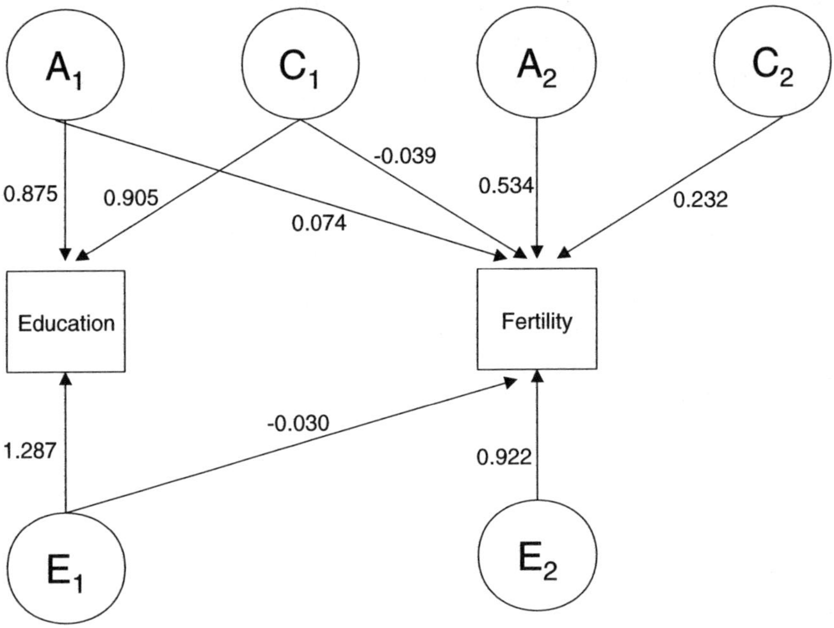

FIGURE 3-2 Bivariate behavioral genetics model for education and fertility, males.

also reveals that there are overlapping sources of genetic and shared environmental factors that affect both education and fertility. For genetic influences, however, this overlap is almost negligible, and only about 0.3 percent [= 0.036^2 / (0.036^2 + 0.617^2)] of the genetic variance in fertility is shared with education. Genetic variance in fertility is therefore almost exclusively due to residual genetic influences that affect fertility but not education. The situation is strikingly different for shared environmental influences, where the results in Figure 3-1 reveal no residual shared environmental influences for fertility; all shared environmental influences on fertility result from factors that also affect education, and shared environmental influences that increase education tend to decrease fertility. The overall effect of the contribution of these shared environmental influences to variance in fertility remains low (c^2 = 0.02 for fertility).

---

sum of all squared coefficients on the paths leading to education (or fertility). For instance, heritability of education in Figure 3-1 is obtained as $0.945^2 / (0.945^2 + 0.690^2 + 1.15^2) = 0.332$ and that of fertility is obtained as $(0.036^2 + 0.617^2) / (0.036^2 + 0.617^2 + (-0.156)^2 + 0 + (-0.020)^2 + 0.837^2) = 0.345$. We note some violations of the additive genetics model among these path coefficients.

The corresponding results for males are shown in Figure 3-2 and imply a heritability of our education measure (years of tertiary education) of h^2 = 0.24 (95 percent CI: 0.07 to 0.40) and a coefficient of shared environmental influences of c^2 = 0.25 (95 percent CI: 0.12 to 0.38). For male fertility the results imply a coefficient of heritability and shared environmental influences equal to h^2 = 0.25 (95 percent CI: 0.04 to 0.36) and c^2 = 0.05 (95 percent CI: 0.0 to 0.20). Similar to females, there is only a very small amount of overlapping genetic influence between education and fertility. In contrast to females, however, there is a substantial amount of residual shared environmental influence that affects fertility but not education, and only small amounts of shared environmental influences are common to both education and fertility.

In summary, the bivariate behavioral genetics model in Figures 3-1 and 3-2 confirms our earlier findings that fertility in low-fertility settings, such as contemporary Denmark, is subject to important genetic influences. A new and somewhat unexpected result of the above analyses is that genetic variance in fertility is not necessarily shared with genetic variance in completed education (measured in years of tertiary education). Instead, our results show that for both males and females most genetic variance in fertility is residual variance that affects the number of children but not educational attainment.[8] Overlapping influences mainly exist for shared environmental factors in female analyses, where all shared environmental factors affecting fertility also affect education.

EDUCATION AND CHANGES IN HERITABILITIES ACROSS COHORTS

The scope for analyzing education and fertility from a behavioral genetics perspective is not restricted to the above bivariate models that decompose the variance in education and fertility into genetic and environmental factors. In addition, our analysis in this section addresses whether changes in education levels across cohorts have contributed to the changing pattern of heritabilities found in our earlier studies. In particular, the hypothesis for our analyses in this section is that the increase in heritabilities for female fertility observed in younger cohorts (Kohler et al., 1999, 2002b) is partly due to increased education for females. That is, we predict that females with higher education in the older cohorts were already subject to the higher heritabilities that became characteristic later for the overall fe-

[8]In additional analyses not reported here, we found similar results using years of primary and secondary education as the education measure in the behavioral genetics model.

male population, and females with lower education were subject to lower heritabilities during the early part of this transition. We also hypothetize that the time trend toward increased heritabilities in younger cohorts is reduced once an interaction between education and heritability is incorporated into the analyses.

To investigate these hypotheses about changing cohort patterns in heritabilities, we extend the data to include all twins born during 1953-1970 for whom we observed fertility until the end of 1998 (see description of the data above). We also choose a slightly different methodology and estimate the polychoric correlation in the latent "propensity" to have children for MZ and DZ twins using bivariate ordered probit models (see Kohler and Rodgers 1999).[9] The advantages of these models are that (1) they are better suited to ordered outcomes, such as fertility, than standard behavioral genetics models and (2) the models can include various twin-pair-specific or individual-specific covariates known to influence the level of fertility. In our application, controlling for cohort trends in fertility is particularly important since there is a marked cohort trend in the average number of children born to respondents (see Table 3-4), due to the fact that younger cohorts had not completed their childbearing as of 1998. We include in the bivariate probit models 2-year cohort dummies that capture cohort trends in fertility and especially the decline in the level of fertility in younger cohorts. In addition, in some analyses we include education as another observed characteristic that affects the level of fertility of individuals. Finally, the

---

[9]The bivariate (ordered) probit model for estimation of heritability is specified as follows (see also Kohler and Rodgers 1999): y_{ij}^* is a latent scalar measuring the propensity to conceive with $y_{ij}^* = x_{ij}\beta + e_{ij}$, where $i = 1, \ldots, N$ denotes twin pairs; $j = 1, 2$ denotes twins within twin pairs; x_{ij} is a $1 \times K_1$ vector of covariates; and e_{ij} is a normally distributed random term that is independent across twin pairs but correlated within pairs. The observed variable (or trait) y_{ij} equals $0, 1, \ldots,$ if the latent variable y_{ij}^* falls into the intervals $(-\infty, c_1], \ldots, (c_\omega, \infty)$, where $c_1, \ldots, c_\omega$ are estimated cut points and $\omega + 1$ is the number of categories. The bivariate probit model is a special case with only two categories and $\omega = 1$. To estimate heritabilities, the correlation of the random terms e_{i1} and e_{i2} in twin pairs is specified as $\rho_i = \delta_1 + \delta_2 R_i$, where R_i is the genetic relatedness of twin pair i. The coefficients δ_1 and δ_2 yield estimates for the shared environment effect, c^2, and the genetic effect, h^2, respectively, while the coefficient β estimates the influence of the covariates x_{ij} on the mean realization of the propensity y_{ij}^* and the trait y_{ij}. In order to estimate the within-twin pair correlation in the random propensity, e_{ij} to have children, as we do in the present analyses, the equation for the correlation is specified as $\rho_i = \delta_1 I_{MZ,i} + \delta_2 I_{DZ,i}$, where $I_{MZ,i}$ and $I_{DZ,i}$ are dummy variables that are equal to 1 if twin pair i is MZ or DZ, respectively. In the analyses that include interactions with birth year and/or education levels, specification of the correlation is extended with interaction effects as $\rho_i = \delta_1 \cdot I_{MZ,i} + \delta_2 \cdot I_{MZ,i} \cdot \text{birth year}_i + \delta_3 \cdot I_{MZ,i} \cdot \text{education}_i + \delta_4 I_{DZ,i} + \delta_5 \cdot I_{DZ,i} \cdot \text{birth year}_i + \delta_6 \cdot I_{DZ,i} \cdot \text{education}_i$, where education$_i$ denotes the average education within a twin pair (in some models one of the two interactions is dropped).

focus of our analyses on polychoric MZ and DZ twin-pair correlations, instead of heritabilities, is advantageous because these analyses do not assume a specific behavioral genetics model that is based on assumptions such as additive genetic influences or the absence of assortative mating. Within-pair correlations therefore provide a more direct assessment of changes in the similarity of fertility patterns of MZ and DZ twins across cohorts, and these correlations do not require assumptions about a specific genetic model that is required in order to translate these correlations into coefficients of h^2 and c^2.[10] In other words, we report statistics more closely related to the raw data and less influenced by assumptions of the additive genetics model.

In contrast to our bivariate behavioral genetics model in the previous section, which focused on completed education and (almost) complete fertility, we characterize education in our subsequent analyses by the number of years of primary and secondary education. This different specification is motivated by two considerations. First, in young cohorts many respondents had not completed their education at the time of the twin omnibus survey in 1994, and there is substantial uncertainty about the level of completed education in young cohorts in our data. Second, primary and secondary education is usually completed prior to fertility, and years of primary and secondary education therefore provide an indicator of educational and professional opportunities in early adulthood that are an important determinant of life course decisions regarding fertility and related decisions. If these opportunities are an important factor affecting the relevance of genetic influences on fertility, as we argued in our earlier studies, our reasoning suggests that primary and secondary education should interact with the genetic etiology of fertility.

In our subsequent bivariate probit analyses of the within-MZ and within-DZ pair correlations in the propensity to have children, we include the above education measure (years of primary and secondary education) in a twofold manner: First, we include individual education as a determinant of the level of fertility. Second, we calculate the average number of years of schooling for each twin pair and estimate interactions between the level of education in a twin pair and the MZ/DZ twin-pair correlation in the propensity to have children. These latter interaction models will be of primary interest since the interaction terms with education reveal whether the pattern of heritability in fertility changes systematically with different levels of educational attainment.

Table 3-5 reports the results of the following analyses:

---

[10]We note, however, that these correlations and corresponding covariances represent exactly the same information used in more sophisticated biometrical fitting routines to estimate h^2 and c^2.

TABLE 3-5 Females—Bivariate Ordered Probit Estimation for Number of Children

Females	Number of Children				
	Model 1	Model 2	Model 3	Model 4	Model 5
Variables influencing mean level					
Cohort (reference category: cohort 1953-54)					
1955-1956	–0.085	–0.056	–0.057	–0.058	–0.058
	(0.092)	(0.091)	(0.090)	(0.091)	(0.090)
1957-1958	–0.109	–0.075	–0.077	–0.075	–0.076
	(0.086)	(0.086)	(0.084)	(0.085)	(0.084)
1959-1960	0.050	0.084	0.082	0.081	0.080
	(0.085)	(0.085)	(0.084)	(0.085)	(0.084)
1961-1962	–0.002	0.040	0.038	0.039	0.038
	(0.083)	(0.083)	(0.082)	(0.083)	(0.082)
1963-1964	–0.104	–0.051	–0.053	–0.051	–0.052
	(0.082)	(0.082)	(0.081)	(0.082)	(0.081)
1965-1966	–0.327	–0.272	–0.273	–0.273	–0.274
	(0.082)**	(0.082)**	(0.081)**	(0.082)**	(0.081)**
1967-1968	–0.667	–0.601	–0.603	–0.599	–0.600
	(0.084)**	(0.084)**	(0.083)**	(0.084)**	(0.083)**
1969-1970	–1.041	–0.968	–0.968	–0.968	–0.968
	(0.089)**	(0.089)**	(0.089)**	(0.089)**	(0.089)**
Years of elementary and secondary	–0.063	–0.063	–0.064	–0.064	
education		(0.010)**	(0.010)**	(0.010)**	(0.010)**
Constant	1.019	1.694	1.695	1.700	1.699
	(0.070)**	(0.128)**	(0.127)**	(0.127)**	(0.126)**

(continues)

TABLE 3-5 Continued

Females	Number of Children				
	Model 1	Model 2	Model 3	Model 4	Model 5
Correlation within twin pairs					
DZ twins	0.164	0.150	0.150	0.152	0.151
	(0.029)**	(0.030)**	(0.030)**	(0.030)**	(0.030)**
DZx (birth year - 1961.5)			0.005		0.005
			(0.007)		(0.007)
DZ x (years of elementary + secondary Education - 11.04)				−0.007	−0.007
				(0.022)	(0.022)
MZ twins	0.486	0.482	0.466	0.465	0.454
	(0.028)**	(0.028)**	(0.030)**	(0.030)**	(0.031)**
MZ x (birth year - 1961.5)			0.013		0.010
					(0.006)*
	(0.007)				
MZ x (years of elementary + secondary Education - 11.04)				0.049	0.043
				(0.017)**	(0.018)*
N (twin pairs)	2,395	2,395	2,395	2,395	2,395

NOTES: p values: + < .1; * < .05; ** < .01. Cut points of the ordered probit model are not reported.

- *Model 1*: bivariate probit estimation with only birth-year dummies.
- *Model 2*: bivariate probit estimation with birth-year dummies and education (years of elementary and secondary schooling).
- *Model 3*: bivariate probit estimation with birth-year dummies, education, and interaction of correlation with birth year (centered around mean birth year).
- *Model 4*: bivariate probit estimation with birth-year dummies, education, and interaction of correlation with twin-pair average years of schooling (centered around overall mean of schooling).
- Model 5: bivariate probit estimation with birth-year dummies, education, and interaction of correlation with birth year and education.

Our first set of analyses in Model 1 reflects the trend in the level of fertility through the increasingly negative size of the cohort dummies that measure the decrease in the latent propensity to have children in the ordered probit models in younger cohorts as compared to the reference category. Moreover, the analyses also reveal a DZ correlation in the propensity to have children of about 0.164 and a MZ correlation of about 0.486. As we have already mentioned above, it is interesting that the MZ correlation is more than twice as large as the DZ correlation, which is suggestive of either genetic dominance (i.e., the presence of gene interactions at the same loci) or epistasis (i.e., genetic interactions across different loci). Focusing on the DZ and MZ twin correlations in our present analyses, instead of heritabilities and shared environmental influences, avoids the need to specify these interactions in more detail at this stage of the analysis.

In further analyses we additionally include education in order to investigate two questions of how human capital formation affects fertility behavior and how these education effects influence the cohort trends in heritability found in our earlier analyses (Kohler et al., 1999). First, in Model 2 we allow for the possibility that education (measured separately for each twin) affects the level of fertility. This is achieved by including years of primary and secondary education of each twin in a pair in the $x_{ij}\beta$ term of the bivariate probit model (see footnote 9), and the respective coefficient is reported under *variables influencing the mean level* in the tables representing our bivariate probit analyses. The results for Model 2 show first that, as expected, higher levels of education are associated with lower fertility levels, with a coefficient suggesting that one additional year of schooling decreases the latent propensity to have children by about 0.06. It is also worth noting these effects of education in Denmark are relatively modest due to institutional arrangements, such as day care provision, that facilitate very high female labor force participation (e.g., see Knudsen, 1993). In addition, the results for Model 2 show that the DZ and MZ correlations are slightly reduced after the direct effect of education on the level of fertility is controlled for, as expected, because part of the similarity in twin pairs is due to correlated education outcomes; however, the effect is relatively modest.

In the third set of analyses (Model 3), we include an interaction of the DZ and MZ correlations with the birth year. Because the interaction is centered around the mean birth year, the coefficients for DZ and MZ twins reflect those correlations for twin pairs born around the mean birth year (1961.5), while the interaction term reveals the change in the DZ or MZ within-pair correlation from one birth cohort to the next (i.e., for a 1-year difference in birth year). The analyses reveal that there is no clear cohort trend in the DZ correlation, although there is a trend for the MZ correlation. This correlation tends to increase by about 0.013 per year from younger to older cohorts. Because the DZ correlation is approximately constant (or only very slightly increasing), this result is consistent with an increasing relevance of genetic factors for variation in fertility outcomes.

In the fourth set of analyses (Model 4), we allow for the possibility that education affects not only the level of fertility but also the relevance of genetic and shared environmental influences on fertility. In particular, we interact the within-twin-pair correlation in the propensity to have children with the average education level in a pair (measured as the mean years of primary and secondary education in a twin pair, centered around the overall mean education) (see footnote 9 for detailed specification). This specification therefore tests whether twin pairs with higher levels of education share higher within-pair correlations and also reveals whether this effect differs by zygosity. The coefficients of these interaction terms are reported under *correlation within twin pairs* in the tables that report our bivariate probit results.[11] Because the interaction is centered around the mean education, the coefficients for DZ twins and MZ twins reflect the correlations for twin pairs with average education (11.04 years). The interaction term indicates the change in the MZ/

[11]Initially an alternative specification that includes individual instead of average twin-pair education in this analysis might seem more plausible because it would allow for the possibility that individual instead of only average twin-pair education affects the similarity of fertility outcomes in twin pairs. In particular, individual specification can be included in the model by specifying the correlation equation in the bivariate probit model $\rho_i = \delta_1 \cdot I_{MZ,i} + \delta_2 \cdot I_{MZ,i} \cdot \text{education}_{i1} + \delta_3 \cdot I_{MZ,i} \cdot \text{education}_{i2} + \delta_4 I_{DZ,i} + \delta_5 \cdot I_{DZ,i} \cdot \text{education}_{i1} + \delta_6 \cdot I_{DZ,i} \cdot \text{education}_{i2}$, where education_{ij} denotes the individual education level of twin j in pair i. Because the assignment of twins 1 and 2 in a pair is random, the coefficients δ_2 and δ_3, as well as the coefficients δ_5 and δ_6, should be equal in this model. The respective terms can therefore be combined as $\rho_i = \delta_1 \cdot I_{MZ,i} + \delta_2 \cdot I_{MZ,i} \cdot (\text{education}_{i1} + \text{education}_{i2}) + \delta_4 I_{DZ,i} + \delta_5 \cdot I_{DZ,i} \cdot (\text{education}_{i1} + \text{education}_{i2})$. As a consequence, the specification with individual-level education is conceptually and formally equivalent to the specification that includes only the average education of twin pairs, and the effect of individual-level education on the within-twin-pair correlation in the propensity to have children cannot be distinguished from the effect of the average twin-pair education.

DZ within-twin-pair correlations for each additional year of education. Most importantly, the analyses show that one additional year of education increases the MZ correlation in the latent propensity to have children by about 0.05, while it has virtually no effect on the DZ correlation. In terms of a heritability model with shared environmental and genetic influences, this suggests that higher education tends to increase the proportion of variance attributed to genetic factors and to decrease the fraction attributed to shared environmental factors. In the final set of analyses (Model 5), we combine both interaction effects to see whether the interaction with birth year or with years of education dominates. Our analyses show that only the interaction of the MZ correlation with years of education remains statistically significant, with an only modestly reduced size at 0.044, while the effect of birth year is reduced and no longer significant.

The results implied for monozygotic twins by Models 3, 4, and 5 in Table 3-5 are visualized in Figure 3-3. Figure 3-3a reports the results of Model 3, which includes only an interaction with birth year in the specification of the within-twin-pair correlation. The horizontal line gives the within-MZ-twin-pair correlation for the birth year 1961.5 ("mean birth year") of 0.47, while the diagonal line gives the cohort trend resulting from the interaction with birth year: cohorts born in the mid-1950s have a within-MZ correlation of below 0.4, while cohorts born in the late 1960s exhibit a within-MZ correlation of above 0.55. The linear relationship in Figure 3-3a is, of course, a consequence of our model specification in Table 3-5, and this linear cohort trend should be interpreted as a first-order approximation to a potentially more complicated cohort pattern that levels off for the youngest and oldest cohorts included in our data. Nevertheless, the figure clearly reveals the changing MZ correlation across cohorts. Whereas the DZ correlation remains approximately constant, there is a marked increase in the within-MZ-twin-pair correlation as we progress from the oldest to the youngest cohorts. This pattern suggests that genetic influences gain in relevance for variations in completed fertility in young cohorts.

Figure 3-3b depicts the results of Model 2, which includes an interaction with education in the specification of the within-twin-pair correlation, and the figure visualizes our earlier discussion. Within-MZ correlations are below 0.4 for twin pairs with relatively low education, while the MZ correlation increases to above 0.5 for twin pairs with relatively high education (years of elementary and secondary schooling). The coefficients in Table 3-5 also reveal that this interaction of the MZ correlation with education is statistically significant. The vertical lines in Figure 3-3b also indicate the mean and mean plus or minus one standard deviation of our education measure. The corresponding values of the MZ correlation reveal that this education effect is sizable and quite relevant: the within-pair corre-

a

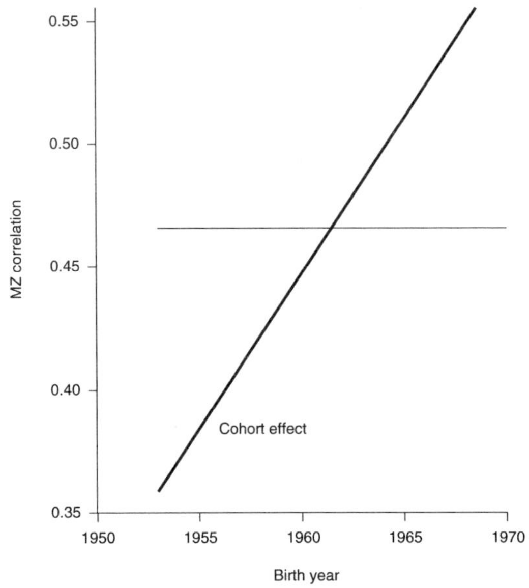
0.55
0.50
0.45
0.40
0.35
MZ correlation
Cohort effect
1950
1955
1960
1965
1970
Birth year

b

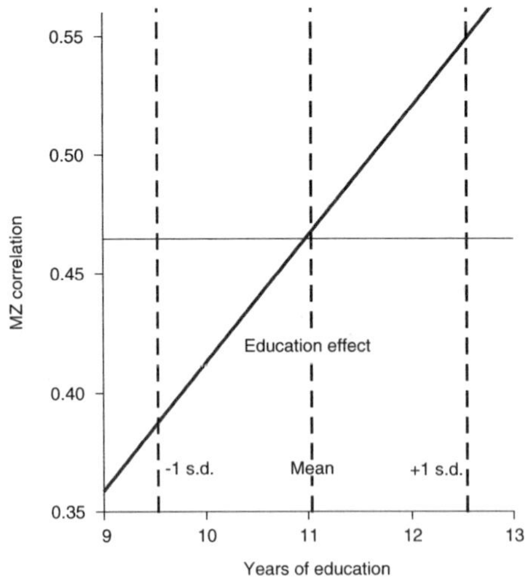
0.55
0.50
0.45
0.40
0.35
MZ correlation
Education effect
-1 s.d.
Mean
+1 s.d.
9
10
11
12
13
Years of education

c

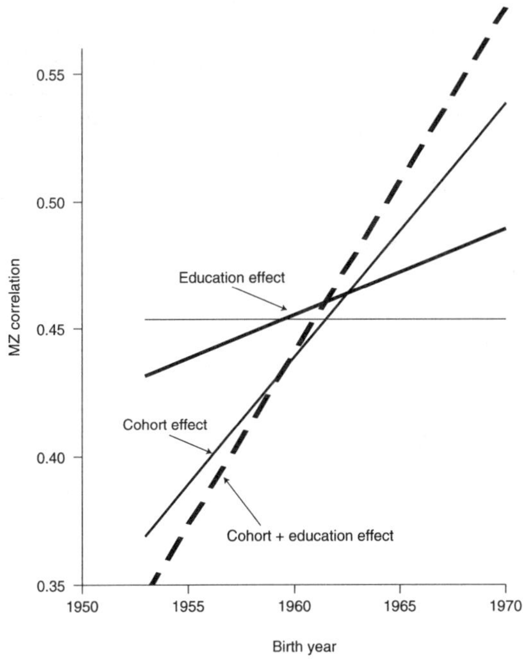

FIGURE 3-3 Cohort and education effects on within-MZ correlation.

lations of MZ twin pairs one standard deviation above and below the mean education differ by almost 0.15.

Figure 3-3c presents the results of Model 5, which includes interaction with birth year as well as education levels and shows the extent to which the within-MZ correlation across the 1953-1970 cohorts increases due to the interaction with birth cohort (holding education constant at 11.04 years) and the interaction with education (holding birth year constant at 1961.5). The former effect is shown by the dashed line. Once education is included in the specification of the MZ correlation, this cohort effect is weakened compared to Model 3 and looses its statistical significance. Nevertheless, the point estimate of the coefficient continues to suggest a relevant increase in heritabilities that occurs due to the interaction of the MZ twin-pair correlation with birth year. The broken line in Figure 3-3c, on the other hand, reveals the increase in the average MZ correlation across cohorts owing to the fact that the mean years of schooling increased from 10.5 to 11.9 years for the 1953-1970 cohorts. While statistically significant at the 5 percent level and quite sizable for a marginal increase in years of education, the change in MZ correlation due to this education effect is modest for the overall cohort trend because mean education increased by only 1.4 years across the cohorts included in our data. The full line in Figure 3-3c represents the combined effect of the increase in the within-MZ-twin-pair correlation due to the joint effect of education and birth-year interactions. The increase in education across cohorts therefore explains a significant part of the increase in within-MZ correlations across the 1953-1970 cohorts. At the same time, the individual-specific effect of education, which changes the within-MZ correlation according to the average education in a pair, seems to be more relevant than the education effect operating through the increased educational attainment of cohorts. The strong education effect in Figure 3-3b is only slightly diminished in Model 5, which includes both interactions, compared to Model 4, which includes only the interaction with education.

The analyses in Table 3-5 and Figure 3-3 therefore suggest that education, as measured by years of primary and secondary schooling, is an important factor mediating the role of genetic variance in fertility outcomes. Within birth cohorts, patterns of heritability tend to vary with education in a manner that seems counterintuitive at first sight: A higher education level in a twin pair tends to imply a higher MZ correlation in the propensity to have children and does not seem to affect the DZ correlation. Within cohorts, higher education therefore is associated with higher heritabilities in fertility outcomes. In addition, the trend toward increased female education across cohorts seems to be an important factor that helps explain the increased relevance of genetic variance in fertility outcomes in younger cohorts found by Kohler et al. (1999).

In robustness tests for the above results, we investigated whether our findings about the interactions between education and patterns of within-twin-pair correlations are sensitive to our specific education measure. In additional analyses, not reported here in detail, we replaced years of schooling with a simple dummy variable indicating whether a respondent has 12 or more years of education. The education level of twin pairs can then be represented by a variable that equals 0 if both twins have less than 12 years of education, 0.5 if one twin has more than 12 years of education, and 1 if both twins have more than 12 years of education. If the analyses in Table 3-5 are replicated using this alternative education measure, the results remain unchanged: Twin pairs with higher education levels are subject to significantly higher MZ (but not DZ) correlations in the propensity to have children, and the increase in educational attainment across cohorts partially explains the cohort trend toward increased heritabilities for fertility in younger cohorts. In addition, it is worth noting that "years of primary and secondary education" (or the derived indicator variable "more than 12 years of schooling") is the only measure of education that yields robust, consistent, and significant interaction effects in the above analyses. Similar estimations with years of tertiary education did not yield systematic interactions (the signs are consistent with the above analyses, but the effects were not sufficiently strong to be significant). Hence, education measures that are determined relatively early in life seem to be the most important for these interactions with MZ and DZ correlations and subsequently also heritabilities.

In additional analyses we also investigated the patterns of DZ and MZ correlations for male twins (see Table 3-6). In earlier studies we found a significant relevance of genetic factors also for male fertility outcomes, but within these male patterns of heritabilites the social conditioning was substantially less relevant than for females. In the long-term cross-cohort comparisons, male heritabilities neither declined nor increased markedly and especially did not increase as strongly in the most recent cohorts as did the female heritabilities.

This pattern is confirmed in the present analyses. In Models 1 through 5 in Table 3-6 we report the bivariate probit estimates of the male DZ and MZ correlations that are analogous to the female models discussed above. Our first set of analyses (Model 1) reveal a DZ correlation of 0.21 and a MZ correlation of 0.32. The difference between MZ and DZ twins is substantially lower than in our analyses for females, and this implies somewhat lower estimates for heritabilities (consistent with our earlier findings). As expected, including education as a covariate that influences the level of fertility reduces these correlations (Model 2), but the effect is relatively small. Most importantly for the present context are again the interactions of the DZ and MZ correlations in the propensity to have children with birth year and education. Our analyses show that both interactions are relevant also for MZ males (Model 3 and 4), and the MZ correlations tend to increase the more recent the birth cohort is and the higher the education level is within a twin pair. These interactions are not statistically significant nor substantively relevant for the within-DZ-pair correlation. In the combined analyses that include both interactions (Model 5), the interaction of birth year with the MZ correlation is the only effect that remains relevant and (weakly) significant. The education effect is in the same direction as in our results for females, but the magnitude and the level of statistical significance are less than for females. In summary, these findings for males are consistent with our earlier findings in Kohler et al. (1999): There seem to be relevant genetic influences on fertility outcomes also for males, but the social conditioning of these heritability patterns is weaker. In particular, education does not seem to have the same strong effect on the MZ and DZ correlations for males as it does for females.

TABLE 3-6 Males—Bivariate Ordered Probit Estimation for Number of Children

	Number of Children				
Males	Model 1	Model 2	Model 3	Model 4	Model 5
Variables influencing mean level					
Cohort (reference category: cohort, 1953-1954)					
1955-1956	0.013	0.032	0.034	0.028	0.030
	(0.079)	(0.079)	(0.078)	(0.079)	(0.078)
1957-1958	0.053	0.077	0.077	0.073	0.073
	0.081)	(0.081)	(0.079)	(0.081)	(0.079)
1959-1960	−0.083	−0.049	−0.050	−0.054	−0.055
	(0.077)	(0.077)	(0.076)	(0.077)	(0.076)
1961-1962	−0.228	−0.197	−0.198	−0.201	−0.201
	(0.082)**	(0.082)*	(0.081)*	(0.082)*	(0.081)*
1963-1964	−0.269	−0.236	−0.235	−0.244	−0.243
	(0.081)**	(0.081)**	(0.080)**	(0.081)**	(0.080)**
1965-1966	−0.626	−0.584	−0.584	−0.592	−0.592
	(0.079)**	(0.080)**	(0.079)**	(0.080)**	(0.079)**
1967-1968	−0.947	−0.892	−0.893	−0.897	−0.899
	(0.085)**	(0.086)**	(0.086)**	(0.086)**	(0.086)**
1969-1970	−1.327	−1.279	−1.276	−1.281	−1.280
	(0.090)**	(0.090)**	(0.090)**	(0.090)**	(0.090)**

Years of elementary and secondary education		−0.055 (0.010)**	−0.054 (0.010)**	−0.055 (0.010)**	−0.054 (0.010)**
Constant	0.830 (0.061)**	1.387 (0.120)**	1.375 (0.119)**	1.398 (0.120)**	1.386 (0.119)**
Correlation within twin pairs					
DZ twins	0.208 (0.032)**	0.202 (0.032)**	0.209 (0.033)**	0.185 (0.035)**	0.192 (0.036)**
DZ x (birth year - 1961.5)			0.006 (0.007)		0.006 (0.007)
DZ x (years of elementary + secondary Education - 11.04)				−0.032 (0.022)	−0.032 (0.023)
MZ twins	0.324 (0.036)**	0.317 (0.036)**	0.327 (0.036)**	0.332 (0.036)**	0.337 (0.036)**
MZ x (birth year - 1961.5)			0.017 (0.008)*		0.015 (0.008)+
MZ x (years of elementary + secondary Education - 11.04)				0.034 (0.021)+	0.027 (0.021)
N (twin pairs)	2073	2073	2073	2073	2073

NOTES: p values: + < .1; * < .05; ** < .01. Cut points of the ordered probit model are not reported.

DISCUSSION

Changes in the levels of and returns to education, especially female education, are central to many theories of demographic and related social changes. For instance, education features prominently in theories about fertility decline, changing female labor force participation, and household allocation modes. Here we investigate whether education, and changes in education, are also an important aspect in biodemographic approaches to fertility. The analyses presented in this chapter investigate these questions from a twofold perspective and provide a clear indication that education constitutes an important aspect related to the biodemography of fertility.

In our first analyses, we applied a multivariate behavioral genetics model to investigate genetic and shared environmental contributions to the variance and covariance in completed education and (almost) completed fertility. These analyses showed that both education and fertility are subject to genetic and shared environmental influences, but the overlapping sources of genetic influences are relatively small. Variation in fertility for both males and females is therefore primarily related to residual genetic variance that is independent of genetic influences on completed education.

Our second analyses focused on the question of whether changes in educational attainment across cohorts provide an explanation for the increased heritabilities in fertility observed in our earlier studies. In particular, our analyses estimated the correlations in the latent propensity to have children in MZ and DZ twins and included tests for interactions of those correlations with birth year and levels of education.

For females these analyses revealed that education and cohorts are two key factors that interact with MZ twin correlations, while DZ twin correlations are almost not affected by including these interactions. This implies that it is primarily the genetic factors consistent with variation in fertility outcomes that are affected by education and cohorts. In particular, our analyses suggested that genetic influences tend to become stronger in twin pairs with a higher level of education and that genetic influences tend to become stronger in more recent cohorts. However, this secular trend across cohorts was substantially reduced once the interaction with education was included, suggesting that increased levels of education constitute an important factor contributing to the increased heritabilities in younger cohorts found in our earlier studies. For males the interaction with education was present but seemed to be weaker in terms of both statistical significance and the magnitude of the effect. Again, this is consistent with our earlier findings that cohort trends in heritabilities are much weaker for males than for females.

An interesting aspect of the above analyses is the fact that years of primary and secondary education, not years of tertiary education, resulted in important interactions with the within-twin-pair correlations in the propensity to have children. This may be due to the fact that years of primary and secondary education are an important determinant of the overall "options" available to young adults in Denmark. Hence, in many ways the primary and secondary years of education are a key determinant of the "life course options" available to young adults, and this finding is consistent with our arguments in Kohler et al. (1999) and Rodgers et al. (2001b): Genetic variation in fertility outcome may become most relevant in societies and contexts where there is a large set of life course options that affect fertility and related demographic outcomes.

Udry (1996) developed this argument on purely theoretical grounds, anticipating these empirical findings. These options increase the set of potential pathways through which genetic influences affect fertility outcome, and increased opportunities—for instance in the labor market—are likely to heighten the implications of endowments for labor market outcomes and therefore indirectly also on fertility. The theoretical framework of fertility behavior that is embedded in a broad context of life cycle decisions and processes provides a basis for analyzing and understanding these changing contributions of genetic factors to variations in fertility outcomes, and future analyses that combine detailed socioeconomic information and multivariate behavioral genetics models can investigate these different pathways in greater detail.

Another interesting aspect of our analyses is that for females the standard additive genetic model does not seem to hold. In particular, the MZ correlations are more than twice as high as the DZ correlations, which indicates that more complicated gene interactions—for instance, due to dominance effects or epistasis—are present. There are several potential interpretations for those types of nonadditive patterns. Genetic interactions are implied by dominance (interaction within alleles) and epistasis (interaction across alleles). Or complex polygenic patterns can be caused by a particular configuration of genes (Lykken et al., 1992), a process called emergenesis. These effects are implied by sizable MZ twin correlations and very small—approximately zero—correlations for all other relatives (because only MZ twins will share a genetic configuration). The presence of such gene interactions is consistent with the evolutionary theory of life history traits, where Fisher's (1930) fundamental theorem of natural selection suggests that additive variance tends to be diminished over time and is reintroduced again only through "perturbing forces," such as mutations, changes in socioeconomic or normative contexts, or contraceptive (or proceptive) technologies (see Rodgers et al., 2001a).

In our analyses we avoided the specification of a specific genetic model by reporting within-pair correlations instead of heritabilities and shared environmental influences. Nevertheless, the presence of such gene interactions is an important question for future research, and we have argued in related research (Christensen et al., 2003) that genetic factors contributing to fecundity, as measured by the waiting time to pregnancy, occur primarily through relatively complicated gene interactions across different loci.

The main conclusion of our analyses that the patterns of genetic variance, whether measured as heritabilities or by comparing MZ and DZ twin correlations, are strongly socially conditioned and that contemporary societies might lead to a strengthening instead of a weakening role of genetic favors for variation of fertility outcomes is supported by recent investigations of the intergenerational transmission of fertility. Studies in a number of countries and time periods (e.g., Anderton et al., 1987; Berent, 1953; Johnson and Stokes, 1976; Pullum and Wolf, 1991) have shown that there is usually a positive correlation between the number of children of parents and their offspring, while there is also the possibility of a negative relation due to cohort size effects (e.g., see Easterlin, 1980). Studies of intergenerational correlation without indicators of genetic relatedness can obviously not identify the contribution of genetic and social factors to this intergenerational transmission of fertility. Nevertheless, because (additive) genetic influences on fertility tend to cause a positive intergenerational correlation (though not necessarily if genetic factors operate through epistatis), findings that intergenerational correlations are also not weakened in posttransitional societies and more recent cohorts is supportive of our behavioral genetics analyses.

Murphy and Wang (2001), for instance, estimated the correlations between number of siblings and children for different contemporary developed countries, including Italy, Great Britain, Australia, Norway, and Germany, and found that the positive intergenerational relationship in fertility is not only substantial and present in all countries investigated but also that this relationship has been increasing in younger cohorts and persists even after controlling for socioeconomic characteristics. Similarly, in a study using Danish register data, Murphy and Knudsen (2002) did not find that the intergenerational fertility transmission weakened in younger cohorts, despite the fact that the socioeconomic and ideational changes experienced by these cohorts during the second demographic transmission would tend to attenuate parental influences and intergenerational transmission.

In summary, our empirical work falls into the category of research encouraged by Rutter and Silberg (2002) of gene-environment interplay. The specification of models in which behavioral genetics design/analysis is complemented by environmental measures is a natural way to formalize the goals of developing consilience between biodemographic and demographic approaches to studying fertility. Further, our empirical finding that the genetic variance implied by analysis of the twin design is strongly conditioned on educational level is an example of how the ultimate result of such efforts toward consilience can be greater than the sum of the parts.

ACKNOWLEDGMENTS

The authors contributed equally to this paper. Much appreciation is extended to Kaare Christiansen, Kirstin Kyvik, and others involved in collecting and managing the Danish Twin Registry in Odense, Denmark.

REFERENCES

Adams, J., A. Hermalin, D. Lam, and P. Smouse
1990 *Convergent Issues in Genetics and Demography*. New York: Oxford University Press.

Anderton, D.L., N.O. Tsuya, L.L. Bean, and G.P. Mineau
1987 Intergenerational transmission of relative fertility and life course patterns. *Demography* 24:467-480.

Becker, G.S.
1981 *A Treatise on the Family*. Cambridge, MA: Harvard University Press.

Behrman, J.R., M.R. Rosenzweig, and P. Taubman
1994 Endowments and the allocation of schooling in the family and in the marriage market: The twins experiment. *Journal of Political Economy* 102(6):1131-1173.
1996 College choice and wages: Estimates using data on female twins. *Review of Economics and Statistics* 73(4):672-685.

Berent, J.
1953 Relationship between family sizes of the successive generations. *Milbank Memorial Fund Quarterly Bulletin* 31:39-50.

Bongaarts, J., and S.C. Watkins
1996 Social interactions and contemporary fertility transition. *Population and Development Review* 22:639-682.

Capron, C., and A. Vetta
2001 Comments on "Why have children in the 21st century?" *European Journal of Population* 17(1):23-30.

Carey, A.D., and J. Lopreato
1995 The evolutionary demography of the fertility-mortality quasi-equilibrium. *Population and Development Review* 21(3):613-630.

Christensen, K., O. Basso, K.O. Kyvik, S. Juul, J. Boldsen, J.W. Vaupel, and J. Olsen
1998 Fecundability of female twins. *Epidemiology* 9(2):189-192.

Christensen, K., H.-P. Kohler, O. Basso, J. Olsen, J.W. Vaupel, and J.L. Rodgers
2003 The correlation of fecundability among twins: Evidence of a genetic effect on fertility? *Epidemiology* 14(1):60-64.

Cleland, J.
2001 Potatoes and pills: An overview of innovation-diffusion contributions to explanations of fertility decline. Pp. 39-65 in *Diffusion Processes and Fertility Transition.* Committee on Population, J. Casterline, ed. Division of Behaviorial and Social Sciences and Education. Washington, DC: National Academy Press.

DeFries, J.C., and D.W. Fulker
1985 Multiple regression analysis of twin data. *Behavior Genetics* 15(5):467-473.

Easterlin, R.A.
1980 *Birth and Fortune: The Impact of Numbers on Personal Welfare*. Chicago: University of Chicago Press.

Falconer, D. S.
1981 *Introduction to Quantitative Genetics.* New York: Longman.
Fisher, R.A.
1930 *The Genetical Theory of Natural Selection.* Oxford: Clarendon Press.
Foster, C.
2000 The limits to low fertility: A biosocial approach. *Population and Development Review* 26(2):209-234.
Frank, R.
2001 The misuse of biology in demographic research on racial/ethnic differences: A reply to van den Oord and Rowe. *Demography* 38:563-568.
Gottleib, G.
2000 Environmental and behavioral influences on gene activity. *Current Directions in Psychological Science* 9:93-97.
Halpern, C.T., J.R. Udry, and C. Suchindran
1997 Testosterone predicts initiation of coitus in adolescent females. *Psychosomatic Medicine* 59(2):161-171.
Halpern, C.T., J.R. Udry, B. Campbell, and C. Suchindran
1999 Effects of body fat on weight concerns, dating, and sexual activity: A longitudinal analysis of black and white adolescent girls. *Developmental Psychology* 35(3): 721-736.
Halpern, C.T., K. Joyner, J.R. Udry, and C. Suchindran
2000 Smart teens don't have sex (or kiss much either). *Journal of Adolescent Health* 26(3):213-225.
Higgins, J.V., E. Reed, and S.C. Reed
1962 Intelligence and family size: A paradox resolved. *Eugenics Quarterly* 9:84-90.
Hill, K., and H. Kaplan
1999 Life history traits in humans: Theory and empirical studies. *Annual Review of Anthropology* 28:397-430.
Johnson, N.E., and C.S. Stokes
1976 Family size in successive generations: The effects of birth order, intergenerational change in lifestyle, and familial satisfaction. *Demography* 13(2):175-187.
Kaplan, H., K. Hill, J. Lancaster, and A.M. Hurtado
2000 A theory of human life history evolution: Diet, intelligence, and longevity. *Evolutionary Anthropology* 9(4):156-185.
Kaplan, H., J. Lancaster, and S. Johnson
1995 Does observed fertility maximize fitness among New Mexican men? *Human Nature* 6(4):325-360.
Kirk, K.M., S.P. Blomberg, D.L. Duffy, A.C. Heath, I.P.F. Owens, and N.G. Martin
2001 Natural selection and quantitative genetics of life history traits in Western women: A twin study. *Evolution* 55:423-435.
Knudsen, L.B.
1993 *Fertility Trends in Denmark in the 1980s: A Register Based Socio-demographic Analysis of Fertility Trends.* Copenhagen: Denmark Statistics.
Kohler, H.-P.
2001 Comments on Morgan and King (2001): Three reasons why demographers should pay attention to evolutionary theories and behavior genetics in the analysis of contemporary fertility. *European Journal of Population* 17(1):31-35.
Kohler, H.-P., L. Knudsen, A. Skytthe, and K. Christensen
2002a The fertility pattern of twins and the general population compared: Evidence from Danish cohorts 1945-64. *Demographic Research* 6(14):383-408.

Kohler, H.-P., J.L. Rodgers, and K. Christensen
2002b Between Nurture and Nature: The Shifting Determinants of Female Fertility in Danish Twin Cohorts 1870-1968. Unpublished document, Max Planck Institute for Demographic Research, Rostock, Germany.

Kohler, H.-P., F.C. Billari, and J.A. Ortega
2002c The Emergence of Lowest-Low Fertility in Europe During the 1990s. *Population and Development Review* 28(4).

Kohler, H.-P., J.L. Rodgers, and K. Christensen
1999 Is fertility behavior in our genes? Findings from a Danish twin study. *Population and Development Review* 25(2):253-288.

Kohler, H.-P., and J.L. Rodgers
1999 DF-like analyses of binary, ordered and censored variables using probit and tobit approaches. *Behavior Genetics* 29(4):221-232.

Kyvik, K.O., K. Christensen, A. Skytthe, B. Harvald, and N.V. Holm
1996 The Danish twin register. *Danish Medical Bulletin* 43(5):465-470.

Kyvik, K.O., A. Green, and H. Beck-Nielsen
1995 The new Danish twin register: Establishment and analysis of twinning rates. *International Journal of Epidemiology* 24:589-596.

Lewontin, R.C., S. Rose, and L.J. Kamin
1984 *Not in Our Genes: Biology, Ideology, and Human Nature*. New York: Pantheon.

Lesthaeghe, R., and D. van de Kaa
1986 Twee demografische transities? Pp. 9-24 in *Bevolking: Groei en Krimp,* R. Lesthaeghe and D. van de Kaa, eds. Deventer: Van Loghum Slaterus.

Loehlin, J.C., and R.C. Nichols
1976 *Heredity, Environment, and Personality*. Austin: University of Texas Press.

Lykken, D.T., M. McGue, A. Tellegen, and T.J. Bouchard
1992 Emergenesis: Genetic traits that may not run in families. *American Psychologist* 12:1565-1577.

MacMurray, J., B. Kovacs, M. McGue, J.P. Johnson, H. Blake, and D.E. Comings
2000 Associations between the endothelial nitric oxide synthase gene (NOS3), reproductive behaviors, and twinning. In *Genetic Influences on Human Fertility and Sexuality*. J.L. Rodgers, D.C. Rowe, and W.B. Miller, eds. Boston: Kluwer Academic Press.

Marini, M.M.
1981 Effects of the timing of marriage and first birth on fertility. *Journal of Marriage and the Family* 43(1):27-46.

Miller, W.B., D.J. Pasta, J. MacMurray, C. Chiu, H. Wu, and D.E. Comings
1999 Dopamine receptors are associated with age at first sexual intercourse. *Journal of Biosocial Science* 31:43-54.

Miller, W.B., D.J. Pasta, J. MacMurray, D. Muhleman, and D.E. Comings
2000 Genetic influences on childbearing motivation: Further testing a theoretical framework. In *Genetic Influences on Human Fertility and Sexuality*. J.L. Rodgers, D.C. Rowe, and W.B. Miller, eds. Boston: Kluwer Academic Press.

Miller, W.B., and J.L. Rodgers
2001 *The Ontogeny of Human Bonding Systems: Evolutionary Origins, Neural Bases, and Psychological Manifestations*. Boston: Kluwer Academic Press.

Montgomery, M.R., and J.B. Casterline
1996 Social learning, social influence, and new models of fertility. *Population and Development Review* 22(Suppl.):151-175.

Morgan, S.P., and R.B. King
2001 Why have children in the 21st century? Biological predispositions, social coercion, rational choice. *European Journal of Population* 17(1):3-20.
Morgan, P.S., and R.R. Rindfuss
1999 Reexamining the link of early childbearing to marriage and to subsequent fertility. *Demography* 36(1):59-75.
Murphy, M., and L.B. Knudsen
2002 The relationship of full and half sibs, birth order and gender with fertility in contemporary Denmark. *Population Studies*.
Murphy, M., and D. Wang
2001 Continuities in childbearing in low fertility societies. *European Journal of Population* 17(1):75-96.
Neale, M.C., S.M., Boker, G. Xie, and H.H. Maes
1999 *Mx: Statistical Modeling*, 5th ed. Richmond, VA: Department of Psychiatry.
Neiss, M., D.C. Rowe, and J.L. Rodgers
2002 Does education mediate the relationship between IQ and age of first birth? A behavioral genetic analysis. *Journal of Biosocial Science* 34:259-275.
Pedersen, N.L., G.E. McClearn, R.Plomin, J.R. Nesselroade, S. Berg, and U. de Faire
1991 The Swedish adoption/twin study of aging. *Acta Geneticae Medicae et Gemmellologiae* 40:7-20.
Plomin, R.
1990 *Nature and Nurture*. Pacific Grove, CA: Brooks/Cole.
Plomin, R., J.C. DeFries, and G.E. McClearn
1990 *Behavioral Genetics: A Primer*. New York: Freeman.
Plomin, R., and R. Rende
1991 Human behavioral genetics. Pp. 161-190 in *Annual Review of Psychology*. M.R. Rosenzweig and L.W. Porter, eds. Palo Alto, CA: Annual Reviews Inc.
Potts, M.
1997 Sex and the birth rate: Human biology, demographic change and access to fertility-regulation methods. *Population and Development Review* 23(1):1-39.
Pullum, T.W., and D.A. Wolf
1991 Correlations between frequencies of kin. *Demography* 28:391-409.
Retherford, R.D., and W.H. Sewell
1988 Intelligence and family size reconsidered. *Social Biology* 35:1-40.
Roberts, J.A.F.
1938 Intelligence and family size. *Eugenics Review* 30:237-247.
Rodgers, J.L., H.H. Cleveland, E. van den Oord, and D.C. Rowe
2000 Resolving the debate over birth order, family size, and intelligence. *American Psychologist* 55:599-612.
Rodgers, J.L., K. Hughes, H.-P. Kohler, K. Christensen, D. Doughty, D.C. Rowe, and W.B. Miller
2001a Genetic influences help explain variation in human fertility outcomes: Evidence from recent behavioral and molecular genetic studies. *Current Directions in Psychological Science* 10:184-188.
Rodgers, J.L., and H.-P. Kohler, eds.
2003 *The Biodemography of Human Reproduction and Fertility*. Boston: Kluwer Academic Press.
Rodgers, J.L., H.-P. Kohler, and K. Christensen
2003 Genetic variance in human fertility: Biology, psychology, or both? Pp. 229-250 in *The Biodemography of Human Reproduction and Fertility*. J.L. Rodgers and H.-P. Kohler, eds. Boston: Kluwer Academic Press.

Rodgers, J.L., H.-P. Kohler, K. Kyvik, and K. Christensen
2001b Behavior genetic modeling of human fertility: Findings from a contemporary Danish twin study. *Demography* 38(1):29-42.
Rodgers, J.L., D.C. Rowe and M. Buster
1999 Nature, nurture, and first sexual intercourse: Fitting behavioral genetic models to NLSY kinship data. *Journal of Biosocial Science* 31:29-41.
Rodgers, J.L., D.C. Rowe, and C. Li
1994a Beyond nature versus nurture: DF analysis of nonshared influences on problem behaviors. *Developmental Psychology* 30:374-384.
Rodgers, J.L., D.C. Rowe, and K. May
1994b DF analysis of NLSY IQ/achievement data: Nonshared environmental influences. *Intelligence* 19:157-177.
Rodgers, J.L., D.C. Rowe, and W.B. Miller
2000 *Genetic Influences on Human Fertility and Sexuality: Theoretical and Empirical Contributions from the Biological and Behavioral Sciences.* Boston: Kluwer Academic Press.
Rose, R.J.
1995 Genes and human behavior. In *Annual Review of Psychology.* J. Spence, J. Darley, and D. Foss, eds. Palo Alto, CA: Annual Reviews.
Rosenzweig, M.R., and T.P. Schultz
1985 The demand for and supply of births: Fertility and its life cycle consequences. *American Economic Review* 75(5):992-1015.
Rutter, M., and J. Silberg
2002 Gene-environment interplay in relation to emotional and behavioral disturbance. In *Annual Review of Psychology.* S. Fiske, D. Schacter, and C. Zahn-Waxler, eds. Palo Alto, CA: Annual Review.
Scarr, J.C., and L. Carter-Salzman
1979 Twin method: Defense of a critical assumption. *Behavior Genetics* 9:527-542.
Turkheimer, E.
1998 Heritability and biological explanation. *Psychological Review* 105:782-791.
2000 Three laws of behavior genetics and what they mean. *Current Directions in Psychological Science* 9:160-164.
Udry, J.R.
1995 Sociology and biology: What biology do sociologists need to know? *Social Forces* 73:999-1010.
1996 Biosocial models of low-fertility societies. In *Fertility in the United States: New Patterns, New Theories.* J.B. Casterline, R.D. Lee, and K.A. Foote, eds. New York: The Population Council.
van de Kaa, D.J.
1987 Europe's second demographic transition. *Population Bulletin* 42:1-57.
van den Oord, E.J., and D.C. Rowe
2000 Racial differences in birth health risk: A quantitative genetic approach. *Demography* 37:285-298.
Wahlsten, C.
1999 Single-gene influences on brain and behavior. In *Annual Review of Psychology.* J. Spence, J. Darley and D. Foss, eds. Palo Alto, CA: Annual Reviews.
Willis, R.J.
1973 A new approach to the economic theory of fertility behavior. *Journal of Political Economy* 81(2, pt. 2):14-64.
Wilson, E.O.
1998 *Consilience: The Unity of Knowledge.* New York: Vintage.

Wood, J.

1994 *Dynamics of Human Reproduction: Biology, Biometry, Demography*. Hawthorne, NY: Aldine.

Yashin, A.I., and I.A. Iachine

1997 How frailty models can be used for evaluating longevity limits: Taking advantage of an interdisciplinary approach. *Demography* 34(1):31-48.

Zuberi, T.

2001 One step back in understanding racial differences in birth weight. *Demography* 38:569-572.

4

The Neural Basis of Pair Bonding in a Monogamous Species: A Model for Understanding the Biological Basis of Human Behavior

Larry J. Young

There is an ongoing debate in psychology as to the relative roles of genes and environment on the development of human behavior. There is little doubt that genes play a significant role in shaping certain innate human behaviors, such as sexual and parental behavior, social bonding, fear, and aggression. As in all animals, genes determine the underlying neurochemistry and circuitry that drive human emotions and behavior, but the manifestation of each of these behaviors is also clearly influenced by culture. Furthermore, the frequencies of various alleles for these genes are subject to selection based on social and ecological factors, which in turn shape behavior. Thus, if we are to fully understand the nature, diversity, and evolution of human behavior, we must understand the socioecological factors that shape behavior and learn more about the ways that genes act in the brain to establish the biological mechanisms underlying behavior. Elsewhere in this volume, Kaplan and Lancaster (Chapter 7), and Gangestad (Chapter 8) provide a theoretical framework for understanding the evolution of mating patterns and parental investments. This chapter discusses in detail the biological mechanisms underlying pair bond formation in monogamous voles. It must be stated at the outset that there has not been enough research to provide evidence that these same mechanisms are involved in homologous human behaviors. Research results for monogamous voles are presented here as a model for understanding how genes can influence the expression of a social behavior critical for reproduction.

The human species is rather unusual among mammals in that we form long-lasting selective social bonds between mates in addition to the parent-child bond resulting in the nuclear family. The precise nature of the nuclear family varies from culture to culture, ranging from strict monogamy reinforced by society and religion to polygyny or polyandry. Whether or not one considers human beings to be truly monogamous, it is clear that the selective bond between mates, manifested in our species as an emotion we call love, is extremely powerful, and is undoubtedly rooted in our biology and genetic heritage.

Controlled experiments on the neurobiological basis of sociosexual behaviors in humans are not possible. Thus, we must rely on animal models to provide principles that might generalize to humans. How might we find a suitable animal model for human bonding? Approximately 90 percent of bird species are considered monogamous, at least over one breeding season. In contrast, only approximately 5 percent of mammals exhibit a monogamous social structure (Kleiman, 1977). The term "monogamy" does not imply lifelong exclusive mating with a single individual. In fact, many birds form pair bonds over a season, raise their offspring together, and then select another partner the following season. For biologists, monogamy implies selective (not exclusive) mating, a shared nesting area, and biparental care. In recent years, genetic analyses of offspring have provided evidence for extra-pair copulations even among species thought to mate exclusively monogamously.

Biomedical research relies heavily on rodent models because rodents are small, breed well in the laboratory, and are suitable for many types of experimental manipulations. The use of behaviorally monogamous rodent species is efficient for investigating the biology of monogamy and social attachment. Several species of voles, genus *Microtus*, fit these criteria and have become rodent models for research on the neurobiological basis of pair bonding (Insel and Young, 2001). This chapter reviews the progress in understanding the molecular, cellular and neurobiological nature of pair bonding emerging from intensive studies of monogamous prairie voles, and discusses the implications of this research for human behavior.

Prairie voles (*Microtus ochrogaster*) are field mice found in the Midwestern prairie of the United States. Studies in the field indicate that prairie voles form long-term social bonds with their mates and produce multiple litters together (reviewed in Carter et al., 1995). In fact, one study reported that in pairs in which one individual disappears, fewer than 20 percent of the survivors took on a new mate. However, despite their social monogamy, not all prairie voles display exclusive mating, since females have been reported to carry mixed-paternity litters. The selective pressures leading to the evolution of monogamy in prairie voles are unclear. In theory, monogamous social structures are thought to be favored under conditions of low food availability, high nest predation, and low population density. Males in monogamous species typically display paternal care of their offspring by contributing food resources and by defending the nest from predators while the mother forages.

Prairie voles are believed to have evolved in the tall-grass prairies, which are very low in food resources and where population densities are likely to be very low. Under these conditions, males may enhance their reproductive success by nesting with a single female and producing multiple litters, rather than risk not finding a fertile mate. An alternative explanation proposes that, since prairie voles utilize a saturated habitat, dispersal opportunities are low. Thus, natural selection favors the production of high-quality, low-quantity offspring reared by two parents. In contrast, polygamous species, such as meadow voles, occupy patchy habitats, where dispersal success is more dependent on high-number, low-quality offspring. Data to support these potential explanations for the evolution of monogamy in prairie voles have been inconclusive. Interestingly, some populations of prairie voles are not monogamous, illustrating that even within a species there is a fair degree of plasticity in the neural circuits underlying pair bonding (Cushing et al., 2001). Thus, prairie voles, along with several other species of voles with various mating patterns, provide an opportunity to test hypotheses regarding mating patterns.

The pair bonding process in voles can be observed in the laboratory using a partner preference paradigm. In this procedure an adult male prairie vole and a female prairie vole are paired under differing experimental manipulations (i.e., duration of cohabitation, presence or absence of mating, antagonist infusions). After the designated time of cohabitation, the pair is separated and then placed in a partner preference testing arena. The arena is constructed of three chambers—the "partner" chamber in which the partner is tethered to restrict its movement to that chamber; the "stranger" chamber in which an unfamiliar animal of equal stimulus value as the partner is tethered; and the neutral chamber, which is connected to the other two chambers via tubing. The experimental subject is placed in the neutral chamber and is observed as it roams freely between the chambers. An animal is said to have developed a partner preference, the laboratory measure of a pair bond, if it spends more than twice as much time in contact with its partner than with the novel stimulus animal.

Data collected during tests of partner preference formation in prairie voles suggest that mating facilitates partner preference formation in both male and female prairie voles. For example, 6 hours of cohabitation without mating was not sufficient for the female to develop a partner preference, while the same duration of cohabitation with mating was sufficient (Williams et al., 1992). Similar results were obtained with males (Insel et al., 1995). However, in some cases, longer periods of cohabitation without mating are sufficient to result in the formation of a pair bond. Thus, it appears that both the quality and the quantity of social interactions between a pair of prairie voles contribute to the likelihood of partner preference formation and that mating acts to strengthen the pair bond. Using the partner preference paradigm in conjunction with pharmacological manipulations, we have begun to understand the chemical triggers and neural circuits underlying this pair-bonding process.

THE NEUROCHEMISTRY OF THE PAIR BOND

What neurotransmitter or hormone systems might be involved in the pair bond process? As mentioned above, social attachment is fairly rare between adult mammals; however, strong attachments between mothers and their offspring are widespread. It is conceivable that similar neural and molecular mechanisms that have evolved for regulating the mother-infant bond have been co-opted to produce the pair bond. This in fact appears to be the case. First, what hormones are involved in mother-infant bonding?

Not surprisingly, maternal nurturing behavior is facilitated by hormones released during pregnancy and parturition (Young and Insel, 2002). For example, in rats the levels of estrogens and progestins rise during pregnancy and then progestins decline at parturition. Maternal behavior is facilitated in virgin rats when estrogen and progestin treatment is followed by progestin withdrawal. Parental behavior in primates appears to be less dependent on hormonal stimulation; however, estrogen treatment in ovariectomized rhesus macaques does increase interaction with infants. In addition to these steroid hormones, oxytocin (OT) is a hormone that has multiple functions in the parturient mother, including the regulation of maternal behavior. OT is a nine amino acid cyclical neuropeptide hormone produced in the hypothalamus, which sends projections to the posterior pituitary as well as the brain (Gainer and Wray, 1994). OT is released into the plasma from the posterior pituitary gland during labor and is thought to play a role in facilitating parturition through its actions on uterine OT receptors. OT is also released into the plasma in a pulsatile manner during nursing, where it stimulates the milk ejection reflex, making breast-feeding possible. Studies in rodents and sheep have suggested that OT released in the brain also plays an important role in initiating maternal behavior as well as facilitating the selective bond between the mother and her offspring (Pedersen et al., 1994; Kendrick et al., 1997).

Several studies have now demonstrated that oxytocin plays a role in the development of the pair bond in the female prairie vole. Injections of an OT antagonist, a drug that blocks activation of the OT receptor, directly into the female prairie vole brain prior to cohabitation and mating inhibits the subsequent development of a partner preference (Insel and Hulihan, 1995). Furthermore, infusion of OT directly into the brain facilitates formation of a partner preference despite the absence of mating (Williams et al., 1994).

Some studies have suggested that OT's role in partner preference formation is specific only for females, while other studies have found similar effects in both sexes (Cho et al., 1999). However, in males there is clear evidence that the peptide arginine vasopressin (AVP) plays a significant role in the formation of the pair bond of the male for its mate. AVP is structurally related to OT, differing from OT in only two amino acids. Like OT, AVP is synthesized in the hypothalamus and transported to the posterior pituitary gland (Gainer and Wray, 1994). However, extrahypothalamic AVP neurons from the amygdala and bed nucleus of the stria terminalis project into the forebrain where they are thought to influence behavior through interactions with the V1a subtype of the AVP receptor (V1aR). These extrahypothalamic AVP projections are sexually dimorphic, with males producing far more AVP than females (DeVries, 1990). Infusion of a compound that blocks V1aR activation prior to cohabitation and mating prevents male prairie voles from displaying a partner preference (Winslow et al., 1993). Conversely, infusion of AVP during an abbreviated cohabitation without mating facilitates formation of a partner preference.

The fact that OT and AVP are involved in the formation of the pair bond does not imply that these factors act alone in this process. Pair bond formation is surely a highly complex process involving multiple brain structures, neurochemicals, and sensory modalities in rodents. However, the knowledge that OT and AVP appear to play a critical role in this process provides investigators with a useful starting point for understanding the molecular basis of the pair bond. This research is further facilitated by the existence of vole species that are genetically very similar to prairie voles yet differ dramatically in their social structure. For example, montane voles, from the Rocky Mountains region of the United States, look very similar to prairie voles but are rather asocial and do not form pair bonds between mates. In fact, males of this species are polygynous. Therefore, the prairie and montane voles provide a comparative approach for understanding the biology of the pair bond.

Since OT and AVP are involved in pair bond formation in the prairie vole and montane voles fail to produce a pair bond, one might hypothesize that montane voles show lower levels of these peptides in the brain. This appears not to be the case, as peptide distribution in the brain appears to be similar between the monogamous and polygamous species (Wang et al., 1996). It is possible that the nonmonogamous species simply do not release these peptides in response to social stimulation and mating, explaining the lack of pair bond formation, and there is some evidence to support this hypothesis (Bamshad et al., 1993; Wang et al., 1994). However, there is another intriguing possibility. Using a technique called receptor autoradiography, it is possible to determine the distribution and density of the receptors for OT and AVP in the brain. Receptors are the molecules on the target cells that transduce the signal of the peptide. Insel found that there are striking species differences in the distribution of OT and V1aR in the brains of the monogamous versus nonmonogamous vole species (Insel and Shapiro, 1992; Insel et al., 1994). Thus, a release of OT or AVP in the brain, which presumably occurs during mating, would activate different neural circuits in a monogamous species compared to a nonmonogamous species.

NEURAL CIRCUITS OF PAIR BOND FORMATION

What are the relevant neural circuits involved in pair bond formation? Comparison of the locations of high-receptor densities in the monogamous prairie and the montane vole provides interesting clues. For example, Insel found that the nucleus accumbens and the prelimbic cortex of the prairie vole are rich in oxytocin receptors, whereas these regions have few receptors in the montane vole. Likewise, the prairie vole ventral striato-pallidal region is rich in vasopressin receptors, while the montane vole ventral striato-pallidal region is not (Young et al., 2001). These regions are excellent candidates for facilitating pair bond formation because they are rich in dopamine, a neurotransmitter associated with reward and addiction. Amphetamines and cocaine are thought to produce their euphoric effects by modulating the dopamine system in these regions (McBride et al., 1999). In fact, injection of cocaine into these regions of the rat brain results in the development of a conditioned *place* preference (Gong et al., 1996). That is, the rat prefers to be in the environment where it received an injection of the drug.

Thus one could hypothesize that activation of the oxytocin and vasopressin receptors in these reward centers might result in the development of a conditioned *partner* preference in prairie voles. Since montane voles have few receptors in these regions, mating and/or the release of peptides in the brain would not result in the formation of a partner preference but may instead elicit other types of behaviors.

Interestingly, comparisons of vasopressin receptors in other species of mammals reveal that monogamous behavior is associated with elevated vasopressin receptors in the ventral striato-pallidum. For example, the monogamous California mouse (*Peromyscous californicus*) has a high density of vasopressin receptors in this region, whereas the closely related but nonmonogamous white-footed mouse (*P. leucopus*) does not (Bester-Meredith et al., 1999). Likewise, this region of the monogamous marmoset, a primate, has a high density of vasopressin receptors, whereas the nonmonogamous rhesus monkey does not (Young, 1999).

There is direct experimental evidence in voles that these reward circuits are involved in pair bonding. First, infusion of an oxytocin receptor blocker into the nucleus accumbens and prelimbic cortex prevents formation of pair bonds in females who have mated (Young et al., 2001). This same drug had no effect when injected into an adjacent area. In another study, Pitkow used a gene therapy approach to increase vasopressin receptors in the ventral striato-pallidum of male prairie voles. In this study a viral vector was used to deliver the prairie vole vasopressin receptor gene into the ventral striato-pallidum of male prairie voles. This modified virus infected the cells around the injection site and inserted the receptor gene into the neurons in the region. This gene was then expressed, leading to a significant increase in vasopressin receptor in the ventral striato-pallidum. Control animals were injected in the same region with a different virus carrying a control gene or with the same virus but in an adjacent brain area. Those animals with artificially elevated vasopressin receptors in the ventral pallidum displayed increased levels of affiliative behavior toward a novel juvenile (i.e., increased investigation and huddling) and readily formed strong pair bonds even in the absence of mating (Pitkow et al., 2001). Both studies examining the OT and AVP receptors strongly suggested that the activation of these receptors in the reward circuitry is important for development of the pair bond.

THE GENETICS OF PAIR BONDING

From the outside, prairie (monogamous) and montane (polygamous) voles look quite similar, and are, in fact, indistinguishable to the untrained eye. Their shared physical characteristics attest to their close genetic relationship, yet their brain neurochemistry and social structure differ dramatically. How can this be explained genetically? The distribution of oxytocin and vasopressin receptors in the brain, not the binding characteristics of the receptors, is different between these species. This suggests that something must be different in the part of the receptor genes that determines in which brain region the genes are expressed. Genes are composed of a coding sequence, which defines the structure of the final protein, and a regulatory sequence, which determines when and in what cells the gene is going to be expressed. Therefore, we hypothesized that there must be species differences in the regulatory regions of these genes that result in the species-specific pattern of receptor.

The vasopressin receptor gene has been characterized in both montane and prairie voles (Young et al., 1999). Not surprisingly, the coding sequences of the vasopressin receptor are virtually identical between these species. However there is a 420-bp stretch of sequence in the 5 prime regulatory region of the prairie vole gene that is absent in the montane vole gene. This sequence is also found in another monogamous vole species, the pine vole, but not in the nonmonogamous meadow vole. This prairie vole sequence is rich in highly repetitive sequences, or microsatellite DNA, which are known to be genetically unstable. Perhaps this instability in the regulatory region of the vasopressin receptor gene, as a result of the microsatellite DNA, results in the rapid evolution of receptor expression patterns, which in turn results in the evolution of social behaviors.

For example, there is an extraordinary amount of individual variation in both microsatellite length and brain vasopressin receptor binding patterns in a single population of prairie voles (Hammock and Young, 2002). Furthermore, there is a significant correlation between microsatellite length and receptor densities in specific brain regions. Thus, within the population there is variation in gene sequence that corresponds with variation in receptor binding. If these individual differences in receptor densities in the brain translate into variations in behavior, natural selection could quickly change social behavior in the population through changes in the frequency of vasopressin receptor alleles.

IS THE VASOPRESSIN RECEPTOR THE "MONOGAMY" GENE?

The data presented above suggest that a single gene can have a profound influence on the expression of complex behaviors defining reproductive strategies. In fact, the data suggest that simple changes in the locations in the brain that express the receptor for vasopressin can have a major impact on behavior. This was demonstrated conclusively by inserting the prairie vole vasopressin receptor gene along with regulatory elements into the mouse genome. Mice transgenic for the prairie vole vasopressin receptor gene displayed a pattern of V1aR binding that was remarkably similar to that of prairie voles but very different from nontransgenic mice (Young et al., 1999). When injected with vasopressin, the mice with a prairie vole pattern of vasopressin receptor expression in the brain responded similarly to prairie voles by exhibiting increased levels of affiliative behavior. Vasopressin injections did not alter social behavior in the nontransgenic mouse. This proves that simple changes in vasopressin receptor expression patterns can alter social behavior. This is certainly not the first study to demonstrate that mutations in a single gene can alter behavior. For example, one study in the nematode *C. elegans* identified a single gene that was responsible for strain differences in social interaction during feeding. When the gene, a homologue of the mammalian neuropeptide Y receptor gene, was transferred from one strain to the other, the recipient strain exhibited the behavior of the donor (de Bono and Bargmann, 1998). In addition, a large number of single-gene mutant mice have been created that have unusual behaviors, ranging from lack of parental care, increased or absent aggression, lack of social recognition, and deficits in mating behavior (Pfaff, 2001).

How can a single gene have such a large impact on a single behavior? In reality there are a multitude of genes involved in pair bonding in monogamous species. For example, pheromones must be detected, social stimuli processed, and a social memory formed. Many genes are involved in the development of the brain circuitry for the senses, cognition, learning, and memory. The V1aR itself cannot function in a vacuum but is coupled to a G-protein that activates the intracellular signaling pathway. Activation of the intracellular signaling pathways then likely modulates the expression of a number of other genes. So the V1aR is simply one protein in a complex of genes and gene products that produce the biochemical and neural circuit underlying social attachment. Every species has a reward circuitry, which evolved to promote certain behaviors beneficial for the reproductive success of the species. Perhaps by placing the V1aR in that pathway, social cues are processed by the addiction circuitry to yield an enduring social attachment. Thus, there is no single monogamy gene, but the V1aR gene, acting in concert with many other factors, profoundly influences social behavior.

In addition to pair bonding, the V1aR appears to alter other aspects of social behavior. For example, infusion of AVP into the prairie vole brain increases general social interaction. It is conceivable that AVP and OT may modulate many types of social bonds, not just parent-infant or pair bonds. Perhaps these neuropeptides play some role in the establishment or maintenance of social bonds or even social hierarchies in nonmonogamous primate species. To date, there is no experimental evidence to support this, but it is an area for future exploration.

IMPLICATIONS FOR HUMANS

Voles have provided a wealth of knowledge on the molecular, cellular, and systems neurobiology underlying pair bond formation. Undoubtedly, these rodents will continue to provide a detailed understanding of how social attachments can form and lead to a better understanding of the formation of social relationships in our own species. However, to the disappointment of many, it is unlikely that this research will result in drugs or gene therapies that ensure fidelity in relationships. That of course, is not the goal of this research. However, it may help us understand the neurobiological underpinnings of love and pair bonding in humans and enhance our understanding of human behavior and the factors associated with intimate human relationships. It may also provide hypotheses regarding the evolution and diversity in social relationships in our species. It must be noted that there is no direct evidence that the hormones oxytocin or vasopressin are actually involved in bonding in *humans*. Such data would be extremely difficult to obtain. These neuropeptides do not efficiently cross the blood-brain barrier, making pharmacological experiments in people difficult. However, there is evidence that oxytocin and vasopressin are released during sexual intercourse. One study demonstrated that plasma oxytocin levels increased at the time of orgasm in males (Carmichael et al., 1987), and another study reported that plasma vasopressin levels were elevated during sexual arousal prior to orgasm (Murphy et al., 1987). However, the relationship between plasma hormone levels and brain levels is unclear, so care must be taken in interpreting these results.

Molecular studies in voles suggest that mutations in the 5 prime regulatory region of the vasopressin receptor could be responsible for the species differences in receptor expression patterns in the brain. Interestingly, the human vasopressin receptor gene also has highly repetitive sequences in the same region of the gene (Thibonnier et al., 2000). As mentioned above, these sequences tend to be highly unstable due to their repetitive nature. The repetitive sequences in the human vasopressin receptor are highly variable among individuals, although not to the degree found between prairie and montane voles. Thus, if vasopressin receptors are important in social relationships in humans and these variations in sequence are associated with variations in expression in the brain, one would predict that some aspects of social attachment may, in fact, be affected by these genetic elements. A recent study found a nominally significant transmission disequilibrium between one allele of the human V1aR gene and autism (Kim et al., 2002). It would be interesting to perform genetic analyses to determine whether social-behavioral traits in the normal range correlate with these variable alleles of the vasopressin receptor. Certainly, if the individual variability in human V1aR sequence translates into individual variability in the distribution of receptor expression as it does in voles, this single gene could be responsible for individual differences in social behavior, which could be subject to natural selection in different ecological and cultural conditions.

Studies in voles suggest that, while sex may not be essential to formation of the pair bond, it does facilitate it. This observation likely has implications for human relationships. Our species is unusual in the animal kingdom in that sexual activity is not always associated with reproduction. In most mammals, a female become sexually receptive only during the period of the ovarian cycle when she can become pregnant, usually just before or after ovulation. In these species, sex has a single purpose—procreation. In human beings, sexual activity does not vary drastically with the ovarian cycle. It is possible that this has important social implications unrelated to fertility, namely strengthening the bond between mates. Perhaps frequent sexual activity stimulates the neural circuits responsible for maintaining the pair bond, preserving the strength of the bond over time.

Studies of voles have produced an exciting hypothesis that suggests pair bond formation is regulated by the same brain regions involved in the actions of drugs of abuse. These so-called reward circuits are regions of the brain that regulate feelings of pleasure and reward. These regions are activated by a neurotransmitter called dopamine, which is increased in the brain after taking cocaine and amphetamines. Those experiencing love often report feelings of euphoria when intimate with their partners, and these feelings are often reported as being similar to being "high." There is some scientific evidence that these reward circuits may in fact be involved in the psychobiology of love. One study examined brain activation in people while viewing photographs of someone to whom the subject reported being deeply in love. Brain activity was also determined while these same subjects viewed photographs of other familiar individuals. The authors reported that viewing photographs of their lovers elicited brain activation that was remarkably similar to that seen in other studies after drug consumption (Bartels and Zeki, 2000). This suggests that perhaps similar neural circuits are used to facilitate pair bonding in voles and humans. Perhaps the saying "love is an addiction" has biological support.

The biological basis of the pair bond in humans may change with time. In the early years of a relationship, love is experienced as an incredibly intense sensation that often drives the behavior of the individual. People experience a euphoria that may be similar to that experienced by drugs of addiction, and this experience undoubtedly has a specific neurochemistry underlying it. The individuals in these relationships are consumed by thoughts of being with their partner, often at the expense of other relationships. However, often in later years of a marriage, the nature of this bond changes and becomes less visceral and more a relationship of codependence. Perhaps for our primitive ancestors, the transition between these two types of love, which would occur after the offspring of the relationship are less dependent on the mother, would mark the dissolution of the relationship. However, for modern humans it is desirable to remain together in marriage as long as possible. Perhaps through understanding the neurobiology of the pair bond and how it is regulated, we may be able to discover strategies to maintain and reinvigorate the pair bond in couples, ultimately leading to strengthening of the nuclear family.

REFERENCES

Bamshad, M., M.A. Novak, and G.J. DeVries

1993 Sex and species differences in the vasopressin innervation of sexually naive and parental prairie voles, *Microtus ochrogaster*, and meadow voles, *M. pennsylvanicus*. *Journal of Neuroendocrinology* 5:247-255.

Bartels, A., and S. Zeki

2000 The neural basis for romantic love. *Neuroreport* 11:3829-3834.

Bester-Meredith, J.K., L.J. Young, and C.A. Marler

1999 Species differences in paternal behavior and aggression in Peromyscus and their associations with vasopressin immunoreactivity and receptors. *Hormones and Behavior* 36:25-38.

Carmichael, M.S., R. Humbert, J. Dixen, G. Palmisano, W. Greenleaf, and J.M. Davidson

1987 Plasma oxytocin increases in the human sexual response. *Journal of Clinical Endocrinology and Metabolism* 64:27-31.

Carter, C., A. DeVries, and L. Getz
1995 Physiological substrates of mammalian monogamy: The prairie vole model. *Neuroscience and Biobehavioral Reviews* 19:303-314.
Cho, M.M., A.C. DeVries, J.R. Williams, and C.S. Carter
1999 The effects of oxytocin and vasopressin on partner preferences in male and female prairie voles (*Microtus ochrogaster*). *Behavioral Neuroscience* 113:1071-1079.
Cushing, B.S., J.O. Martin, L.J. Young, and C.S. Carter
2001 The effects of peptides on partner preference formation are predicted by habitat in prairie voles. *Hormones and Behavior* 39:48-58.
de Bono, M., and C. Bargmann
1998 Natural variation in a neuropeptide Y receptor homolog modifies social behavior and food response in *C. elegans*. *Cell* 94:697-689.
DeVries, G.J.
1990 Sex differences in the brain. *Journal of Neuroendocrinology* 2:1-13.
Gainer, H., and W. Wray
1994 Cellular and molecular biology of oxytocin and vasopressin. Pp. 1099-1129 in *The Physiology of Reproduction*. E. Knobil and J.D. Neill, eds. New York: Raven Press.
Gong, W., D. Neill, and J.B. Justice
1996 Conditioned place preference and locomotor activation produced by injection of psychostimulants in ventral pallidum. *Brain Research* 707:64-74.
Hammock, E.H.D., and L.J. Young
2002 Variation in the vasopressin V1a receptor promoter and expression: Implications for inter- and intra-specific variation in social behavior. *European Journal of Neuroscience* 16:399-402.
Insel, T.R., and T. Hulihan
1995 A gender-specific mechanism for pair bonding: Oxytocin and partner preference formation in monogamous voles. *Behavioral Neuroscience* 109:782-789.
Insel, T.R., S. Preston, and J.T. Winslow
1995 Mating in the monogamous male: Behavioral consequences. *Physiology & Behavior* 57:615-627.
Insel, T.R., and L.E. Shapiro
1992 Oxytocin receptor distribution reflects social organization in monogamous and polygamous voles. *Proceedings of the National Academy of Sciences* 89:5981-5985.
Insel, T.R., Z. Wang, C.F. and Ferris
1994 Patterns of brain vasopressin receptor distribution associated with social organization in microtine rodents. *Journal of Neuroscience* 14:5381-5392.
Insel, T.R., and L.J. Young
2001 Neurobiology of social attachment. *Nature Neuroscience* 2:129-136.
Kendrick, K.M., A.P.C.D. Costa, K.D. Broad, S. Ohkura, R. Guevara, F. Levy, and E.B. Keverne
1997 Neural control of maternal behavior and olfactory recognition of offspring. *Brain Research Bulletin* 44:383-395.
Kim, S., L.J. Young, D. Gonen, J. Veenstra-VanderWeele, R. Courchesne, E. Courchesne, C. Lord, B.L. Leventhal, E.H. Cook, and T.R. Insel
2002 Transmission disequilibrium testing of arginine vasopressin receptor 1A (AVPR1A) polymorphisms in autism. *Molecular Psychiatry* 7:503-507.
Kleiman, D.G.
1977 Monogamy in mammals. *Quarterly Review of Biology* 52:39-69.

McBride, W.J., J.M. Murphy, and S. Ikemoto
1999 Localization of brain reinforcement mechanisms: Intracranial self-administration and intracranial place-conditioning studies. *Behavioral Brain Research* 101:129-152.

Murphy, M.R., J.R. Seckl, S. Burton, S.A. Checkley, and S.L. Lightman
1987 Changes in oxytocin and vasopressin secretion during sexual activity in men. *Journal of Clinical Endocrinology and Metabolism* 65:738-741.

Pedersen, C.A., J.D. Caldwell, C. Walker, G. Ayers, and G.A. Mason
1994 Oxytocin activates the postpartum onset of rat maternal behavior in the ventral tegmental and medial preoptic area. *Behavioral Neuroscience* 108:1163-1171.

Pfaff, D.
2001 Precision in mouse behavior genetics. *Proceedings of the National Academy of Sciences* 98:5957:5960.

Pitkow, L.J., C.A. Sharer, X. Ren, T.R. Insel, E.F. Terwilliger, and L.J. Young
2001 Facilitation of affiliation and pair-bond formation by vasopressin receptor gene transfer into the ventral forebrain of a monogamous vole. *Journal of Neuroscience* 21:7392-7396.

Thibonnier, M., M.K. Graves, M.S. Wagner, N. Chatelain, F. Soubrier, P. Corvol, H.F. Willard, and X. Jeunemaitre
2000 Study of V(1)-vascular vasopressin receptor gene microsatellite polymorphisms in human essential hypertension. *Journal of Molecular and Cellular Cardiology* 32:557-564.

Wang, Z., W. Smith, D.E. Major, and G.J. DeVries
1994 Sex and species differences in the effects of cohabitation on vasopressin messenger RNA expression in the bed nucleus and stria terminalis in prairie voles (*Microtus orchogaster*) and meadow voles (*Microtus pennsylvanicus*). *Brain Research* 650:212-218.

Wang, Z., L. Zhou, T.J. Hulihan, and T.R. Insel
1996 Immunoreactivity of central vasopressin and oxytocin pathways in microtine rodents: A quantitative comparative study. *Journal of Comparative Neurology* 366:726-737.

Williams, J., K. Catania, and C. Carter
1992 Development of partner preferences in female prairie voles (*Microtus ochrogaster*): The role of social and sexual experience. *Hormones and Behavior* 26:339-349.

Williams, J.R., T.R. Insel, C.R. Harbaugh, and C.S. Carter
1994 Oxytocin administered centrally facilitates formation of a partner preference in prairie voles (*Microtus ochrogaster*). *Journal of Neuroendocrinology* 6:247-250.

Winslow, J., N. Hastings, C.S. Carter, C. Harbaugh, and T.R. Insel
1993 A role for central vasopressin in pair bonding in monogamous prairie voles. *Nature* 365:545-548.

Young, L.J.
1999 Oxytocin and vasopressin receptors and species-typical social behaviors. *Hormones and Behavior* 36:212-221.

Young, L.J., and T.R. Insel
2002 Hormones and parental behavior. In *Behavioral Endocrinology*. J. Becker, M. Breedlove, and D. Crews, eds. Cambridge, MA: MIT Press.

Young, L.J., M.M. Lim, B.Gingrich, and T.R. Insel
2001 Cellular mechanisms of social attachment. *Hormones and Behavior* 40:133-138.

Young, L.J., R. Nilsen, K.G. Waymire, G.R. MacGregor, and T.R. Insel
1999 Increased affiliative response to vasopressin in mice expressing the vasopressin receptor from a monogamous vole. *Nature* 400:766-768.

5

Hormonal Mediation of Physiological and Behavioral Processes That Influence Fertility

Judy L. Cameron

This chapter reviews the complex and diverse roles that hormones play in mediating the physiological and behavioral processes that influence human fertility. Much of the focus is on hormones of the reproductive axis, which mediate the physiological processes governing fertility and provide powerful modulation of sexual behavior. Secretion of these hormones changes over the life span. Reproductive hormones are secreted in surprisingly high levels in prenatal development and at this time help set the stage for later development of normal reproductive physiology and behavior in adulthood. There is then a period of childhood quiescence, when the reproductive axis is essentially "turned off", followed by a cascade of hormonal changes that occur with puberty. In males, reproductive hormone secretion is rather stable in the adult years, with a slow decline in levels occurring with aging. In contrast, much greater fluxes in hormone secretion occur throughout adulthood in women, with large changes in hormone secretion occurring over the course of each menstrual cycle, followed by a period of irregular hormone secretion during the transition to menopause and ultimately a marked decline in reproductive hormone levels in the postmenopausal period. Understanding the changes in reproductive hormone secretion across the life span has implications for the design of biodemographic studies with regard to how and when reproductive function and sexual behavior are assessed and understanding the factors that influence these measures.

Many lifestyle choices and life events can modulate activity of the reproductive axis and thus impact significantly on both reproductive physiology and behavior. In the modern world, pharmacological modulation of reproductive hormone levels is common. Large numbers of women take exogenous hormones in the form of contraceptives, and even greater numbers of women are given estrogen replacement therapy in the postmenopausal period. A more limited but rapidly expanding subset of individuals consume steroid hormones to regulate body strength and endurance, particularly individuals who participate in competitive sports. And with the more widespread consumption of foods that contain phytoestrogens, environmental exposure to hormones is becoming an issue of greater importance.

A variety of events that occur over the course of a normal life can also significantly influence activity of the reproductive axis. Pregnancy and lactation are associated with profound changes in the functioning of the reproductive axis, fertility, sexual behavior, and maternal behavior. Common life stresses, including metabolic stresses associated with undernutrition or the increased energy expenditure of participation in chronic vigorous exercise can suppress the activity of the reproductive axis. And psychosocial stresses provide an even more common inhibition to the reproductive axis. Even if reproductive hormone secretion is maintained, these life events can markedly alter circulating levels of reproductive hormones and thus influence fertility and sexual behavior. Biodemographic studies need to track lifestyle choices and life events to allow an accurate conceptualization of factors influencing fertility outcomes in human relationships.

Lastly, it is important to keep in mind that there are dramatic individual differences in normal circulating levels of reproductive hormones, the amount of hormone needed to maintain normal reproductive physiology and sexual behavior, and the sensitivity of individuals to the various forms of stress-induced reproductive dysfunction. We are just beginning the daunting task of elucidating the systems in the brain that underlie these individual differences. However, it is likely that the task of understanding the role that individual differences play in contributing to fertility outcomes will be even more complex.

HORMONES INFLUENCING REPRODUCTIVE FUNCTION AND BEHAVIOR

Physiological Regulation by Reproductive Hormones

This section provides an overview of the hormones that comprise the reproductive axis, how they are regulated and secreted, and their physiological actions in the body (for more detailed information see Steiner and Cameron, 1989; and Griffin and Ojeda, 2000). Particular attention is given to issues that influence the types of measurements made in the field of biodemography.

Although many people think of reproductive function as a bodily function governed by endocrine organs of the pelvis, testes, and ovaries, specialized neurons in the brain and hormones secreted by the "master endocrine organ," the pituitary, located just beneath the brain, play critical roles in governing reproductive function (see Figure 5-1). Not only do the brain and pituitary coordinate and provide the "central drive" to the reproductive axis throughout life, the brain is also the primary site where environmental factors that modulate reproductive function act.

The region of the brain involved in the regulation of reproductive function as well as many of the body's other basic homeostatic functions (i.e., control of food intake, growth, response to stress, water balance, metabolic rate) is the hypothalamus. The hypothalamus sits at the base of the brain and is connected by a specialized portal blood system to the pituitary, just below. A population of specialized neurons in the hypothalamus produce the neurotransmitter, gonadotropin-releasing hormone (or GnRH, named for its ability to release the hormones in the pituitary that provide trophic support to the ovaries and testes—the gonadotropins—luteinizing hormone, LH and follicle-stimulating hormone, FSH). GnRH travels via the portal capillaries to the anterior pituitary, where it stimulates the synthesis and release of the pituitary hormones, LH and FSH.

Many neurotransmitter systems from the brainstem, limbic system, and other areas of the hypothalamus convey information to GnRH neurons (Kordon et al., 1994). These afferent systems include neurons that contain neurotransmitters that are generally stimulatory to GnRH neurons, such as norepinephrine, dopamine, serotonin, glutamate, neuropeptide Y, and galanin, as well as neurotransmitters that are generally inhibitory to GnRH neurons, such as gamma aminobutyric acid (GABA), endogenous opiate peptides, and the central hypothalamic hormone that governs the adrenal axis, corticotropin-releasing hormone (CRH). Importantly, both in normal physiological conditions and in response to environmental signals (such as changes in nutrition, exercise, and psychosocial stress) the activity of the reproductive axis is changed by modulation of the neural inputs into GnRH neurons. For example, various forms of stress can lead to a suppression of reproductive function by acting to increase inhibitory drive to GnRH neurons by increasing either ß-endorphin or CRH input into the GnRH neuronal system (Feng et al., 1991; Norman and Smith, 1992). Decreased firing of GnRH neurons leads to less GnRH stimulation of pituitary LH and FSH release and thus less stimulation of ovarian and testicular function. It is also important to understand that changes in neuronal function in a number of neurological and psychiatric diseases can be associated with alterations in both reproductive physiology and behavior. For example, changes in both reproductive function and sexual behavior are commonly reported by patients suffering from depression, anxiety disorders, and obsessive-compulsive disorders (Clayton, 2002; Shabsigh et al., 2001). The

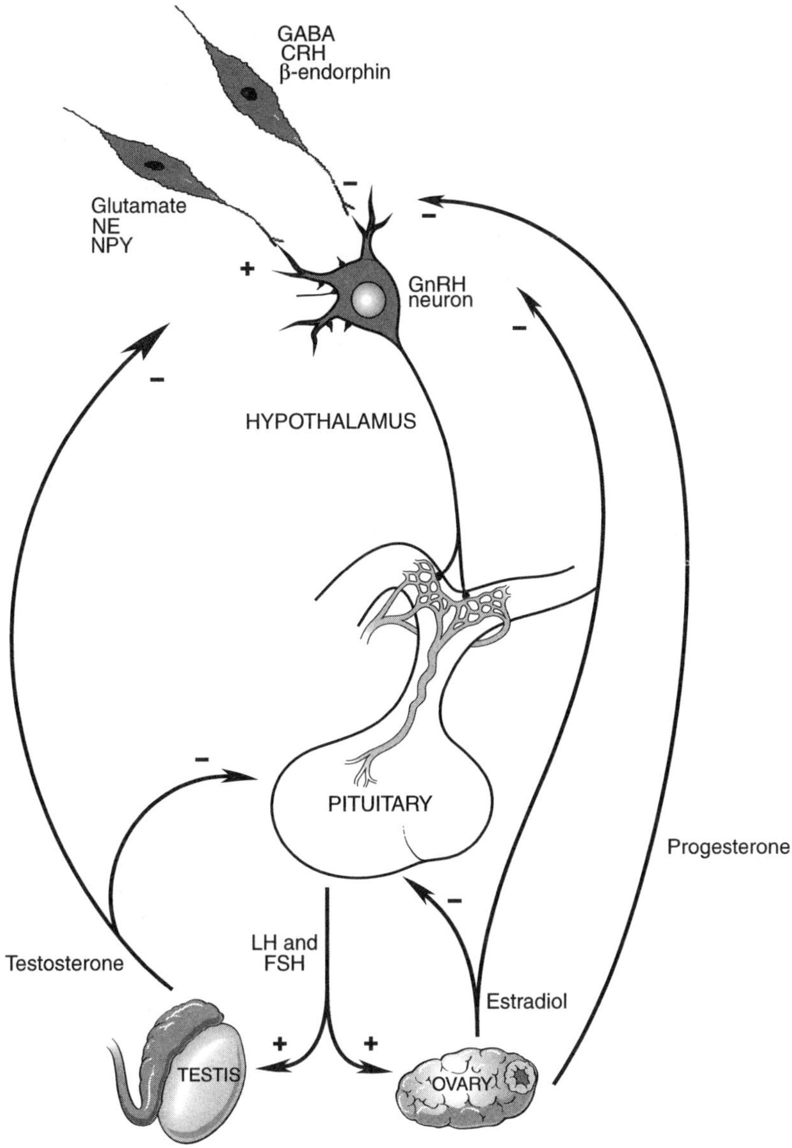

FIGURE 5-1 Schematic diagram of the hypothalamic-pituitary-gonadal axis. Interrelationships between hormones and neurotransmitters are shown as stimulatory (+) or inhibitory (–).

drugs used to treat these disorders have the potential to impact reproductive function because they can affect neural input into GnRH neurons as well as treat neurotransmitter imbalances in higher cortical areas (Clayton, 2002; Montgomery et al., 2002).

GnRH is a small 10 amino acid peptide that is rapidly metabolized, so although it reaches the pituitary in adequate concentrations to stimulate the synthesis and secretion of LH and FSH, it is usually not detectable in the peripheral circulation. However, GnRH can be given systemically to stimulate activity of the reproductive axis in a number of situations where reproductive function is suppressed. In such circumstances it is important to provide GnRH in a "pulsatile" fashion (a pulse every 1 to 3 hours), in that continuous administration of GnRH will down-regulate pituitary GnRH receptors and lead to a suppression of pituitary LH and FSH release, rather than a stimulation of release (Belchetz et al., 1978). However, as one can imagine, administration of pulses of GnRH is difficult and inconvenient, usually requiring the patient to have an in-dwelling subcutaneous catheter and wear an electronic pump. Thus, restoration of normal reproductive function in individuals in which normal activity of the reproductive axis is compromised can be a fairly arduous undertaking. The converse situation, where the reproductive axis is active at an inappropriate time, such as in cases of precocious puberty, is much more easily resolved by giving a long-acting GnRH-analog (many orally active forms are available) that will provide continuous activity at the pituitary, down regulate GnRH receptors, and thus essentially shut off pituitary LH and FSH synthesis and secretion and all functions of the reproductive axis downstream from the pituitary (Moghissi, 1990).

LH and FSH are glycoprotein hormones originally named for their action at the level of the ovary in the female, but the same hormones are produced in the male and govern testicular function (Griffin and Ojeda, 2000; Steiner and Cameron, 1989). The gonadotropins are released into the peripheral bloodstream and act at cells that have specific LH and FSH receptors, primarily at the gonads. In the male, LH binds to testicular cells (Leydig cells) and stimulates the synthesis and secretion of testosterone. FSH binds to Sertoli cells in the seminiferous tubules and along with testosterone stimulates the process of spermatogenesis. In the female, FSH acts on ovarian follicles to stimulate their growth and the production of estrogen. LH acts on the fully developed follicle to stimulate ovulation and then to support the function of the transient endocrine tissue formed during the last 2 weeks of each menstrual cycle, the corpus luteum (see Figure 5-2 for an overview of hormonal changes during the female menstrual cycle). The corpus luteum secretes both estrogen and progesterone, which play a critical role in preparing the uterine endometrium for implantation of a developing embryo should fertilization occur. Not surprisingly, in that both LH

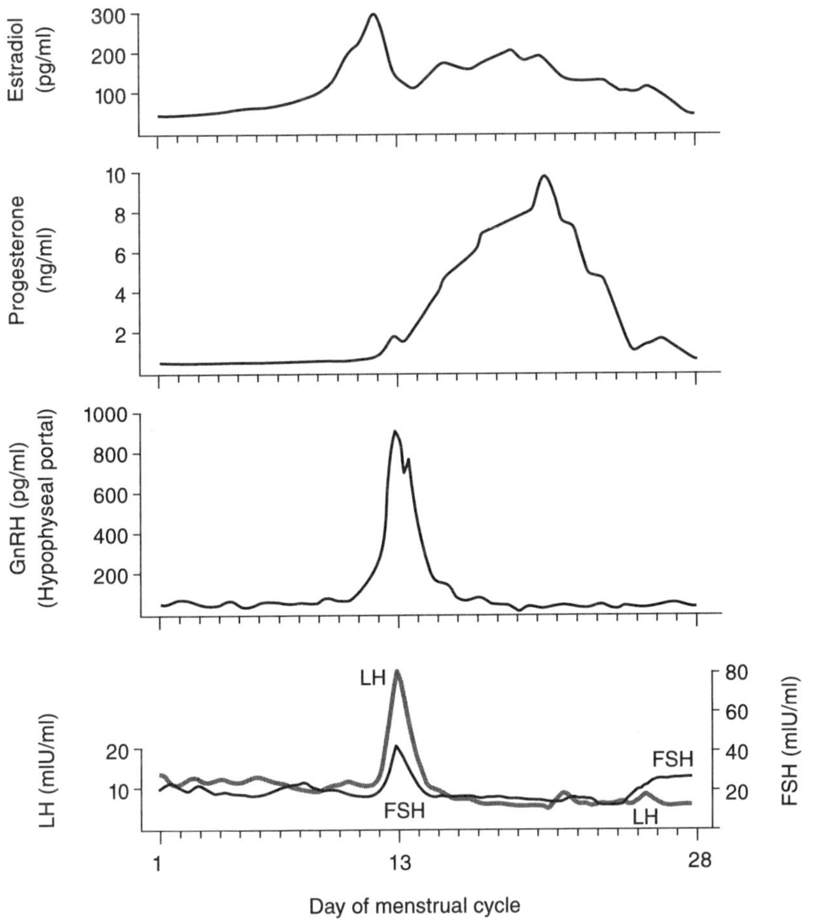

FIGURE 5-2 Diagrammatic representation of changes in plasma levels of estradiol, progesterone, LH, FSH, and portal levels of GnRH over the human menstrual cycle.

and FSH secretion are stimulated by GnRH, both hormones are released into the bloodstream in a pulsatile manner, at rates of about one pulse every 2 to 3 hours in males and at rates that vary in females from one pulse every hour to one pulse every 8-12 hours at various stages of the menstrual cycle (Soules et al., 1984; see Figure 5-3). The pulsatile nature of LH and FSH secretion can be a confound when hormone measures are collected as part of large population studies, in that a single blood sample may be collected when hormone levels are at the peak or nadir of a pulse; thus, variation

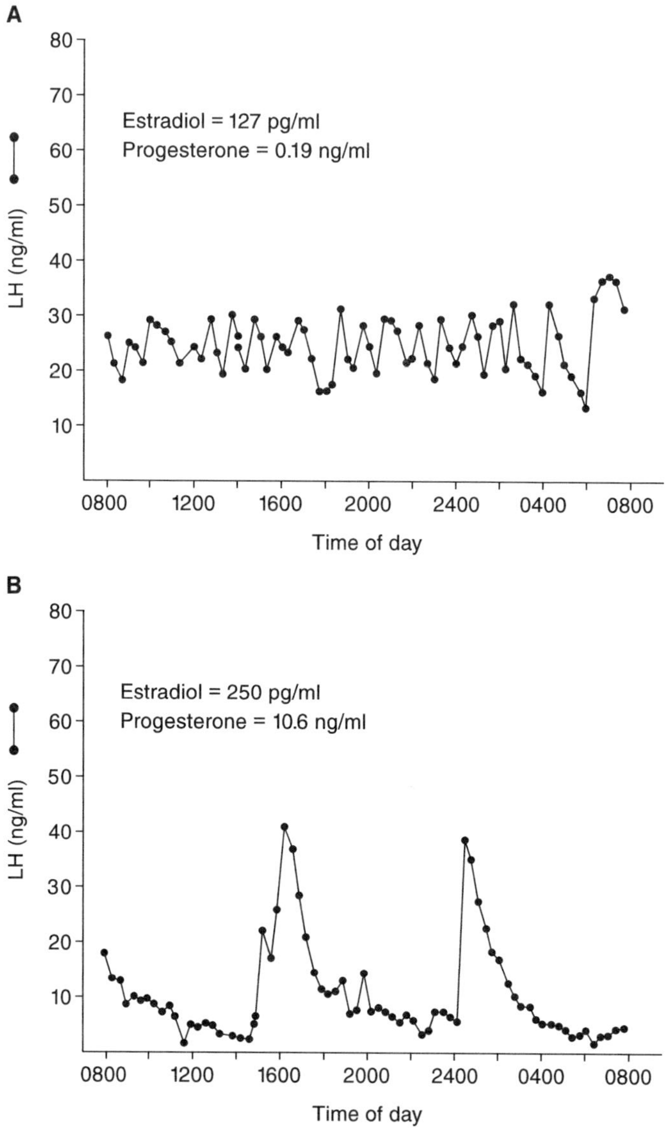

FIGURE 5-3 Examples of the pulsatile pattern of LH secretion in a woman during the late follicular phase (A) and midluteal phase (B) of the menstrual cycle. Steroid hormone levels on the day of each study are indicated on each graph. Note the dramatic slowing of pulsatile LH secretion as a result of gonadal steroid hormone negative feedback during the luteal phase. (Redrawn from Soules et al., 1984.)

within an individual can be great, making it difficult to detect group differences or changes in hormone levels in response to environmental or social conditions.

The gonadal steroid hormones are produced in a common synthetic pathway, all of them derived from the same precursor, cholesterol. Although androgens are commonly thought of as male hormones, they are produced in both the male and the female, and likewise the female hormone, estrogen, is present in the male and the female. In males, testosterone produced by the Leydig cells of the testes can act at its target tissues by binding to testosterone receptors, or first being converted to a more potent androgen, dihydrotestosterone, by the enzyme 5 α-reductase, or by being converted to estrogen by the enzyme aromatase and acting by binding to estrogen receptors. In females the pathway for estradiol production involves an intermediate step of androgen production, and thus the ovary is a source of low levels of androgens, principally androstenedione. The body produces three forms of estrogen: estradiol, which is the principal form of estrogen produced by the ovary; estrone; and estriol, which is produced predominantly by aromatization of androgens in peripheral fat tissue. Estriol production is thus related to body fat composition and is an important source of estrogen in the postmenopausal woman, once production of estradiol by the ovaries has ceased. Steroid hormones primarily travel through the bloodstream bound to proteins (>70 percent bound). In conditions where there is a change in the concentration of binding proteins in the circulation (i.e., with long-term changes in nutritional status, changes in either the level of energy availability or the ratio of protein to carbohydrate consumed; pregnancy, liver disease), the amount of steroid hormone in the circulation and its delivery to tissues are also affected. Assay procedures are generally available to measure both free and total (free + protein bound) steroid hormone concentrations in the blood, and it is important to distinguish between these.

The gonadal steroid hormones have important actions in a number of reproductive tissues. In the male, testosterone acts to stimulate development of male secondary sexual characteristics, including enlargement of the penis and testes, increased muscle mass, deepening of the voice, and stimulation of adult hair growth patterns. In the ovaries, estrogen acts to stimulate proliferation of follicular cells and maturation of the oocyte, preparing it for ovulation. At the uterus, estrogen acts during both the follicular and luteal phases of the menstrual cycle to stimulate development of the uterine lining and prepare it for implantation of a fertilized ovum. During the late follicular phase, rising levels of estrogen also act on the cervical mucosa to stimulate the elaboration of a thin, watery mucus that is amenable to sperm penetration. At the breast, estrogen stimulates development at puberty and further development during pregnancy and plays an important role in stimulating milk production during lactation. Estrogen receptors are also found in many other organs, including bone, pancreas, fat, and blood vessels.

Progesterone is secreted in large quantities during the last 2 weeks of each menstrual cycle. Under the influence of progesterone, the uterine glands in the endometrium enter a secretory phase and produce large amounts of glycogen, which provides nutritional support for early development of an embryo. Withdrawal of progesterone at the end of the luteal phase leads to shedding of the uterine endometrium and menses, which marks the termination of one menstrual cycle and the initiation of the next cycle. Progesterone also acts at the cervix to thicken cervical mucus, making it hostile to sperm penetration, and at the breast in late pregnancy working in concert with estrogen to prepare for lactation. All three gonadal steroid hormones also act at receptors in the brain, as will be discussed in more detail in the section below. One of the actions of these hormones in the brain is to provide feedback regulation to the hypothalamic GnRH neurons and the pituitary gonadotropin-secreting cells.

Steroid hormone secretion is relatively stable in the adult years in males, although it must be remembered that the gonadotropins and testosterone are secreted in a pulsatile fashion. However, in the female there are marked changes in the circulating concentrations of gonadotropins and gonadal steroid hormones across the menstrual cycle (Erickson, 1978; Figure 5-2). The menstrual cycle is commonly divided into two phases, each of which is approximately 2 weeks in length. The first 2 weeks constitute the follicular phase. During this time small groups of ovarian follicles, each of which is a layer of cells surrounding an ovum, are developing and maturing, and as they do so under the trophic influence of FSH and LH, they secrete increasing concentrations of estradiol. Thus, over this 2-week time span, estradiol levels are very low during the first week and then increase exponentially in the second week. The rising secretion of estradiol by a fully developed follicle provides a positive feedback signal to the brain and pituitary, resulting in a massive release of LH and FSH at midcycle, and this "surge" of gonadotropins triggers ovulation, so that the mature follicle bursts and the ovum is released into the nearby fallopian tube and can travel to the uterus. The follicular cells that surrounded the developing ovum reorganize into a transient endocrine tissue, the corpus luteum, which produces both estradiol and progesterone in the last 2 weeks of the cycle, the luteal phase. Unless pregnancy occurs, the corpus luteum spontaneously regresses after about 2 weeks, and the withdrawal of progesterone support to the uterine lining leads to menstruation, which marks the beginning of a new cycle. Population studies that track reproductive hormone secretion must take these rather marked cyclic fluctuations in hormone levels into account in order to adequately examine how changes in hormone secretion in females of reproductive age are linked to fertility outcomes, behavior, or environmental conditions.

Measurement of reproductive hormone levels in large field studies can be a challenge. Many of these studies are conducted at some distance from medical or laboratory facilities, where collection of blood samples, centrifugation of the samples to collect plasma, and immediate transfer to frozen storage to prevent deterioration of hormones are not possible. Fortunately, considerable advances have been made in the last decade in the development of techniques for measuring reproductive hormone levels in more easily obtainable body—fluids, saliva and urine (Campbell, 1994; Ellison, 1994; Lasley et al., 1994; Lasley and Shidleler, 1994). Improvement of the sensitivity of assay methods makes it possible to detect the low levels of hormones that are present in these fluids (Clough et al., 1992; Ellison, 1988; Stanczyk et al., 1980;). Moreover, development of collection and storage techniques that can be utilized in remote areas of the world (Lipson and Ellison, 1989; Young and Bermes, 1986) has facilitated the study of the relationship between activity of the reproductive axis and many other parameters measured in demographic population studies. Salivary samples can reflect acute changes in plasma hormone levels, while urinary measures provide an integrated assessment of steroid hormone secretion over a number of hours. Salivary samples are useful for detection of gonadal steroid hormones. Salivary steroid hormone levels reflect the levels of free hormone present in the blood (i.e., steroid that is not bound to plasma proteins). Saliva can be easily collected at frequent intervals and can be stored at room temperature for several weeks without significant deterioration of hormones. However, it is not useful for measurement of the gonadotropins, LH and FSH, and will not provide an index of changes in plasma protein levels that may be responsible for changes in free steroid hormone concentrations. Gonadotropin metabolites, as well as steroid hormones, can be measured in urine samples. And urine is particularly useful for the early detection of human chorionic gonadotropin, a placental hormone that serves as a useful indicator of early pregnancy (Canfield and O'Connor, 1991).

Behavioral Regulation by Reproductive Hormones

Sexual behavior can be divided into distinct aspects, in both males and females, which include attractiveness, sexual desire, arousal, orgasm, and reinitiation. Here we will not focus on detailed information about how each of these sexual behaviors is influenced by hormones but rather on two broad areas—sexual desire and sexual behavior. There is evidence that most aspects of sexual behavior, particularly in males, are influenced by gonadal steroid hormones. Steroid hormone receptors are abundant in the brain. Classical estrogen receptors (now called estrogen α-receptors) are strongly concentrated in the hypothalamus but are also found in areas of the brain with strong connections to the hypothalamus (Simerly et al., 1990). More recently, a second form of estrogen receptor (estrogen ß-receptors) was identified and found to be present throughout the rostral-caudal extent of the brain, including the cerebral cortex (Shughrue et al., 1997). Specific receptors for progesterone are induced by estrogen in hypothalamic regions of the brain, and there is also some evidence for constitutive expression of progesterone receptors (Bethea et al., 1992). Androgen receptor mapping studies have shown considerable overlap in the distribution of androgen and estrogen receptors throughout the brain (Michael et al., 1995; Simerly et al., 1990). Our discussion here will focus on the effects of gonadal steroid hormones on sexual behaviors, although there is evidence that they modulate a variety of other behaviors (Cameron, 2001).

Recognition of an important link between sexual behavior and hormones arose originally from the finding that castration of adult males often results in diminished sexual activity and erectile difficulty (Luttge, 1971). In hypogonadal or castrated men, withdrawal of testosterone has been reported to result in a rapid decrease in sexual interest and activity that is reinstated with testosterone replacement (Davidson et al., 1982; Kwan et al., 1983). There are similar findings in nonhuman primate species, such that as the breeding season comes to an end and the annual cycle of testicular regression occurs, male sexual activity falls off sharply (Gordon et al., 1976). However, there is also clear evidence of tremendous variability among individuals in the rate of loss of sexual activity and the degree of diminution of sexual activity with loss of testosterone. The 1959 study by Bremer followed 244 men castrated for medical reasons and found that a third of them retained sexual interest and activity for over a year, some for up to 10 years. Similarly, in male macaques castration has been associated with a gradual reduction but not an elimination of male sexual behavior (Michael and Wilson, 1974; Phoenix et al., 1973). In normal men there is no correlation between testosterone levels and individual differences in sexual desire or behavior (Schiavi and White, 1976). This finding supports the concept that there is a threshold for testosterone actions on sexual behavior in males over which no further effects of testosterone are apparent (Meston and Frohlich, 2000). Studies in macaques suggest that other social factors interact with circulating testosterone concentrations to impact on sexual behavior. Wallen (1999) showed that suppression of testicular hormones decreased sexual activity in low-ranking male monkeys but that sexual behavior in high-ranking males was not measurably affected.

In women the factors regulating sexual desire and activity, and the role that hormones play in this regard, are even less well understood. Studies of surgical ovariectomy generally report that these women have a decrease in sexual desire from presurgical levels (Dennerstein et al., 1977; Lieblum et al., 1983). Both estrogen therapy and androgen therapy have been shown to have some effect on the restoration of sexual behavior after surgical ovariectomy (Lieblum et al., 1983; Sherwin et al., 1985). Estrogen replacement in ovariectomized female monkeys has been shown to increase female initiation of sexual behavior (Zehr et al., 1998). At menopause, when there is a naturally occurring decrease in reproductive hormone levels (both estrogens and androgens), a decrease in sexual desire has been generally reported (McCoy and Davidson, 1985). There have been several reports of a general correlation between androgen levels and sexual interest in postmenopausal women (Lieblum et al., 1983; McCoy and Davidson, 1985), but these studies have not determined whether fluctuations in androgen levels in individuals correlate with changes in sexual interest. Estrogen treatment can also lead to an increase in sexual activity in postmenopausal women, but it is difficult to determine if this is an action at the level of the brain or is secondary to increased comfort with intercourse due to increased lubrication of the vagina (Sherwin, 1991). Studies looking for correlations in premenopausal females with circulating levels of androgens and estrogens have been somewhat confusing.

In macaques there is a clear increase in sexual behavior in midcycle (Goy, 1979; Wallen, 1990). Although this could be due to an increase in attractiveness of females to males as estrogen levels rise (Czaja et al., 1977), there is evidence that, when the male's mobility is limited and the female can control proximity, there is a cyclic increase in the female's approach to males (Czaja and Bielert, 1975; Pomerantz and Goy, 1983), and females will work harder on an operant task to gain access to males at midcycle (Bonsall et al., 1978). However, whether these cyclic changes in sexual interest are governed by estrogens or androgens is difficult to determine because they rise in concert, androgens being a precursor to the ovarian synthesis of estrogen. A study by Zehr et al. (1998) showing that estrogen replacement alone to ovariectomized female monkeys can stimulate female sexual initiation and earlier studies showing that in the normal menstrual cycle changes in circulating estradiol but not androgen correlate with changes in female sexual initiation (Wallen et al., 1986) support a role for estrogen in governing female sexual behavior.

Several studies in ovariectomized, estrogen-treated monkeys have suggested that adrenal androgens may play a role in modulating female sexual behavior (Baum et al., 1977; Everitt et al., 1972), but such an effect has not been seen in ovary-intact macaques (Lovejoy and Wallen, 1990). Moreover, Wallen et al. (1986) found that ovarian suppression eliminated female sexual initiation, even though the adrenals were intact and functioning. As reviewed by Wallen (2001), hormonal influences on women's sexuality have been difficult to demonstrate and to interpret due to unwillingness of subjects to be sampled either physiologically or behaviorally and strong influences of male partners on women's sexual activity. However, there is evidence for changes in the level of female sexual desire in women with a peak at midcycle (Bancroft et al., 1983; Dennerstein et al., 1994; Stanislaw and Rice, 1988; Van Goozen et al., 1997). Thus, although hormones are not necessary for female sexual behavior, there is accumulating evidence that hormones modulate sexual desire (Meston and Frolich, 2000; Wallen, 2001). Further studies are needed to understand the differential roles of estrogens and androgens in this regard. As discussed for the male, there is also evidence that social factors interact with hormonal influences with regard to sexual behavior in females. Adams et al. (1997) showed that women who used less reliable contraceptives showed less pronounced midcycle increases in heterosexual initiation, but much greater midcycle increases in autosexual behavior.

HORMONAL CHANGES THROUGH THE LIFE SPAN

Early-Life Activation of the Reproductive Axis

Early in embryonic development the components of the reproductive axis are formed and become functional. GnRH neurons, which provide the central drive to the reproductive axis, are an unusual neuronal population in that they originate from outside the central nervous system, coming originally from the epithelial tissue of the nasal placode (Schwanzel-Fukuda and Pfaff, 1989; Wray et al., 1989). During embryonic development, GnRH neurons migrate across the surface of the brain into the hypothalamus. Migration is dependent on a scaffolding of neurons and glial cells along which the GnRH neurons move, with chemical signals guiding the process (Silverman et al., 1994). Failure of GnRH neurons to properly migrate leads to a clinical condition, Kallman's syndrome, in which GnRH neuroendocrine neurons do not reach their final destination and thus do not stimulate pituitary gonadotropin secretion (Schwanzel-Fukuda et al., 1989). Patients with Kallman's syndrome do not spontaneously enter puberty. Administration of exogenous GnRH effectively treats this form of hypothalamic hypogonadism, although, as discussed above, this requires pulsatile administration of GnRH.

Functional activity of the reproductive axis as a whole is initiated during fetal development, and surprisingly by midgestation circulating levels of LH and FSH reach values similar to those found in adulthood (Ellinwood and Resko, 1984; Kaplan et al., 1976). Later in gestational development the gonadotropin levels decline, restrained by rising levels of circulating gonadal steroids (Kaplan et al., 1976; Resko and Ellinwood, 1985). The steroids having this effect are likely placental in origin, in that following parturition there is a rise in circulating gonadotropin levels that is apparent for the first 12 to 18 months of life (Winter et al., 1975). The decline in reproductive hormone secretion between ages one and two appears to be due to a decrease in GnRH stimulation of the reproductive axis. This decrease occurs even in agonadal individuals, and the period of elevated gonadotropin and gonadal steroid secretion can be extended by treating with administration of pulses of GnRH (Plant, 2001).

Steroid hormone secretion has effects on both primary sexual differences between males and females (i.e., differentiation of the sexual organs) and the development of secondary sexual differences (i.e., body fat distribution, muscle development, breast development, differences in hair distribution; Cooke et al., 1998; Cameron, 2001). In the case of sexual differentiation of the body, it is clear that exposure of males to various testicular secretory products, especially testosterone, during early prenatal development leads to sexual differentiation of the internal and external genitalia. Later activation of the reproductive axis at puberty, with a sustained increase in circulating testosterone then leads to the development of secondary sexual characteristics. Thus, testosterone has both "organizational" and "activational" influences on the sexual differentiation of the body. The organizational effects of gonadal hormones are conceptualized as resulting from the early influence of gonadal hormones on structural development, which do not require continued hormone exposure to maintain sexual differentiation. Activational effects are conceptualized as later stimulation of reversible influences on sexual differentiation that require continued exposure to gonadal hormones to maintain sex differences.

The concept that sex steroid hormones have important and permanent organizational effects on the developing brain was originally postulated based on experimental findings that treatment of developing mice with testosterone produced permanent effects on reproductive capacity (Barraclough and Leathem, 1954), with early treatment with testosterone blocking later activation of ovulation by estradiol. A similar coordination of early and later influences of gonadal steroid hormones on reproductive behavior also occurs in many species studied to date (Cooke et al., 1998; MacLusky and Naftolin, 1981; Phoenix et al., 1959). In general, exposure of males to testicular hormones during prenatal and early postnatal periods leads to both masculinization of some tissues and functions (i.e., masculine changes in genital structure, copulatory behavior, and other behaviors characteristic of males) and defeminization of other tissues and functions (i.e., ovulatory competence, feminine sexual behaviors like lordosis, and other behaviors characteristic of females). In rodents the critical period for steroid-hormone-mediated organization of brain regions and sexually dimorphic behaviors appears to be postnatal, with most effects occurring during the first 10 days of life. In primates, sexual differentiation of the brain occurs prenatally, over an extended period in midgestation (Phoenix et al., 1968). There is also recent evidence in male macaques that neonatal exposure to testosterone may play a role in determining the extent of adult sexual behavior (Mann et al., 1998).

Pubertal Activation of the Reproductive Axis

Pubertal reawakening of the reproductive axis occurs in late childhood and is marked by a cascade of hormonal, physical, psychological, and behavioral changes. One of the earliest signs of puberty is an elevation of gonadotropin and gonadal steroid hormone levels specifically at night (Boyar et al., 1974), although because detection of this rise requires collecting blood samples at night it is virtually never examined in demographic studies. Investigation into the mechanisms controlling the pubertal reawakening of the GnRH pulse generator has been an area of intense investigation for the past two decades (Ojeda and Bilger, 2000; Plant, 2001). Although the mechanisms are not fully understood, significant progress has been made in identifying central changes in the hypothalamus that appear to play a role in this process. There is strong evidence of both increases in stimulatory neural input into GnRH neurons and decreases in inhibitory input. Despite an increased understanding of the neural changes occurring at puberty, the question of what signals trigger the pubertal awakening of the reproductive axis is unanswered at this time. Availability of food and nutritional status have been shown to affect the timing of puberty; however, these signals appear to be only modulators of the pubertal process in that puberty can only be moderately advanced by increasing food availability (Frisch and MacArthur, 1974). Whether there is a genetic timing mechanism that regulates puberty or whether other signals from the body are responsible for timing the reactivation of the reproductive axis awaits further research.

Changes in body habitus are the first signs of puberty detected by most individuals, although these emanate from increased levels of gonadal steroid hormones and are thus relatively late events in the reawakening of the reproductive axis. Likewise, in girls, menarche is a very late event, heralding the point where the adult cyclic interplay between the hypothalamic-pituitary-ovarian axis is initiated. As described in the section above, the increase in testosterone at puberty in males leads to development of the secondary sexual characteristics, including increased growth of facial, axillary, and pubic hair; deepening of the voice; increase in muscle mass; enlargement of the testes and penis; increased incidence of erections and ejaculations; and attainment of fertility. Sexual behavior is also dramatically increased in males at puberty, and there is a strong correlation at this age between plasma testosterone levels and degree of sexual desire and sexual activity (Halpern et al., 1998; Udry et al., 1985).

In females the rising tide of estrogen at puberty is the primary stimulus for development of most of the secondary sexual characteristics, including breast development, widening of the hips, and increased deposition of subcutaneous body fat. The growth of axillary and pubic hair is under androgenic control and is stimulated by an increase in dehydroepiandrosterone (DHEA) from the adrenal gland. This developmental increase in DHEA is referred to as adrenarche and generally precedes puberty by several months to several years. Increases in sexual desire and sexual behavior also occur in girls at puberty. And, as in adulthood, there is controversy as to which hormones may be mediating these increases. There are correlations between androgen levels in adolescent girls and sexual interest (Udry et al., 1986) and the initiation of coitus (Halpern et al., 1997). However, the role of estrogens, which tend to covary with androgens in females, has not been adequately examined. Moreover, there is evidence that social factors can be as important as hormonal factors in determining a girl's sexual behavior (Udry et al., 1986).

Changes with Aging

In males, testosterone levels decrease slightly with aging and there is a mean decrease in sexual behavior, although again there are large individual variations (Meston and Frohlich, 2000). Although there have been a number of reports showing an improvement in libido and erectile function in older men with testosterone and dihydrotestosterone treatment (Bain, 2001; Kunelius et al., 2002; Morley, 2001; Nolten, 2000), these have been uncontrolled open studies, with no large-scale multicenter prospective studies performed to date. Moreover, although there is fairly consistent data showing that decreases in libido and sexual activity can occur with progressive age in males (Bain, 2001; Morales and Heaton, 2001; Nolten, 2000), there is a large degree of individual variability, and within individuals who have normal testosterone levels there is no correlation between libido and testosterone levels (Rhoden et al., 2002). Most men continue to produce sperm and remain fertile well into old age. In recent years recognition that the adrenal androgen DHEA decreases with aging has led to the popular notion that DHEA treatment may increase libido and erectile function. However, several controlled double-blind studies have failed to show significant effects of DHEA supplementation on sexual function (Flynn et al., 1999; Hermann and Berger, 2001; Reiter et al., 1999).

Changes in reproductive physiology with aging are much more dramatic in females (Burger et al., 2002). The term "menopause" refers to a woman's last menstrual cycle. During the transition to ovarian quiescence at menopause, there is a gradual diminution of ovarian hormone production, with the earliest apparent decline occurring in ovarian inhibin production, which leads to a rise in FSH. With elevated FSH, estradiol production remains elevated in the early phases of menopause, but eventually there is a depletion of ovarian follicles and steroid hormone production falls below that necessary for stimulating the endometrium, and menopause occurs. The loss of ovarian cyclicity results from the gradual depletion of ovarian follicles, such that eventually there are no follicular cells to respond to elevated FSH levels. Thus, as menopause nears, plasma levels of estradiol are maintained initially or can actually be somewhat stimulated, but this is followed by a dramatic decline in circulating estrogen. The decline in estrogen levels leads to a number of other physiological changes, including a decrease in hormonal support of female secondary sexual characteristics, vasomotor instability known as hot flashes, increased loss of bone density, and loss of the protective effects of estrogen on the cardiovascular system. As discussed in the section above, a decrease in sexual desire in females after menopause has been generally reported, as well as a decrease in the frequency of sexual activity (McCoy and Davidson, 1985). Some studies have shown an increase in sexual interest in postmenopausal women taking estrogen (Dennerstein et al., 1980; Iatrakis et al., 1986; Sherwin, 1991), but other studies suggest that estrogen therapy alone has little effect on sexual behavior (Campbell and Whitehead, 1977; Furuhjelm et al., 1984; Sherwin et al., 1985). And, as in premenopausal women there are studies suggesting that androgen, not estrogen, levels correlate with sexual interest (Bachman et al., 1985; Bachmann and Leiblum, 1991; McCoy and Davidson, 1985).

ENVIRONMENTAL EXPOSURE TO HORMONES

Intentional consumption of steroids in the form of hormonal contraceptives, steroid hormones taken to increase muscle strength and fitness, and hormone replacement therapy in postmenopausal women are significant, particularly in Western countries. In the case of the first two, the amount of steroids consumed can be quite significant. Although not discussed in detail here, exogenous steroids have many of the same effects as endogenous steroids on target tissues (discussed in detail above). This includes both the positive effects to stimulate secondary sexual characteristics and the inhibitory effects of providing increased negative feedback support to the hypothalamus and pituitary, and thus essentially turning off or at least turning down the central drive to the reproductive axis. As a result, exogenous steroid exposure at high levels inhibits fertility. This is, in fact, the desired action in the case of contraceptives, but it is an unintended side effect of steroid hormones used to promote fitness. It is also possible for exogenous steroid hormones to influence sexual behavior; however, these effects can be complex and are poorly understood at this time. For example, for oral contraceptives one could have concern that the increased doses of estradiol and progesterone that provide increased negative feedback to the reproductive axis and thus decrease ovarian production of androgens could potentially decrease sexual drive in women. However, studies that have examined this have generally shown no effect of oral contraceptives on female sexual behavior (Meston and Frohlich, 2000). Moreover, as discussed above, there is a report by Adams et al. (1997) suggesting that sexual behavior can be increased in women using reliable contraception, most likely due to loss of fear of becoming pregnant. This reiterates a general theme discussed throughout this chapter—that hormones and many other factors interact to determine behavioral outcomes. That is, hormone exposure modulates behavior but does not determine human reproductive behavior (Wallen, 2001).

In the past decade the concept that significant exposure to exogenous estrogen can come from environmental sources has gained increased attention (Golden et al., 1998). Concerns have arisen because of the theoretical potential for exogenous sources of estrogen to influence many aspects of reproductive biology and behavior, including altering reproductive physiology in females; altering reproductive behavior in both females and males, increasing reproductive pathologies in females, such as endometriosis, by providing additional stimulation to uterine endometrial tissue; increasing the incidence of breast, testicular, and prostate cancer by providing extra trophic support to these steroid-sensitive tissues; and increasing male fertility problems by providing negative feedback to the brain and pituitary and thus leading to a decrease in endogenous testosterone production.

The two sources of environmental estrogens that have received the greatest attention are from ingestion of PCBs (polychlorinated hydroxybiphenyls), found in plastic containers that are used more and more frequently to store beverages and from consumption of phytoestrogens found in food products such as soy. Tests of estrogenic activity of a number of PCBs have shown that the most potent is 80 times less potent than estradiol in binding to estrogen receptors, and most others are at least 100 times less potent than estradiol (Korach et al., 1988). When toxic equivalency is calculated, dietary exposure to these environmental estrogens is calculated as being no more than 0.0000025 percent of the daily intake of naturally occurring estrogenic flavonoids in the diet (Safe, 1995), and these in turn are much less potent than endogenous estradiol. Thus, it seems unlikely that exogenous estrogen exposure from PCBs in food and drink containers has any significant impact on reproductive physiology or behavior in most human populations.

In contrast, there seems little doubt that human consumption of phytoestrogens, either due to naturalistic consumption of foodstuffs high in phytoestrogens or because women intentionally consume foods with high phytoestrogen content for their estrogenic effect, has a greater potential to have an impact on reproductive physiology. About 200 different naturally occurring phytoestrogens have been identified to date (Golden et al., 1998). These compounds vary in structure and can act as either estrogen agonists or estrogen antagonists, with their action sometimes switching as a function of dose. Of these, coumestrol, found in soy protein, has been shown to have the greatest estrogenic potency, 0.03 to 0.2 times that of estradiol. Coumestrol binds competitively to the estrogen receptor and at low doses has an estrogenic effect, but at high doses it has an antiestrogen effect in studies examining its action in cell culture. In some cultures, such as in Japan, relatively high levels of phytoestrogen metabolites of soy protein are found in the urine (Mackey and Eden, 1998). Epidemiological studies show that the Japanese have a lower incidence of such diseases as breast, endometrial, and prostate cancer, which can be aggravated by estrogen. However, whether consumption of soy phytoestrogens plays a causal role in the lower incidences of these cancers remains to be determined (Mackey and Eden, 1998). In recent years there have been several well-controlled intervention studies, in both women and men, examining the effects of soy intervention on reproductive function (Kurzer, 2002). The studies in women provide evidence for very weak effects of increased soy intake on estrogen-sensitive tissues, such as the breast, and reproductive hormone levels. The studies in men have not validated the concerns of adverse effects of phytoestrogen consumption on reproductive hormone levels or sperm production.

LIFE EVENTS THAT ALTER HORMONE LEVELS

Life events that impact the functioning of the reproductive axis are often those that produce various forms of stress. Many physical forms of stress, including energy restriction, increased energy expenditure with exercise, temperature stress, infection, pain and injury, and psychosocial stress have been associated with suppression of reproductive hormone secretion and, if sustained, a suppression of fertility (Cameron, 1997, 1998; Lachelin and Yen, 1978; Pirke et al., 1989). Stress-induced reproductive dysfunction can occur in both females and males. In adulthood, reproductive impairment in females is characterized by suppression of ovulation, a lengthening of the menstrual cycle, followed eventually by a loss of ovarian cyclicity and amenorrhea. As ovarian steroid production is decreased, there is also a decline in secondary sexual characteristics, including breast size and amount of subcutaneous fat. In males the reproductive impairment is characterized by a loss of libido, a decrease in testosterone secretion, and thus a decrease in spermatogenesis and hormonal support for secondary sexual characteristics. Chronic stress, occurring during the process of pubertal development, can impair the progression of puberty in both females and males, leading in some cases to a very marked delay in the pubertal development of reproductive capacity and the accompanying development of secondary sexual characteristics (Carpenter, 1994).

The primary site of disruption of the reproductive axis, with all forms of stress studied in detail to date, appears to be at the level of the GnRH neurons, which provide the central neural drive to the reproductive axis. Using animal models of various stresses, it has been shown that for at least some stresses GnRH secretion is impaired (I'Anson et al., 2000). However, more typically, it is inferred that GnRH secretion is impaired in stress conditions, when a suppression of pituitary gonadotropin secretion is measured. This is further supported by the finding that, in all conditions of stress-induced reproductive dysfunction studied to date, administration of exogenous GnRH can stimulate the function of the reproductive axis, indicating that stress is not acting to directly suppress pituitary or gonadal activity (Hotchkiss and Knobil, 1994). In some forms of acute stress a fall in gonadotropin secretion can be noted within minutes to hours. With more subtle stresses, impairment of gonadotropin secretion is generally noted when the stress is present on a chronic basis.

The mechanisms by which various forms of stress impair activity of the reproductive axis appear to have some common elements, but there also appear to be mechanisms specific to each type of stress. For example, many forms of stress can activate the hypothalamic-pituitary-adrenal axis (HPA), and experimental studies have shown several mechanisms by which activation of the HPA axis can impair the central neural drive to the reproductive axis. On the other hand, certain aspects of stress, such as decreased fuel availability, only occur with some forms of stress and are likely to impair the activity of the reproductive axis via relatively specific mechanisms.

Energetic Stresses

Much of what we know about the mechanisms by which nutritional status modulates activity of the reproductive axis comes from the clinical study of patients with the psychiatric disorder anorexia nervosa (Aono et al., 1975; Marshall and Kelch, 1979; Warren and Vande Wiele, 1973). This disorder involves an obsessive fear of being fat and leads to a profound decrease in food intake, which causes extreme weight loss and can become life-threatening. Nearly all females who develop anorexia nervosa show a loss of ovarian cyclicity and amenorrhea. Amenorrhea is often apparent for great lengths of time, with normal menstrual cycles sometimes returning when patients regain weight but often lasting long after weight recovery. Measurement of circulating levels of LH and FSH show that gonadotropin secretion during the weight loss phase of anorexia nervosa is very low and often nonpulsatile in nature or pulsatile only during the nighttime period, as it is in the early pubertal period (Boyar et al., 1974). Anorexia can often start in the teenage years and, if it does so prior to menarche, can delay menarche for many years, holding the girl in a prepubertal state long beyond the normal time of puberty (Biederman et al., 1986). This delay in activation of adult-like gonadotropin secretion and ovarian function is accompanied by minimal secretion of the ovarian steroid hormones, and thus development of secondary sexual characteristics is delayed. Such a prolongation of childhood and maintenance of a girlish body can be advantageous in certain activities, such as ballet, and the prevalence of anorexia in girls participating rigorously in such exercises is much higher than in the normal population (Warren and Stiehl, 1999). Other conditions in which there are profound changes in energy availability, such as with highly competitive exercise training, can lead to a similar suppression of the reproductive axis (Loucks et al., 1992).

While there is no doubt that severe or chronic decreases in energy availability can lead to a suppression of reproductive hormone secretion and a loss of fertility, a question that is more relevant to most demographic studies is whether mild-to-moderate changes in energy availability impact significantly on reproductive hormone secretion and fertility. Indeed, there are a number of studies with experimental animals showing that brief periods of undernutrition can lead to a suppression of reproductive hormone secretion (Cagampang et al., 1990; Cameron and Nosbisch, 1991). And brief periods of undernutrition have also been documented to decrease reproductive hormone secretion in humans (Cameron et al., 1991). However, fertility would not be expected to be compromised during brief periods of undernutrition, particularly in females who seem to be somewhat protected from the effects of mild undernutrition in the follicular phase of the menstrual cycle, the period leading up to ovulation (Berga et al., 2001; Olson et al., 1995).

The relationship between long-term mild undernutrition and activity of the reproductive axis is more controversial (Wood, 1994). There is generally little animal research addressing this question, probably because maintaining animals on diets for a prolonged period of time would be a rather inefficient method of determining the mechanisms by which energy availability modulates reproductive function, in terms of both time and money. Livestock that are maintained with suboptimal nutritional support have compromised fertility, but, again, most of the experimental work examining this subject involves rather severe undernutrition (Foster et al., 1986). In human populations, where mild-to-moderate undernutrition is relatively common, minimal impact on adult fertility has been reported (Bongaarts, 1980; Gray, 1983; Menken et al., 1981). However, there are stronger correlations between moderate nutritional compromise and later timing of puberty onset (Bhalla and Shrivatava, 1974; Chowdhuray et al., 1978;

Foster et al., 1986). Moderate levels of exercise are also associated with little impact on the reproductive axis (Rogol et al., 1992). Overall, it would appear that, although prolonged periods of mild-to-moderate undernutrition can have some impact on reproductive function and likely on fertility, the impact is relatively weak compared to the other complex of factors that modulate human reproductive ecology.

Energetic stress occurring during lactation is also an important regulator of fertility. Breast-feeding has the potential to profoundly suppress the activity of the reproductive axis (Kennedy and Visness, 1992; McNeilly, 1993). Suppression of the hypothalamic-pituitary-gonadal axis stems from both the energetic drain associated with milk production and other neuroendocrine signals that occur with lactation, including increased prolactin and oxytocin release (McNeilly et al., 1994; McNeilly, 2001). The controversy in this area has not been about whether lactation can suppress the activity of the reproductive axis but rather to what degree it suppresses reproductive processes in a wide variety of naturally occurring conditions (Lunn, 1994). It is interesting in this regard that the percentage of a mother's daily energy intake that is required to support an infant is relatively low for humans compared to other species (Lunn, 1994). Thus, the degree of energy compromise due to lactation is less. Other important variables that impact the effects of breast-feeding on reproduction include the frequency of nursing, whether supplementation of nutritional sources for the infant is available, and the degree of food available to the mother. The role of hormones released during lactation on maternal behavior is discussed in more detail by Young (Chapter 4, this volume). It is also probable that the shift in hormonal milieu during the postpartum period of lactation has effects on sexual behavior. The relatively few studies examining sexual behavior in women in the puerperium indicate that sexual interactions are relatively lower in the first few months after the birth of a child compared to prepregnancy levels (Alder et al., 1986; al Bustan et al., 1995; Byrd et al., 1998; Kayner and Zagar, 1983). However, the reasons for the drop in frequency of intercourse are complex and include many factors other than hormonal changes, including fatigue, episiotomy discomfort, vaginal bleeding, dyspareunia, insufficient lubrication, fears of awakening the infant or not hearing the infant, and a decreased sense of attractiveness.

Psychosocial Stress

The effects of behaviorally-induced stresses—that is, psychological and social stresses—on the activity of the reproductive axis have received less attention, and their impact on the reproductive axis appears to be more variable. Moreover, in human populations it is difficult to selectively study the impact of psychosocial stress on reproductive function because this stress rarely occurs in isolation from other stresses or in a timely fashion so that it can be easily studied. One of the best characterized forms of psychosocial-stress-induced reproductive dysfunction comes from studies of women who present to infertility clinics with functional hypothalamic amenorrhea (FHA). By definition, FHA is a state of subfertility that is not associated with substantial undernutrition or exercise, does not involve lactation, and is not associated with any organic or structural causes for decreased fertility (Berga et al., 1989; Reame et al., 1985). Studies of women with FHA show that they experience more psychological stress than other women, although they do not experience more stressful life events but rather react more profoundly to the stressful events they do experience (Giles and Berga, 1993). They also show increased activation of physiological systems that respond to stress, including increased HPA axis activity (Berga et al., 1997). Treatment of these patients with cognitive behavioral therapy or with drugs that reduce the activity of some central neural systems activated by stress can restore fertility, although not in all cases (Berga et al., 1991, 1997).

Although the majority of studies examining the effects of psychosocial stress on reproduction have documented stress-induced suppression of reproductive function, there are a handful of human studies which have reported that girls who have grown up under conditions of family stress, such as an absent father in a home, with family conflict, a girl whose parents have divorced, enter puberty at a significantly earlier age (Belsky et al., 1991; Moffitt et al., 1993; Wierson et al., 1993). However, the mechanisms by which such stress exposure would advance the onset of puberty have not been established. Moreover, there is the possibility that early stress exposure does not *cause* advancement of puberty but rather that the likelihood of early puberty and exposure to early life family stresses may simply be correlated because they are both influenced by a common factor(s). For example, one of the factors governing the age of menarche in a girl is her mother's age at menarche (Graber et al., 1995). Thus, it is possible that mothers who experienced early menarche are more likely to have family conflict or divorce when their children are young as well as to have daughters who will have early menarche themselves.

A more detailed understanding of how psychosocial stress can impact reproduction comes from animal studies, with investigations in nonhuman primates having particular relevance to understanding this human condition. Nonhuman primates live in complex social groups and have higher cortical brain areas similar to humans. Moreover, the anatomical and functional organization of their reproductive axes is very similar to humans. A number of studies have shown that acute stresses, such as placing monkeys in restraint chairs (Norman and Smith, 1992), receiving aggressive attacks from other monkeys (Rose et al., 1972), and pairing with unfamiliar partners (Coe et al., 1982), can rapidly suppress reproductive hormone secretion. However, not all psychological stresses have this effect. For example, exposing captive monkeys to the sight of "leather capture gloves" will lead to an increase in heart rate and cortisol, and a suppression of immune cell function, but will not suppress circulating levels of reproductive hormones (Helmreich and Cameron, 1992; Rogers et al., 1998). It seems likely that monkeys perceive the sight of capture gloves as being less threatening than a stress such as an aggressive attack by other monkeys. Thus, the perception of severity of stress is likely to be important in determining whether the stress will lead to a suppression of reproductive hormone secretion.

In nonhuman primates a number chronic social stresses have been associated with a marked and sustained suppression of reproductive hormone secretion. These include prolonged restraint stress (Goncharov et al., 1984) and troop reorganization (Sapolsky, 1983). Interestingly, in the Sapolsky study of baboon troop reorganization, several social factors appeared to modulate the response of the reproductive axis to stress in these animals. There was a high degree of correlation between aggressiveness and testosterone titers, with the more aggressive males showing higher circulating levels of testosterone. There was also an interaction between social status and the level of environmental stress, such that in periods of social stability there was no difference in plasma testosterone levels between dominant and subordinate animals, but in the period of social instability the dominant animals showed higher plasma testosterone levels than did the subordinate males. Similar findings were reported by Rose et al. (1972) in a study of male rhesus monkeys living together in a large outdoor compound, showing that plasma testosterone levels were correlated both with the number of aggressive interactions an animal experienced and the animal's dominance rank. It has also been posited that social status (i.e., dominance rank) plays an important role in determining lifetime reproductive success in primates, with subordinate animals experiencing a greater degree of social stress and having a lesser degree of reproductive success (Cowlishaw and Dunbar, 1991; Dittus, 1979; Drickamer, 1974; Dunbar, 1980; Dunbar and Dunbar, 1977; Sade et al., 1976; Wilson et al., 1978). However, support for this hypothesis is not uniform, and this remains a controversial notion.

Some light may be shed on this issue by reports indicating a correlation between dominance rank and reproductive success in some years but not others (Cheney et al., 1988; deWaal, 1982; Duvall et al., 1976; Nishida, 1983; Witt et al., 1981). It would appear that multiple factors, including dominance rank, time of year, magnitude of stress, aggressiveness of the animal, and level of activity of the reproductive axis prior to stress exposure can all play roles in modulating the response of the reproductive axis to both acute and chronic stresses (see Figure 5-4). Thus, although it is pos-

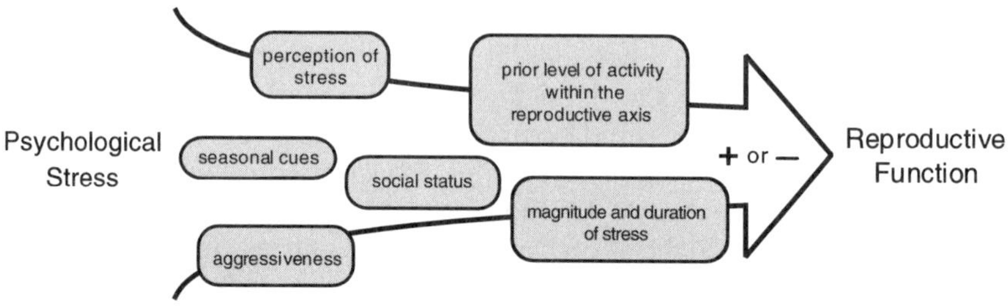

FIGURE 5-4 Schematic diagram of factors that mediate the effects of psychological stress on the activity of the hypothalamic-pituitary-gonadal axis.

sible to measure group mean responses to specific stresses and make conclusions about the effect of a stress on a species' reproductive axis, such a mean assessment may be of little use in determining whether an individual will experience a suppression of reproductive function in response to that stress. An increased understanding of the mechanisms by which psychological and social stresses suppress the activity of the reproductive axis may well be achieved by focusing future studies on these individual differences in response to stress.

SUMMARY AND FUTURE DIRECTIONS

It is becoming clear that to fully understand the multiplicity of factors that come together to regulate and modulate reproductive physiology and reproductive behavior will require integration of demographic and biomedical approaches to these research issues. Many aspects of reproductive biology are difficult to study from the perspective of population biology approaches because of the great variation in function within an individual over a short course of time, such as with fluctuations in hormone levels over the menstrual cycle or even the fluctuation in reproductive hormone levels on an hour-to-hour basis. Biomedical approaches of studying individuals in more detail will be able to define relationships more clearly but are limited by the low power of examining relatively few individuals. What is needed is a twofold approach, first of developing studies that nest demographic and biomedical approaches together and second of using biomedical studies to inform the design of demographic studies.

The first approach would involve performance of large demographic studies to understand the relationships between variables on a global scale, with a select subset of individuals studied in much more detail to test specific hypotheses or to differentiate between possible mechanisms underlying the general relationship. The second approach simply requires further communication between the fields of demography and biomedical sciences, such that methodologies are well understood, where possible similar measurements are made and at the least complexities understood by examining individuals are considered in the design of demographic studies. But it is also important that the information flow go in the opposite direction, so that the field of demography can play a larger role in guiding biomedical scientists toward interesting questions for detailed study.

There are a number of areas in need of further investigation to fully understand the role that hormones play in fertility outcomes. In many areas, studies with more frequent measurements are needed to more accurately assess the hormonal function that may underlie physiology and behavior. In a number of areas there is also a need for more accurate quantification of other measures. For example, in the case of assessing the actual role of undernutrition on fertility in much of the developing world, more accurate measures of the level of nutritional intake and the duration of the undernourished period would help sort out why there seems to be disagreement between demographers and biomedical scientists as to whether energetic status is an important regulator of reproductive ecology. A stronger recognition of the tremendous role that individual differences play in both reproductive physiology and behavior is needed to accurately design and interpret studies. This is true in terms of both normal functioning and reactions to various stresses and environmental conditions. Measurement of a greater number of variables in a given study is going to be essential to fully understand the interactions between hormones and other variables, such as dominance, temperament, and stress sensitivity, in determining both reproductive physiology and behavior. In the end, achieving this complex understanding will likely require a multidisciplinary approach—teams of investigators with different backgrounds working together to design studies that take into account the nuances of physiology, psychology, and population biology.

REFERENCES

Adams, D.B., A.R. Gold, and A.D. Burt
1997 Rise in female-initiated sexual activity at ovulation and its suppression by oral contraceptives. *The New England Journal of Medicine* 299:1145-1150.

al Bustan, M.A., N.F. el Tomi, M.F. Faiwalla, and V. Manav
1995 Maternal sexuality during pregnancy and after childbirth in Muslim Kuwaiti women. *Archives of Sexual Behavior* 24:207-215.

Alder, E.M., A. Cook, D. Davidson, C. West, and J. Bancroft
1986 Hormones, mood and sexuality in lactating women. *British Journal of Psychiatry* 148:74-79.

Aono, T., T. Kinugasa, T. Yamamoto, A. Miyake, and K. Kuracki
1975 Assessment of gonadotropin secretion in women with anorexia nervosa. *Acta Endocrinologica (Copenhagen)* 80:630-641.

Bachmann, G.A., and S.R. Leiblum
1991 Sexuality in sexagenarian women. *Maturitas* 13:43-50.

Bachmann, G.A., S.R. Leiblum, B. Sandler, W. Ainsley, R. Narcesian, R. Shelden, and H.N. Hymans
1985 Correlates of sexual desire in post-menopausal women. *Maturitas* 7:211-216.

Bancroft, J., D. Sanders, D. Davidson, and P. Warner
1983 Mood, sexuality, hormones and the menstrual cycle. III. Sexuality and the role of androgens. *Psychosomatic Medicine* 45:509-516.

Bain, J.
2001 Andropause: Testosterone replacement therapy for aging men. *Canadian Family Physician* 47:91-97.

Barraclough, C., and J. Leathem
1954 Infertility induced in mice by a single injection of testosterone propionate. *Proceedings of the Society for Experimental Biology and Medicine* 85:673-674.

Baum, M.J., B.J. Everitt, J. Herbert, and E.B. Keverne
1977 Hormonal basis of proceptivity and receptivity in female primates. *Archives of Sexual Behavior* 6:173-192.

Belchetz, P.E., T.M. Plant, Y. Nakai, E.J. Keogh, and E. Knobil
1978 Hypophysial responses to continuous and intermittent delivery of hypothalamic gonadotropin-releasing hormone. *Science* 202:631-633.

Belsky, J., L. Steinberg, and P. Draper
1991 Childhood experience, interpersonal development and reproductive strategy: An evolutionary theory of socialization. *Child Development* 62:671-675.

Berga, S.L., T.L. Daniels, and D.E. Giles
1997 Women with functional hypothalamic amenorrhea but not other forms of anovulation display amplified cortisol concentrations. *Fertility and Sterility* 67:1024-1030.

Berga, S.L., T.L. Loucks, and J.L. Cameron
2001 Endocrine and chronobiological effects of fasting in women. *Fertility and Sterility* 75:926-932.

Berga, S.L., A.B. Loucks, W.G. Rossmanith, L.M. Kettel, G.A. Laughlin, and S.S. Yen
1991 Acceleration of luteinizing hormone pulse frequency in functional hypothalamic amenorrhea by dopaminergic blockade. *Journal of Clinical Endocrinology and Metabolism* 72:151-156.

Berga, S.L., J.F. Mortola, L. Girton, B. Suh, G. Laughlin, P. Pham, and S.S. Yen
1989 Neuroendocrine aberrations in women with functional hypothalamic amenorrhea. *Journal of Clinical Endocrinology and Metabolism* 68:301-308.

Bethea, C.L., W.H. Fahrenbach, S.A. Sprangers, and F. Freesh
1992 Immunocytochemical localization of progestin receptors in monkey hypothalamus: Effect of estrogen and progestin. *Endocrinology* 130:895-905.

Bhalla, M., and J.R. Shrivatava
1974 A prospective study of the age of menarche in Kampur girls. *Indian Pediatrics* 11:487-493.

Biederman, J., R.J. Baldessarini, J.S. Harmatz, T.M. Rivinus, G.W. Arana, D.B. Herzog, and U. Schildkrout
1986 Heterogeneity in anorexia nervosa. *Biological Psychiatry* 21:2113-216.

Bongaarts, J.
1980 Does malnutrition affect fecundity? A summary of evidence. *Science* 208:564-569.

Bonsall, R.W., D. Zumpe, and R.P. Michael
1978 Menstrual cycle influences on operant behavior of female rhesus monkeys. *Journal of Comparative Physiological Psychology* 92:846-855.

Boyar, R.M., J. Katz, J.W. Finkelstein, S. Kapen, H. Weiner, E.D. Weitzman, and L. Hellman
1974 Anorexia nervosa: Immaturity of the 24-hour luteinizing hormone secretory pattern. *New England Journal of Medicine* 291:861-865.

Boyar, R.M., R.S. Rosenfeld, S. Kapen, J.W. Finkelstein, H.P. Roffwarg, E.D. Weitzman, and L. Hellman
1974 Human puberty. Simultaneous augmented secretion of luteinizing hormone and testosterone during sleep. *Journal of Clinical Investigation* 54:609-618.

Bremer, J.
1959 *Asexualization, A Follow-up Study of 244 Cases*. New York: Macmillan.

Byrd, J.E., J.S. Hyde, J.D. DeLamater, and E.A. Plant
1998 Sexuality during pregnancy and the year postpartum. *Journal of Family Practice* 47:305-308.

Burger, H.G., E.C. Dudley, D.M. Robertson, and L. Dennerstein
2002 Hormonal changes in the menopause transition. *Recent Progress in Hormone Research* 57:257-275.

Cagampang, F.R., K. Maeda, A. Yokoyama, and K. Ota
1990 Effect of food deprivation on the pulsatile LH release in the cycling and ovariectomized female rat. *Hormone and Metabolic Research* 22(5):269-272.

Cameron, J.L.
1997 Stress and behaviorally-induced reproductive dysfunction in primates. *Seminars in Reproductive Endocrinology* 15(1):37-45.
1998 Fasting and reproduction in non-human primates. Pp. 95-109 in *Pennington Center Nutrition Series: Nutrition and Reproduction*. W. Hansel, G. Bray, and D.H. Ryan, eds. Baton Rouge: University of Louisiana Press.
2001 Effects of sex hormones on brain development. Pp. 59-78 in *Developmental Cognitive Neuroscience*. C.A. Nelson and M. Luciana, eds. Cambridge: The MIT Press.

Cameron, J.L., and C. Nosbisch
1991 Slowing of pulsatile LH and testosterone secretion during short-term fasting in adult male rhesus monkeys (*Macaca mulatta). Endocrinology* 128:1532-1540.

Cameron, J.L., T. Weltzin, C. McConaha, D.L. Helmreich, and W.H. Kaye
1991 Suppression of reproductive axis activity in men undergoing a 48 hour fast. *Journal of Clinical Endocrinology and Metabolism* 73:35-41.

Campbell, K.L.
1994 Blood, urine, saliva and dip-sticks: Experiences in Africa, New Guinea and Boston. *Annals of the New York Academy of Sciences* 709:312-330.

Campbell, S., and M. Whitehead
1977 Oestrogen therapy and the menopausal syndrome. *Clinical Obstetrics and Gynecology* 4:31-47.

Canfield, R.E., and J.F. O'Connor
1991 Biological markers of human pregnancy. *Biomedical and Environmental Sciences* 4:56-68.

Carpenter, S.E.
1994 Psychosocial menstrual disorders: Stress, exercise and diet's effect on the menstrual cycle. *Current Opinion in Obstetrics & Gynecology* 6:536-539.

Cheney, D.L., R.M. Seyfarth, S.J. Andelman, and P.C. Lee
1988 Factors affecting reproductive success in vervet monkeys. Pp. 384-402 in *Lifetime Reproductive Success*. T.H. Clutton-Brock, ed. Chicago: Chicago University Press.

Clayton, A.H.
2002 Female sexual dysfunction related to depression and antidepressant medications. *Current Women's Health Reports* 2:182-187.

Chowdhury, A.K.M.A., S.L. Huffman, and G.T. Curlin
1978 Malnutrition, menarche and age at marriage in Bangladesh. *Social Biology* 24:316-325.
Clough, K.M., F.X. Cole, S.S. Seaver, A. Vesprini, A.Y. Kuo, and B.L. Lasley
1992 Enzyme immunoassay method for total alpha gonadotropin in human urine samples. *Fertility and Sterility* 57:1241-1246.
Coe, C.L., D. Franklin, E.R. Smith, and S. Levine
1982 Hormonal responses accompanying fear and agitation in the squirrel monkey. *Physiological Behavior* 29:1051-1057.
Cooke, B., C.D. Hegstrom, L.S. Villeneuve, and S.M. Breedlove
1998 Sexual differentiation of the vertebrate brain: Principles and mechanisms. *Frontiers in Neuroendocrinology* 19:323-362.
Cowlishaw, G., and R.I. M. Dunbar
1991 Dominance rank and mating success in male primates. *Animal Behavior* 41:1045-1056.
Czaja, J.A., and C. Bielert
1975 Female rhesus sexual behavior and distance to a male partner: Relation to stage of the menstrual cycle. *Archives of Sexual Behavior* 4:583-597.
Czaja, J.A., J.A. Robinson, S.G. Eisele, G. Scheffler, and R.W. Goy
1977 Relationship between sexual skin colour of female rhesus monkeys and the midcycle plasma levels of oestradiol and progesterone. *Journal of Reproduction and Fertility* 49:147-150.
Davidson, J.M., M. Kwan, and W.J. Greenleaf
1982 Hormonal replacement and sexuality. *Clinical Endocrinology & Metabolism* 11:599-623.
Dennerstein, L., G.D. Burrows, C. Wood, and G. Hyman
1980 Hormones and sexuality: Effect of estrogen and progestogen. *Obstetrics and Gynecology* 56:316-322.
Dennerstein, L., C. Wood, and G.D. Burrows
1977 Sexual response following hysterectomy and oophorectomy. *Obstetrics and Gynecology* 49:92-96.
Dennerstein, L., G. Gotts, J.B. Brown, C.A. Morse, T.M. Farley, and A. Pinol
1994 The relationship between the menstrual cycle and female sexual interest in women with PMS complaints and volunteers. *Psychoneuroendocrinology* 19:293-204.
deWaal, R.B.M.
1982 *Chimpanzee Politics*. London: Allen and Unwin.
Dittus, W.P.J.
1979 The evolution of behavior regulating density and age-specific sex rations in a primate population. *Behaviour* 69:265-302.
Drickamer, L.C.
1974 A ten-year summary of reproductive data for free-ranging *Macaca mulatta*. *Folia Primatologica* 21:61-80.
Dunbar, R.I.M.
1980 Determinants and evolutionary consequences of dominance among female gelada baboons. *Behavioral Ecology and Sociobiology* 7:253-265.
Dunbar, R.I.M., and E.P. Dunbar
1977 Dominance and reproductive success among gelada baboons. *Nature* 266:351-352.
Duvall, S.W., I.S. Bernstein, and T.P. Gordon
1976 Paternity and status in a rhesus monkey group. *Journal of Reproduction and Fertility* 47:25-31.

Ellinwood, W.E., and J.A. Resko
1984 Sex differences in biologically active and immunoreactive gonadotropins in the fetal circulation of rhesus monkeys. *Endocrinology* 107:902-907.

Ellison, P.T.
1988 Human salivary steroids: Methodological considerations and applications in physical anthropology. *Yearbook of Physical Anthropology* 31:115-142.
1994 Salivary steroids and natural variation in human ovarian function. *Annals of the New York Academy of Sciences* 709:287-298.

Erickson, G.F.
1978 Normal ovarian function. *Clinical Obstetrics and Gynecology* 21:31-52.

Everitt, B.J., J. Herbert, and J.D. Hamer
1972 Sexual receptivity of bilaterally adrenalectomised female rhesus monkeys. *Physiology & Behavior* 8:409-415.

Feng, Y.J., E. Shalts, L. Xia, J. Rivier, C. Rivier, W. Vale, and M. Ferin
1991 An inhibitory effect of interleukin-1 on basal gonadotropin release in the ovariectomized rhesus monkey: Reversal by a corticotropin-releasing factor antagonist. *Endocrinology* 128:2077-2082.

Flynn, M.A., D. Weaver-Osterholtz, K.L. Sharpe-Timms, S. Allen, and G. Krause
1999 Dehydroepiandrosterone replacement in aging humans. *Journal of Clinical Endocrinology & Metabolism* 84:1527-1533.

Foster, A., J. Menken, A Chowdhury, and J. Trussell
1986 Female reproductive development: A hazards model analysis. *Social Biology* 33:183-198.

Frisch, R., and J. MacArthur
1974 Menstrual cycles: Fatness as a determinant of minimum weight for height for their maintenance or onset. *Science* 185:949-951.

Furuhjelm, M., E. Karlgren, and K. Carstrom
1984 The effect of estrogen therapy on somatic and psychical symptoms in post-menopausal women. *Acta Obstetricia et Gynecologica Scandinavica* 63:655-661.

Giles, D.E., and S.L. Berga
1993 Cognitive and psychiatric correlates of functional hypothalamic amenorrhea: A controlled comparison. *Fertility & Sterility* 60:486-492.

Golden, R.J., K.L. Noller, L. Titus-Ernstoff, R.H. Kaufman, R. Mittendorf, R. Stillman, and E.A. Reese
1998 Environmental endocrine modulators and human health: An assessment of the biological evidence. *Critical Reviews in Toxicology* 28:109-227.

Goncharov, N.P., D.S. Tavadyan, J.E. Powell, and V.C. Stevens
1984 Levels of adrenal and gonadal hormones in rhesus monkeys during chronic hypokinesia. *Endocrinology* 115:129-135.

Gordon, T.P., R.M. Rose, and I.S. Bernstein
1976 Seasonal rhythm in plasma testosterone levels in the rhesus monkey (*Macaca mulatta*): A three year study. *Hormones and Behavior* 7:229-243.

Goy, R.W.
1979 Sexual compatibility in rhesus monkeys: Predicting sexual behavior of oppositely sexed pairs of animals. Pp. 227-255 in *Ciba Foundation Symposium. Sex, Hormones and Behavior*. Amsterdam: Elsevier-North Holland.

Graber, J.A., J. Brooks-Gunn, and M.P. Warren
1995 The antecedents of menarcheal age: Heredity, family environment and stressful life events. *Child Development* 66:346-359.

Gray, R.H.
1983 The impact of health and nutrition on natural fertility. Pp. 139-162 in *Determinants of Fertility in Developing Countries.* R.A. Bulatao and R.D. Lee, eds. New York: Academic Press.

Griffin, J.E., and S. R. Ojeda
2000 *Textbook of Endocrine Physiology*, 4th ed. London: Oxford University Press.

Halpern, C.R., J.R. Udry, and C. Suchindran
1997 Testosterone predicts initiation of coitus in adolescent females. *Psychosomatic Medicine* 59:161-171.
1998 Monthly measures of salivary testosterone predict sexual activity in adolescent males. *Archives of Sexual Behavior* 27:445-465.

Helmreich, D.L., and J.L. Cameron
1992 Effects of an acute stressor on LH and cortisol secretion in rhesus monkeys: Comparison to hormone secretory responses induced by fasting. Proceedings of the 22nd annual meeting of the Society for Neuroscience, *Abstract* 55.14:118. Anaheim, CA (October 25-30).

Hermann, M., and P. Berger
2001 Hormonal changes in aging men: A therapeutic indication? *Experimental Gerontology* 36:1075-1082.

Hotchkiss, J., and E. Knobil
1994 The menstrual cycle and its neuroendocrine control. Pp. 711-749 in *The Physiology of Reproduction*, vol. 2. E. Knobil and J.D. Neill, eds. New York: Raven Press.

I'Anson, H., J.M. Manning, G.C. Herbosa, J. Pelt, C. R. Friedman, R.I. Wood, D.C. Bucholtz, and D.L. Foster
2000 Central inhibition of gonadotropin-releasing hormone secretion in the growth-restricted hypogonadotropic female sheep. *Endocrinology* 141:520-527.

Iatrakis, G., N. Haronis, G. Sakellaropoulos, A. Kourkoubas, and M. Gallos
1986 Psychosomatic symptoms of postmenopausal women with or without hormonal treatment. *Psychotherapy and Psychosomatics* 46:116-121.

Kaplan, S.L., M.M. Grumbach, and M.L. Aubert
1976 The ontogenesis of pituitary hormones and hypothalamic factors in the human fetus: Maturation of central nervous system regulation of anterior pituitary function. *Recent Progress in Hormone Research* 32:161-234.

Kayner, C.E., and J.A. Zagar
1983 Breast-feeding and sexual response. *Journal of Family Practice* 17:69-73.

Kennedy, K.I., and C.M. Visness
1992 Contraceptive efficacy of lactational amenorrhoea. *Lancet* 339:227-230.

Korach, K.S., P. Sarver, K. Chae, J.A. McLachlan, and J.D. McKinney
1988 Estrogen receptor-binding activity of polychlorinated hydroxybiphenyls: Conformationally restricted structural probes. *Molecular Pharmacology* 33:120-126.

Kordon, C., S.V. Drouva, G. Martinez de la Escalera, and R.I. Weiner
1994 Role of classic and peptide neuromediators in the neuronedocrine regulation of luteinizing hormone and prolactin. Pp. 1621-1681 in *The Physiology of Reproduction*, vol. 1. E. Knobil and J.D. Neill, eds. New York: Raven Press.

Kunelius, P., O. Lukkarinen, M.L. Hannulksela, O. Itkonen, and J.S. Tapanainen
2002 The effects of transdermal dihydrotestosterone in the aging male: A prospective, randomized, double blind study. *Journal of Clinical Endocrinology & Metabolism* 87:1462-1466.

Kurzer, M.S.
2002 Hormonal effects of soy in premenopausal women and men. *Journal of Nutrition* 132:570S-575S.

Kwan, M., W.J. Greenleaf, J. Mann, L. Crapo, and J.M. Davidson
1983 The nature of androgen action on male sexuality: A combined laboratory/self-report study on hypogonadal men. *Clinical Endocrinology & Metabolism* 57:557-562.
Lasley, B.L., K. Mobed, and E.B. Gold
1994 The use of urinary hormonal assessments in human studies. *Annals of the New York Academy of Sciences* 709:299-311.
Lasley, B.L., and S.E. Shidleler
1994 Methods for evaulating reproductive health in women. *Occupational Medicine* 9:423-433.
Lachelin, G.C., and S.S. Yen
1978 Hypothalamic chronic anovulation. *American Journal of Obstetrics and Gynecology* 130:825-831.
Lieblum, S., G. Bachmann, E. Kemmann, D. Colburn, and L. Schwartzman
1983 Vaginal atrophy in the post-menopausal woman: The importance of sexual activity and hormones. *Journal of the American Medical Association* 249:2195-2198.
Lipson, S.F., and P.T. Ellison
1989 Development of protocols for the application of salivary steroid analyses to field conditions. *American Journal of Human Biology* 1:249-255.
Loucks, A.B., J. Vaitukaitis, J.L. Cameron, A.D. Rogol, G. Skinar, and M.P. Warren
1992 The reproductive system and exercise: A state-of-the-art review. *Medicine and Science in Sports and Exercise* 24:S288-S293.
Lovejoy, J.C., and K. Wallen
1990 Adrenal suppression and sexual initiation in group-living female rhesus monkeys. *Hormones and Behavior* 24:256-269.
Lunn, P.G.
1994 Lactation and other metabolic loads affecting human reproduction. *Annals of the New York Academy of Sciences* 709:77-83.
Luttge, W.B.
1971 The role of gonadal hormones in the sexual behavior of the rhesus monkey and human: A literature survey. *Archives of Sexual Behavior* 1:61-88.
Mackey, R., and J. Eden
1998 Phytoestrogens and the menopause. *Climacteric* 1:302-308.
MacLusky, N.J., and F. Naftolin
1981 Sexual differentiation of the central nervous system. *Science* 211:1294-1303.
Mann, D.R., M.A. Akinbami, K.G. Gould, K. Paul, and K. Wallen
1998 Sexual maturation in male rhesus monkeys: Importance of neonatal testosterone exposure and social rank. *Journal of Endocrinology* 156:493-501.
Marshall, J.C., and R.P. Kelch
1979 Low dose pulsatile gonadotropin-releasing hormone in anorexia nervosa: A model for human pubertal development. *Journal of Clinical Endocrinology & Metabolism* 49:712-718.
McCoy, N.L., and J.M. Davidson
1985 A longitudinal study of the effects of menopause on sexuality. *Maturitas* 7:203-210.
McNeilly, A.S.
1993 Lactational amenorrhea. *Endocrinology and Metabolism Clinics of North America* 22:59-73.
2001 Lactational control of reproduction. *Reproduction, Fertility and Development* 13:583-590.

McNeilly, A.S., C.C.K. Tay, and A. Glasier
1994 Physiological mechanisms underlying lactational amenorrhea. *Annals of the New York Academy of Sciences* 709:145-155.

Menken, J., J. Trussell, and S. Watkins
1981 The nutrition-fertility link: An evaluation of the evidence. *Journal of Interdisciplinary History* 9:425-441.

Meston, C.M., and P.F. Frohlich
2000 The neurobiology of sexual function. *Archives of General Psychiatry* 57:1012-1030.

Michael, R.P., A.N. Clancy, and D. Zumpe.
1995 Distribution of androgen receptor-like immunoreactivity in the brains of cynomolgus monkeys. *Journal of Neuroendocrinology* 7:713-719.

Michael, R.P., and M. Wilson
1974 Effects of castration and hormone replacement in fully adult male rhesus monkeys (*Macaca mulatta*). *Endocrinology*. 95:150-159.

Moffitt, T.E., A. Caspi, J. Belsky, and P.A. Silva
1993 Childhood experience and the onset of menarche: A test of a sociobiological model. *Child Development* 63:47-58.

Moghissi, K.S.
1990 Gonadotropin releasing hormones. Clinical applications in gynecology. *Journal of Reproductive Medicine* 35:1097-1107.

Montgomery, S.A., D.S. Baldwin, and A. Riley
2002 Antidepressant medications: A review of the evidence for drug-induced sexual dysfunction. *Journal of Affective Disorders* 69:119-140.

Morales, A., and J.P. Heaton
2001 Hormonal erectile dysfunction. Evaluation and management. *Urologic Clinics of North America* 28:279-288.

Morley, J.E.
2001 Testosterone replacement in older men and women. *Journal of Gender-Specific Medicine* 4:49-53.

Nishida, T.
1983 Alpha status and agonistic alliance in wild chimpanzees (*Pan troglodytes schweinfuthii*). *Primates* 24:318-336.

Nolten, W.E.
2000 Androgen deficiency in the aging male: When to evaluate and when to treat. *Current Urology Reports* 1:313-319.

Norman, R.L., and C.J. Smith
1992 Restraint inhibits luteinizing hormone and testosterone secretion in intact male rhesus macaques: Effects of concurrent naloxone administration. *Neuroendocrinology* 55:405-415.

Olson, B.R., T. Cartledge, N. Sebring, R. Defensor, and L. Nieman
1995 Short-term fasting affects luteinizing hormone secretory dynamics but not reproductive function in normal-weight sedentary women. *Journal of Clinical Endocrinology & Metabolism* 65:262-267.

Ojeda, S.R., and M. Bilger
2000 Neuroendocrine regulation of puberty. Pp. 197-224 in *Neuroendocrinology in Physiology and Medicine*. P.M. Conn and M.E. Freeman, eds. Ottowa: Humana Press.

Phoenix, C.H., R.W. Goy, A.A. Gerall, and W.C. Young
1959 Organizing action of prenatally administered testosterone propionate on the tissues mediating mating behavior in the female guinea pig. *Endocrinology* 65:369-382.

Phoenix, C.H., R.W. Goy, and J.A. Resko
1968 Psychosexual differentiation as a function of androgenic stimulation. Pp. 33-49 in *Perspectives in Reproduction and Sexual Behavior*. M. Diamond, ed. Bloomington: Indiana University Press.

Phoenix, C.H., A.K. Slob, and R.W. Goy
1973 Effects of castration and replacement therapy on sexual behavior of adult male rhesus. *Journal of Comparative Physiological Psychology* 84:472-481.

Pirke, K.M., W. Wuttke, and U. Schweiger
1989 *The Menstrual Cycle and Its Disorders*. Berlin: Springer-Verlag.

Plant, T.M.
2001 Neurobiological bases underlying the control of the onset of puberty in the rhesus monkey: A representative higher primate. *Frontiers in Neuroendocrinology* 22:107-139.

Pomerantz, S.M., and R.W. Goy
1983 Proceptive behavior of female rhesus monkeys during tests with tethered males. *Hormones and Behavior* 17:237-248.

Reame, N.E., S.E. Sauder, G.D. Case, R.P. Kelch, and J.C. Marshall
1985 Pulsatile gonadotropin secretion in women with hypothalamic ameonorrhea: Evidence that reduced frequency of gonadotropin-releasing hormone secretion is the mechanism of persistent anovulation. *Journal of Clinical Endocrinology & Metabolism* 61:851-858.

Reamy, K.J., and S.E. White
1987 Sexuality in the puerperium: A review. *Archives of Sexual Behavior* 16:165-186.

Reiter, W.J., A. Pycha, G. Schatzl, A. Pokorny, D.M. Gruber, J.C. Huber, and M. Marberger
1999 Dehydroepiandrosterone in the treatment of erectile dysfunction: A prospective, double-blind, randomized, placebo-controlled study. *Urology* 53:594-595.

Resko, J.A., and W.E. Ellinwood
1985 Negative feedback regulation of gonadotropin secretion by androgens in fetal rhesus macaques. *Biology of Reproduction* 33:346-352.

Rhoden, E.L., C. Teloken, P.R. Sogari, and C.A. Souto
2002 The relationship of serum testosterone to erectile function in normal aging men. *Journal of Urology* 167:1745-1748.

Rogol, A.D., A.Weltman, J.Y. Weltman, R.L. Seip, D.B. Snead, S. Levine, E.M. Haskvitz, D.L. Thompson, R. Schurrer, and E. Dowling
1992 Durability of the reproductive axis in eumenorrheic women during 1 year of endurance training. *Journal of Applied Physiology* 72:1571-1580.

Rogers, C.J., C.S. Brissette-Storkus, L.A. Hayes, J.L. Cameron, and W.H. Chambers
1998 Selective reduction in CD2 expression on $CD2^{bright}/CD8^{+}$ lymphocytes from cynomolgus monkeys (*Macaca fascicularis*) in response to acute stress. *Journal of Neuroimmunology* 86:61-72.

Rose, R.M., T.P. Gordon, and I.S. Bernstein
1972 Plasma testosterone levels in the male rhesus: Influences of sexual and social stimuli. *Science* 178:643-645.

Sade, D.S., K. Cushing, P. Cushing, J. Dunaif, A. Figueroa, J.R. Kaplan, C. Lauer, D. Rhodes, and J. Schneider
1976 Population dynamics in relation to social structure on Cayo Santiago. *Yearbook of Physical Anthropology* 20:253-262.

Safe, S.H.
1995 Environmental and dietary estrogens and human health—Is there a problem? *Environmental Health Perspectives* 103:346-351.

Sapolsky, R.M.
1983 Endocrine aspects of social instability in the olive baboon (*Papio anubis*). *American Journal of Primatology* 5:365-379.

Schiavi, R.C., and D. White
1976 Androgens and male sexual function: A review of human studies. *Journal of Sex & Marital Therapy* 2:214-228.

Schwanzel-Fukuda, M., D. Bick, and D.W. Pfaff
1989 Luteinizing hormone-releasing hormone (LHRH)-expressing cells do not migrate normally in an inherited hypogonadal (Kallmann) syndrome. *Molecular Brain Research* 6:311-326.

Schwanzel-Fukuda, M., and D.W. Pfaff
1989 Origin of luteinizing hormone-releasing hormone neurons. *Nature* 338:161-163.

Shabsigh, R., L. Zakaria, A.G. Anastasiadis, and A.S. Seidman
2001 Sexual dysfunction and depression: Etiology, prevalence, and treatment. *Current Urology Reports* 2:463-467.

Sherwin, B.B.
1991 The impact of different doses of estrogen and progestin on mood and sexual behavior in postmenopausal women. *Journal of Clinical Endocrinology & Metabolism* 72:336-343.

Sherwin, B.B., M.M. Gelfand, and W. Brender
1985 Androgen enhances sexual motivation in females: A prospective, crossover study of sex steroid administration in the surgical menopause. *Psychosomatic Medicine* 47:339-351.

Shughrue, P.J., M.V. Lane, and I. Merchenthaler
1997 The comparative distribution of estrogen receptor-α and β mRNA in rat central nervous system. *Journal of Comparative Neurology* 388:507-525.

Silverman, A.J., I. Livne, and J.W. Witkin
1994 The gonadotropin-releasing hormone (GnRH) neuronal systems: Immunocytochemistry and in situ hybridization. Pp. 1683-1709 in *The Physiology of Reproduction*, vol. 1. E. Knobil and J.D. Neill, eds. New York: Raven Press.

Simerly, R.B., C. Chang, M. Muramatsu, and L.V. Swanson
1990 Distribution of androgen and estrogen receptor mRNA-containing cells in the rat brain: An in situ hybridization study. *Journal of Comparative Neurology* 294:76-95.

Soules, M.R., R.A. Steiner, D.K. Clifton, N.L. Cohen, S. Aksel, and W.J. Bremner
1984 Progesterone modulation of pulsatile luteinizing hormone secretion in normal women. *Journal of Clinical Endocrinology & Metabolism* 58:378-383.

Stanczyk, F.Z., I. Miyakawa, and U. Goebelsmann
1980 Direct radioimmunoassay of urinary estrogen and pregnanediol glucuronides during the menstrual cycle. *American Journal of Obstetrics and Gynecology* 137:443-450.

Stanislaw, H., and F.J. Rice
1988 Correlation between sexual desire and menstrual cycle characteristics. *Archives of Sexual Behavior* 17:499-508.

Steiner, R.A., and J.L. Cameron
1989 Endocrine control of reproduction. Pp. 1289-1342 in *Textbook of Physiology*. H.D. Patton, A.F. Fuchs, B. Hille, A.M. Scher, and R.A. Steiner, eds. Philadelphia: W.B. Saunders.

Udry, J.R., J.O. Billy, N.M. Morris, T.R. Groff, and M.H. Raj
1985 Serum androgenic hormones motivate sexual behavior in adolescent boys. *Fertility & Sterility* 43:90-94.

Udry, J.R., L.M. Talbert, and N.M. Morris
1986 Biosocial foundations for adolescent female sexuality. *Demography* 23:217-230.

Van Goozen, S., V. Wiegant, E. Endert, F. Helmond, and N. Van de Poll
1997 Psychoendocrinological assessment of the menstrual cycle: The relationship between hormones, sexuality and mood. *Archives of Sexual Behavior* 26:359-382.

Wallen, K.
1990 Desire and ability: Hormones and the regulation of female sexual behavior. *Neuroscience and Biobehavioral Reviews* 14:233-241.
1999 Risky business: Social context and hormonal modulation of primate sexual desire. Pp. 289-323 in *Reproduction in Context.* K. Wallen and J. Schneider, eds. Cambridge, MA: MIT Press.
2001 Sex and context: Hormones and primate sexual motivation. *Hormones and Behavior* 40:339-357.

Wallen, K., D.R. Mann, M. Davis-DaSilva, S. Gaventa, J.C. Lovejoy, and D.C. Collins
1986 Chronic gonadotropin-releasing hormone agonist treatment suppresses ovulation and sexual behavior in group-living female rhesus monkeys. *Physiological Behavior* 36:369-375.

Warren, M.P., and A.L. Stiehl
1999 Exercise and female adolescents: Effects on the reproductive and skeletal system. *Journal of the American Medical Women's Association* 54:115-120.

Warren, M.P., and R.L. Vande Wiele
1973 Clinical and metabolic features of anorexia nervosa. *American Journal of Obstetrics and Gynecology* 117:435-449.

Wierson, M., P.J. Long, and R.L. Forehand
1993 Toward a new understanding of early menarche: The role of environmental stress in pubertal timing. *Adolescence* 28:913-924.

Wilson, M.E., T.P. Gordon, and I.S. Bernstein
1978 Timing of births and reproductive success in rhesus monkey social groups. *Journal of Medical Primatology* 7:202-212.

Winter, J.S.D., C. Faiman, W.C. Hobson, A.V. Prasad, and F.I. Reyes
1975 Pituitary-gonadal relations in infancy. I. Patterns of serum gonadotropin concentrations from birth to four years of age in man and chimpanzee. *Journal of Clinical Endocrinology & Metabolism* 40:545-551.

Witt, R., G. Schmidt, and J. Schmidt
1981 Social rank and Darwinian fitness in a multimale group of Barbary macaques (*Macaca sylvanus L.*). *Folia Primatologica* 36:201-211.

Wood J.W.
1994 Maternal nutrition and reproduction: Why demographers and physiologists disagree about a fundamental relationship. *Annals of the New York Academy of Sciences* 709:101-116.

Wray, S., A. Nieburgs, and S. Elkabes
1989 Spatiotemporal cell expression of luteinizing hormone-releasing hormone in the prenatal mouse: Evidence for an embryonic origin in the olfactory placode. *Developmental Brain Research* 46:309-318.

Young, D.S., and E.W. Bermes, Jr.
1986 Specimen collection and processing: Sources of biological variation. Pp. 478-518 in *Textbook of Clinical Chemistry*. N.W. Tietz, ed. Philadelphia: W.B. Saunders.

Zehr, J.L., D. Maestripieri, and K. Wallen
1998 Estradiol increases female sexual initiation independent of male responsiveness in rhesus monkeys. *Hormones and Behavior* 33:95-103.

6

Intraspecific Variability in Fertility and Offspring Survival in a Nonhuman Primate: Behavioral Control of Ecological and Social Sources

Jeanne Altmann and Susan C. Alberts

The great variability and complexity of human vital rates (age-specific survival and fertility rates) and of behaviors affecting these rates are topics of major investigation in many disciplines. The extent and nature of such variability for our closest nonhuman relatives are only beginning to be elucidated. Our goal in the present chapter is to investigate fertility and family behavior from the perspective of life histories—the schedules of vital rates—in a natural primate population. We do this by evaluating the potential fitness consequences, magnitude, and sources of variability in life histories, particularly of females, and in the behaviors affecting them.

Before doing so, we pause to place the life histories of both baboons (the focus of this chapter) and humans in a comparative mammalian perspective. Most evolutionary studies of life histories have been comparative within or among orders of mammals or even at higher taxonomic levels, and the answers to questions about life history variability and the behaviors affecting it are often quite different depending on the taxonomic level being investigated—vertebrates, mammals, primates, or a single species such as baboons or humans. Our brief comparative notes below are restricted to mammals. (In addition to the references that follow, the interested reader is referred to chapters in Boyce, 1988; Stearns, 1992; Charnov, 1993; Lee, 1999; many in Kappeler and Pereira, 2003; and references therein.)

INTERSPECIFIC, COMPARATIVE VARIABILITY IN MAMMALIAN LIFE HISTORIES

In studies that take a classical comparative approach, patterns of variability or constancy among species or higher taxonomic levels such as

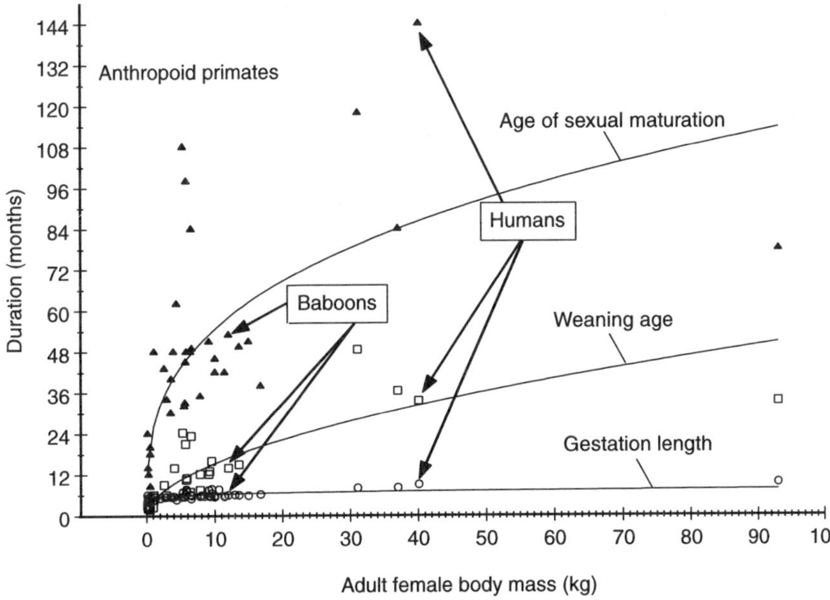

FIGURE 6-1 Duration of several life history stages as a function of body size in anthropoid primates.
SOURCE: Data primarily from compilations in Smuts et al. (1987), updated in Lee (1999) and references therein.

genera are analyzed. Consequently, single species such as humans or baboons represent at most a single point in the analyses. From that coarse perspective, several generalities can be made about the life history traits of various mammals. First, these traits covary and cluster along a continuum, such that some species have "fast" life histories—rapid offspring growth rates, early maturation, high rates of reproduction, and short reproductive spans (high adult mortality). At the other extreme are species with "slow" life histories—low rates of offspring growth, late maturation, low rates of reproduction and adult mortality. Second, large-bodied mammals tend to have slow life histories, small-bodied ones fast life histories (see Figure 6-1 for anthropoid primates). Third, although this pattern of a fast-slow continuum can be seen in all orders of mammals, the tendency toward slow or fast life histories also differs greatly among the various orders of mammals—carnivores versus primates, for example. Mammals of the same size in different orders differ fairly consistently in slow or fast life history style, and primates, mainly anthropoid primates, have particularly slow life histories. Finally, another interesting feature of the fast-slow continuum is that many life history traits, such as growth rates and adult mortality rates

(Charnov, 1993), remain strongly related to each other even when the effects of body size are removed; that is, constraints of size are not what lead to the correlation among traits, as was often assumed in many studies prior to the mid-1980s (see historical review in Harvey and Purvis, 1999).

Both humans and baboons exhibit slow life histories; those of baboons are basically as expected for a primate of their size, whereas some aspects of human life histories tend to be slower than expected (but see, e.g., Hrdy, 1999, and Hawkes, 2002, regarding human "hyperfertility"). That is, primates in general and anthropoid primates in particular have life histories characteristic of much larger nonprimate mammals. They also have particularly long periods of immaturity. Our human quality-based lifestyle runs deep in our phylogenetic history, and we come from a lineage, a family tree, that has at each branch exaggerated or extended the slow lifestyle—to a considerable extent a trade-off of quantity for quality. What explains these patterns, the differences among mammalian orders and the correlations found among life history variables at higher taxonomic levels? Diverse answers to those questions have been proposed, both historically and currently, and the interested reader is referred to Charnov (1993, 2001), Kozlowski and Weiner (1997), the historical review and perspective provided by Harvey and Purvis (1999), and an application to human life history evolution based on Charnov's approach in Hawkes (2002) and Hawkes et al. (2003).

Most important, however, from the perspective of the current volume and the topic of this chapter—variability within a species, whether humans or baboons—is that good explanations of life history variability and correlations are not necessarily the same for all taxa or at all levels of investigation. The relationship among life history variables within species or populations often is, and is expected to be, different in direction, as well as strength, from that among orders (see, e.g., Lande, 1979; Harvey and Clutton-Brock, 1985; Emerson and Arnold, 1989; Lee et al., 1991; Worthman, this volume, for humans). For example, as a result of ecological sensitivity within, rather than among, species, large body size is often associated with large litters, early maturation, high reproductive rates, and low adult mortality rates, in striking contrast to the relationship of these variables among species of a given mammalian order. Life history theories that apply at one level cannot simply be extrapolated from that level to another—for example, from across mammalian orders or from differences among species within an order to variability within species (see, e.g., Lande, 1979; Emerson and Arnold, 1989; Kozlowski and Weiner, 1997).

BABOON LIFE HISTORIES: LIFE HISTORY PATTERN AND VARIABILITY

Comparative studies serve to anchor our perception of human or nonhuman primate traits to our shared biological history and some basic relationships such as those among body size, phylogeny, and life histories. They leave unanswered, however, questions about current dynamic patterns that are shaping behavior, life history variability, ecological responses, and evolutionary potential within species. These require analyses of lifetimes and of the factors that influence them. Here we present two analyses of life history variability in savannah baboons. First, we use matrix demography models to examine the relative strength of selection on different vital rates. In particular, we examine the sensitivity of fitness to comparable changes in infant survival and adult fertility. Second, we evaluate the variability existing in a natural population and the extent to which behavior, particularly choice of habitat and social environment, affects vital rates for both females and males.

Until recently, humans were the only primate species for which the requisite life history data were available for detailed analysis of life history variability (see Blurton-Jones et al., 1999, and Kaplan and Lancaster, this volume, and references in both). However, for a small handful of species, these data are accumulating for at least some life history components, and we provide here one of the first such analyses for the large, sexually dimorphic, predominantly terrestrial and highly social baboon, *Papio cynocephalus*. Selective omnivores, baboons are widespread throughout Africa and occupy a broad range of habitats from mountain through woodland and savannah to semidesert. The data presented here derive primarily from a study underway for more than three decades of the Amboseli baboon population, which resides in the basin to the north and west of Mount Kilimanjaro.

Baboons

Baboons live in discrete social groups. Members of a group forage during the day and sleep at night in much closer proximity to each other than to members of other groups, and virtually all social interactions are among members of the group of residence. A female usually spends her whole life in the group into which she was born, whereas a male leaves his natal group around the time he attains full adulthood at 8 years. Although groups are sometimes in close proximity, the boundaries are usually very clear, spatially as well as behaviorally. The amount of time that groups spend in close proximity is of relatively short duration and can be somewhat tense, even in habitats or years in which these encounters are relatively more frequent (e.g., Cheney and Seyfarth, 1977; Shopland and Altmann, 1987). Within groups, adult females form clear dominance hierarchies that are predominantly stable both within and across generations as juvenile daughters assume the "family rank" about a year before menarche. Dominance rank in males, in contrast, is much more highly dependent on size and strength and is highly age dependent and unstable (Alberts et al., in press; Packer, 1979; Packer et al., 2000).

The larger African carnivores—leopards, lions, and hyenas—prey on baboons and are a particular a risk at night. In each habitat where they are found, members of a baboon group sleep close together either on cliff edges or high in those trees in their habitat that would be the most difficult for a predator to climb. Of the two major tree species in Amboseli, for example, baboons prefer fever trees, *Acacia xanthopholea*, to umbrella trees, *A. tortilis*; fever tree branches are higher off the ground, smoother, and more vertical. For baboons the distribution of sparsely scattered nighttime roosts, as well as of potable water and food resources, affects patterns of encounters between groups, daily travel, and seasonal variability in these patterns. In Amboseli, baboons of the fully wild-foraging groups awaken and descend from their sleeping trees shortly after dawn. For the next 11 to 12 hours, they spend almost 75 percent of their time foraging—feeding or traveling to food—across their short-grassland savannah habitat, approximately 10 percent socializing, and the remainder resting, often in a midday siesta.

Baboon infants weigh a little less than 1 kg at birth. In the first few months of life the infant clings to its mother's ventrum and thereby obtains continuous nipple access and transportation during the 8 to 10 km of daily travel. Gradual nutritional and locomotor independence develops during the next year until the infant's mother conceives again when the infant is about 18 months old and weighs approximately 3 to 4 kg. Although adult male baboons are approximately double the body mass of adult females, infant and juvenile females are very close in size to their male age peers, and almost all of the sexual dimorphism in body size arises during an adolescent growth spurt in males after females reach menarche between 4 and 5 years of age.

Life History Patterns in Amboseli

To analyze baboon life histories and life history variability, we used data collected from 1971 to 1999 for approximately 600 individuals living in completely wild-foraging groups of baboons (Alberts and Altmann, 2003). We constructed life tables with 1-year age classes and the corresponding survivorship and fertility entries of a population projection matrix, shown for females in Table 6-1 and males in Table 6-2. The tables also

TABLE 6-1 Per Annum Vital Rates for Wild-Foraging Amboseli Baboon Females (1971-1999) by One-Year Age Classes for Analysis in Projection Matrix Models

Female Age Class	Entries in Population Projection Matrix		Elasticity		Age-Specific Birth Rate
	Survivorship	Fertility[a]	Survival	Fertility	
1	0.7910	0	0.0972	0	0
2	0.8884	0	0.0972	0	0
3	0.9366	0	0.0972	0	0
4	0.9688	0	0.0972	0	0
5	0.9529	0.1281	0.0906	0.0066	0.0083
6	0.9439	0.2719	0.0778	0.0128	0.3056
7	0.9481	0.2747	0.0661	0.0117	0.3500
8	0.9483	0.2639	0.0558	0.0103	0.3085
9	0.9427	0.2590	0.0466	0.0092	0.3256
10	0.9233	0.2230	0.0395	0.0072	0.2973
11	0.8910	0.1975	0.0338	0.0057	0.2429
12	0.8943	0.2303	0.0281	0.0057	0.2459
13	0.9419	0.2607	0.0226	0.0055	0.3273
14	0.9160	0.2588	0.0177	0.0050	0.3000
15	0.8701	0.2833	0.0129	0.0048	0.3333
16	0.8731	0.3000	0.0086	0.0042	0.3784
17	0.7880	0.2647	0.0055	0.0032	0.3704
18	0.6329	0.2162	0.0035	0.0020	0.3158
19	0.6278	0.2433	0.0022	0.0013	0.3000
20	0.8648	0.1832	0.0016	0.0006	0.4286
21	0.7455	0.2391	0.0009	0.0007	0.0000
22	0.5517	0.3207	0.0003	0.0006	0.7500
23	0.6090	0.1302	0.0001	0.0001	0.0000
24	0.4174	0.2138	0	0.0001	0.5000
25	0.3796	0	0	0	0
26	0.5000	0	0	0	0
27	0	0	0	0	0

[a] The fertility entries in the third column are the elements in the first row of the Leslie matrix, computed from the age-specific birth rates in the last column along with the person-years-lived entries from the estimated life table. The fertility entries take into account both adult survival in the interval and birth rate to individuals in that interval; it is based on the full cohort that *enters* an age class, whether they survive the age class or not. Because baboons, like humans, do not have a distinct birth season, our calculations are based on a birth flow model. For details, see Caswell, (2001), Alberts and Altmann (2003).

contain age-specific birth rates and elasticities, which will be discussed shortly. As evident in the tables, Amboseli baboons experience high infant mortality, much lower female mortality during the late juvenile and early adult years, and then gradually increasing mortality in the latter portion of

TABLE 6-2 Per Annum Vital Rates for Wild-Fraging Amboseli Baboon Males (1971-1999) by One-Year Age Classes for Analysis in Projection Matrix Models

Male Age Class	Entries in Population Projection Matrix		Elasticity		Age-Specific Birth Rate[b]
	Survivorship	Fertility[a]	Survival	Fertility	
1	0.7825	0	0.1066	0	0
2	0.9122	0	0.1066	0	0
3	0.9337	0	0.1066	0	0
4	0.9167	0	0.1066	0	0
5	0.9588	0	0.1066	0	0
6	0.9427	0.3734	0.0948	0.0117	0
7	0.9390	0.7759	0.0743	0.0205	0
8	0.9416	0.7791	0.0570	0.0173	0.0667
9	0.9311	0.7663	0.0428	0.0143	0.5754
10	0.9112	0.7423	0.0313	0.0115	0.8155
11	0.8944	0.7221	0.0222	0.0091	0.6493
12	0.8820	0.7074	0.0151	0.0071	0.8176
13	0.8456	0.6652	0.0099	0.0052	0.5543
14	0.8295	0.6467	0.0060	0.0038	0.4919
15	0.7816	0.5950	0.0034	0.0026	0.3007
16	0.6665	0.4747	0.0020	0.0015	0.3326
17	0.6251	0.4334	0.0012	0.0008	0.0776
18	0.8002	0.6252	0.0005	0.0006	0.0647
19	0.7500	0.5859	0.0001	0.0004	0.0485
20	0.3333	0.2131	0	0.0001	0.0776
21	0	0	0	0	0

[a] The fertility entry takes into account both adult survival in the interval and birth rate to individuals in that interval; it is based on the full cohort that *enters* an age class, whether they survive the age class or not. Because baboons, like humans, do not have a distinct birth season our calculations are based on a birth flow model. For details, see Caswell (2001) and Alberts and Altmann (2003).

[b] Our calculation of birth rate (and therefore fertility) for males is based on the proportion of mating attributable to males of that age class (see text and Alberts and Altmann, 2003, especially p. 78 and Appendix 4.1 for reproductive rate terminology).

the second decade of life (see also Bronikowski et al., 2002). Only a small proportion of individuals live into their third decade. At all three long-term field sites—Gombe and Mikumi, Tanzania, and Amboseli—maximum recorded longevity is 26 to 27 years (Gombe: Packer et al., 1995, and Bronikowski et al., 2002; Mikumi, estimated: Rhine et al., 2000; Amboseli: Bronikowski et al., 2002, and Alberts and Altmann, 2003). Mortality rates for subadult and adult males are somewhat higher than those for like-aged females, reflecting a common mammalian sex difference. For the Amboseli baboons, this sex difference probably derives from a combination of intrinsic and extrinsic causes of senescence and mortality, including the mortality risk of dispersal (Alberts and Altmann, 1995). Known-age males of 15 to 18 years look much older and more frail than their female age peers.[1]

Menarche in baboons is followed by a period of somewhat abnormal sexual cycles and adolescent sub-fertility, followed by several normal cycles, conception, and then a 6-month gestation period; as a result, females produce their first offspring (Table 6-1) approximately 18 months after menarche. A long period of relatively steady birth rates follows until early in the third decade of life for the few females who live that long. These patterns are identifiable from near-daily records of menstruation, probabilistic visual correlates of ovulation, and other aspects of reproduction that are readily observed in baboons (Altmann et al., 1977, and references therein). Interbirth intervals after a surviving offspring are almost 2 years at various sites; if an infant dies, the interval is much shorter as its mother resumes cycling within a month and conceives after only one or two cycles.

Estimating male offspring production is more problematic and requires more caution in interpretation. In baboons, male dominance status is highly age related, dominance is a good predictor of mating behavior when a female is fertile, and observed mating behavior is a good predictor of genetic paternity (Altmann et al., 1996; Alberts et al., in press, and references therein). We used age-specific mating behavior to make proportional paternity assignments for males of each age; the total conception rate of males is constrained to and determined by that of females. Male offspring production declines much more rapidly with age than do birth rates of females, and the sex difference in this decline is much greater than that for survival (Tables 6-1 and 6-2).

A General Approach to Evaluating the Relative Strength of Selection on Different Vital Rates: Perturbations of Female Life Histories Using Matrix Models

If one were to compare two family lineages within a population, one lineage in which investment is successfully directed toward increasing infant survival and another in which it is successfully devoted to increasing birth rates, which would be more effective in enhancing population growth

[1]The estimate of person-years lived in the first year of life used to construct the projection matrix entries is 0.8551 years for females, and the net reproduction ratio—the usual NRR known to demographers, but also referred to as the net reproductive rate (Caswell, 2001)—is 1.50. This large an NRR could not have been sustained over evolutionary time and reflects only immediately prevailing conditions.

or lineage fitness? Would enhanced parental care be favored or enhanced mating effort? The answer depends in part on the species' basic schedule of mortality and birth rates, on the extent and style of fast or slow life history. Focusing the question on anthropoids, given the general pattern of age-specific mortality and fertility found in humans and other large primates (a slow life history), what would be the relative impact on biological fitness of two different behavioral changes, each of which appeared in some individuals, one a behavioral change that produced a small proportional change in infant mortality, the other a behavioral change that produced a small proportional change in birth rates? Demographic matrix models are a useful tool for exploring this question. (For a fuller discussion of these models, see references; below, and Alberts and Altmann, 2003, for an introduction to matrix models in the context of primate life history analysis.)

A matrix model is based on age-specific survival and fertility rates (from life tables). The model used is the usual Leslie matrix projection model, with one-year-wide age groups, familiar to demographers. Notation follows Caswell (2001). The model generates two results that are of particular interest for our purposes. The first result, λ, is a measure of the projected population growth rate. This measure equals e^r, where r is Lotka's intrinsic rate of natural increase. The measure is also equivalent to the relative fitness of the life history described by the vital rates (Lande, 1982a, 1982b; see also McDonald and Caswell, 1993, and Caswell, 2001). The second result is elasticity (or sensitivity) measures, which provide a simple means to explore effects on λ of variability or small perturbations in the initial vital rates. These analyses are of particular relevance to a consideration of the life history consequences of fertility and parental behavior. Each vital rate (each age-specific mortality or fertility rate) in a matrix model will have a characteristic sensitivity, which is an estimate of the impact on λ of a small change in that vital rate (the slope of the vital rate function at that point) with all others held constant. Sensitivities cannot be compared directly because they are based on different rates. Elasticities are more useful; they are sensitivities that have been scaled so that their sum for both fertility and survival across all age classes is 1; they can be directly compared (see, e.g., Benton and Grant, 1999). A vital rate (in our case fertility or survival in a 1-year interval) with large elasticity is one for which small changes result in a relatively large change in λ compared to the effect on λ of a small change in the other vital rates. During the past two decades, matrix models have been greatly extended and many constraining assumptions have been relaxed (Caswell, 2001, and chapters in Heppel et al., 2000, and references therein). Concurrently these models have increasingly been applied to natural populations in studies of population viability and conservation (e.g., Heppel et al., 1994; Crooks et al., 1997; Mills et al.,

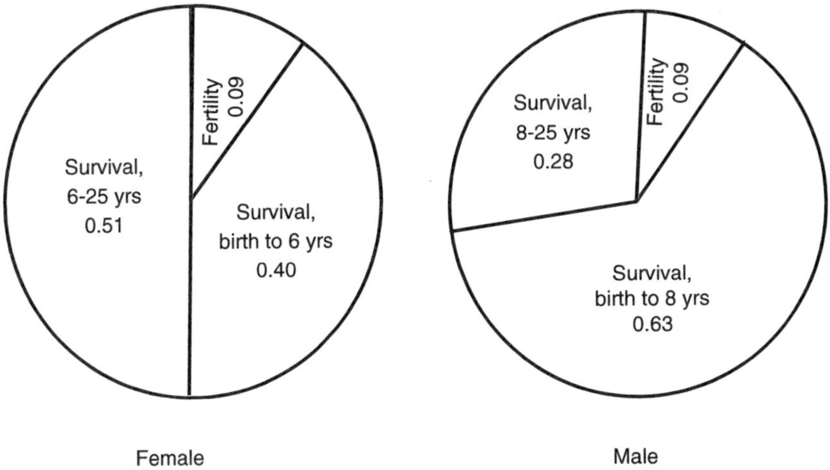

FIGURE 6-2 Proportion of elasticity in the matrix model attributable to immature survival, fertility, and adult survival.
NOTE: The greater proportion attributable to immature versus mature survival for males derives solely from the later maturity of males than females.
SOURCE: Data from Tables 6-1 and 6-2. See text and Alberts and Altmann (2003) for details.

1999), ecology (e.g., chapters in Heppell et al., 2000), and the evolution of behavior (McDonald, 1993; McDonald and Caswell, 1993).

If we return to the two lineages, one that invests in effective infant care versus the other that invests in an effective increase in fertile matings, we can compare—for example, in the Amboseli case—survival elasticities of young infants (age class 1) to fertility elasticities of adults (Table 6-1, Figure 6-2). For baboon females in Amboseli, a small increase in an infant's survival during the first year of life will have a much greater impact on λ—up to two orders of magnitude greater—than a proportional increase in female fertility in any age during adulthood. Specifically, the elasticity of survival for age class 1 is 0.0972, whereas the elasticity of fertility is 0.0128 at its highest, in age class 6, and declines to an order of magnitude less, 0.0013, by age 19. The importance of survival versus fertility is evidenced by the fact that, for Amboseli baboons, survival accounts for 91 percent of the total elasticities and fertility for only 9 percent, for both males and females (Figure 6-2; see also Alberts and Altmann, 2003), a common pattern in long-lived species (discussion in McDonald, 1993, for avian species). The implication of these results for, say, an individual making alternative behavioral or investment decisions is complicated. Interpretation depends partially on whether these are lifetime decisions affecting at once fertility or offspring survival for all years, flexible year-to-year options, or perhaps age-specific decisions (e.g., by young adult or old females). Interpretation also depends on the mechanisms and costs of each type of change; and on whether a key assumption of sensitivity analysis, independence among vital rates, is violated.

One example illustrates some of the potential issues in the case of baboons, although it is applicable to many other species. For an older female, the balance would always seem to favor investment in a current infant's survival rather than in increased fertility (producing another infant). In contrast, for a young adult female in a particular year, a small increase in fertility that year might seem to balance an increase in survival of that single year's infant; however, if infant survival is dependent on maternal care, that is, the independence assumption of sensitivity analysis is violated, the mother's increase in fertility is likely to produce a *decrease* in the current infant's survival rather than leaving it unchanged. For wild-foraging baboons, this is the case even if the current infant is in its second year of life. If the current infant is less than a year old, its death is almost assured if its mother dies or is caring for another infant. Moreover, as we shall see in the next section, the calculus may vary by ecological and social conditions (see also Hrdy, 1999; Ellison, 2001; Worthman and Kaplan and Lancaster chapters in this volume, for discussion of this topic in humans).

This example highlights several limitations or cautions that apply to interpretation of this simple matrix model and of sensitivity analyses in particular. One is the aggregate approach to the vital rates; that is, age classes are treated as groups of homogeneous individuals. Another is that vital rates are assumed to be independent of each other. Both of these assumptions are surely violated to varying degrees. A particularly important example of lack of independence is the case of male fertility rates; male fertility has been calculated by apportioning total female fertility across male age classes according to observed age-specific patterns of mating. Thus, an increase in fertility for one male age class is necessarily accompanied by a decrease in fertility for another. Another example is the situation in which trade-offs between female survival and reproduction or between future reproduction and survival of current offspring (example above) are significant. A third concern about sensitivity analysis is that infinitesimal, independent changes from one set of initial values may not be predictive of responses to larger and otherwise more realistic changes or for changes from a different set of initial vital rates because the fitness function for a vital rate is often not linear (e.g., Pfister, 1998; see also papers in Heppel et al., 2000).

An important complement to sensitivity analysis is direct perturbations of the matrix. Direct perturbation permits manipulation of a matrix to create hypothetical scenarios that are within the range, magnitude, and

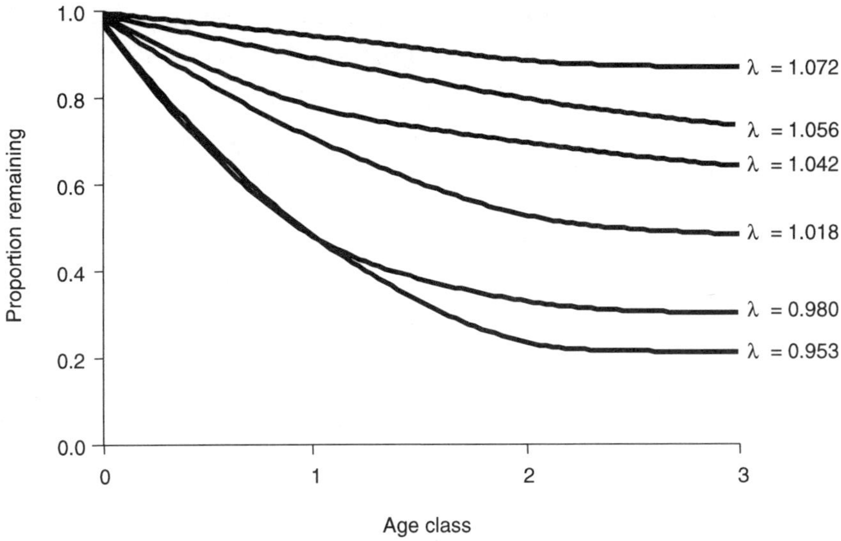

FIGURE 6-3 Projected population growth (or relative fitness) for different levels of first-year survivorship holding all other survival and fertility values to those in Table 6-1 (Amboseli fully wild-foraging groups, 1971-1999).
NOTE: The curve producing $\lambda = 1.042$ results from first-year survival in Table 6-1. The lowest value, $\lambda = 0.953$, results from 0.5 first-year survival obtained in a small sample of wild-foraging individuals during a period leading to a decline in the Amboseli population in the 1960s and early 1970s. The highest value, $\lambda = 1.072$, results from 0.9 first-year survival, obtained during a decade-long study of the lodge group, a "food-enhanced" group that obtained much of its nutrition from a tourist lodge grounds and the discarded foodstuffs at a lodge garbage pit. Published data for first-year survival from other sites fall within the range of survival explored here.

correlation structure realistic for the population of interest (see discussion and application in Mills et al., 1999). We implemented such a perturbation for females by using the basic model built from the female survival and fertility values in Table 6-1 and then simply changed first-year survival within a range from 0.5 through 0.9. This range of values includes all those reported for baboons or observed in Amboseli (see caption for Figure 6-3). This perturbation alone produced a large range of estimates of fitness, or λ, from a value below replacement to an appreciable expansion rate. That is, variability solely in first-year infant survival that is within the observed range for baboons has major consequences for estimates of relative fitness of both sexes and for the future of the population.

Clearly, the fitness potential is great for variability in effective family and fertility behaviors. Is such variability realized and, if so, how?

Variability in a Natural Population: Life History Plasticity and the Behavioral Ecology of Fertility, Offspring Survival, and Offspring Quality in Amboseli Baboons

What magnitude of variability is observed in the different components of the Amboseli baboons' life histories, and what are the social and ecological sources of this variability? For our first analysis, we consider not just the fully wild-foraging baboon groups in Amboseli but also individuals from a group in the Amboseli population that has established its range and does some of its foraging around a nearby tourist lodge in the park (lodge group, Figure 6-4). In the subsequent analyses we again restrict analyses to data for the fully wild-foraging groups. All the analyses below require partitioning of the overall dataset in varying ways by time periods or subsets of individuals. Therefore, to retain reasonable sample sizes, we collapse the vital rates from 1-year age intervals into a few meaningful and manageable

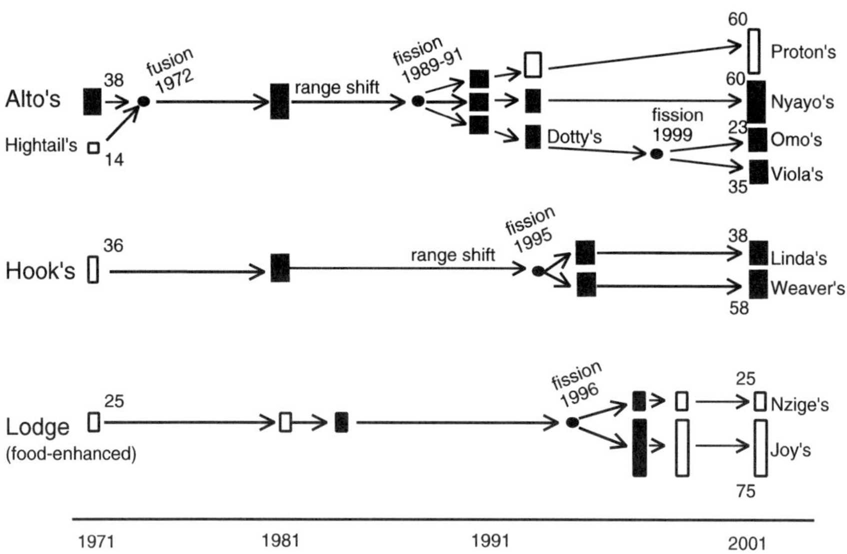

FIGURE 6-4 Amboseli study groups that contributed data to the present analyses. NOTE: Although some demographic data are available for all groups in all years, detailed estimates of all vital rates are available only for years in which a group is indicated as a study group (darkened boxes). Approximate dates that Alto's group and Hook's group made major shifts in home range are indicated; years of group fusion and fission are indicated by arrows. The lodge group and its fission products are food-enhanced groups; all other study groups are completely wild-foraging.

components—infant survival, age at reproductive maturity, and reproductive rate throughout adulthood.

Furthermore, we focus on females for reproductive analyses. Data are better for females than males, because females are the nondispersing sex and because maternity can be assigned with greater certainty than can paternity. We examine variability in two reproductive parameters: reproductive maturity (measured as age at menarche) and fertility or reproductive rate (measured as interbirth interval for mothers with surviving offspring). Infant survival in this analysis is taken as survival through 2 years because interbirth intervals, and maternal investment, are approximately 1.5 to 2 years in duration in fully wild-foraging groups. As in the life tables and basic matrix model, for this first exploration and for consistency with the matrix model, data are aggregate, treated as independent, and pooled across all births in the subsets being compared. In addition, for simplicity and because of power limitations, interactions between ecological and social environments are not explored in the present analyses.

Choosing a Place to Live: Fertility, Offspring Survival, and Offspring Quality Are Food Limited

Home ranges differ in the resource base they provide for individuals or groups. Yet an individual's home range is not something completely outside its control, a condition in which it must just do its best given the circumstances (Worthman, this volume, emphasizes this point for humans). In a heterogeneous environment, groups or individuals can move, for example, and thereby alter their foraging opportunities for the foreseeable future; that is, they may simultaneously alter many age-specific vital rates. Such an action has potential costs and benefits. The costs include short-term ones, such as dealing with a new environment in which the habits of predators and the locations of food and water are poorly known, and also perhaps long-term ones when, for example, a move may entail a trade-off between higher rates of predation and improved foraging. The benefits may outweigh the costs, however, and the move may in the balance be worthwhile if vital rates are highly food limited and if a move can improve foraging conditions.

For evaluating the extent to which offspring survival, offspring quality, and adult fertility are food limited for the Amboseli baboons, we made comparisons for two instances in which baboon groups chose living situations that changed food availability. First, we compared the totally wild-foraging groups in the Amboseli population with a group of baboons that moved into an area near the park's tourist lodges and supplemented their diet with discarded food scraps from the lodge (Altmann et al., 1993; Altmann and Muruthi, 1988; Hahn et al., 2003; Kemnitz et al., 2002;

Muruthi et al., 1991). This situation is common wherever cercopithecine primates live near human habitation (see, e.g., Fa and Southwick, 1988). Second, we compared the fully wild-foraging groups in two time periods—the 1970s and the 1990s—before and after, respectively, the groups moved from an area of low food availability into a richer natural habitat, one in which baboon foods and shelter were more abundant (see Figure 6-4).

Food-Enhanced Groups

Adult females in the lodge group, the group that established a range near human habitation, experienced higher rates of reproduction and their offspring experienced much higher rates of survival and earlier menarche (Table 6-3, rows 1and 2; Table 6-4, row 1). The greatest proportional increase was in offspring survival. The home range and consequent lifestyle chosen by these females required tolerance of close association with humans, of higher density of baboons in close proximity, and of higher rates of aggressive interactions (Altmann et al., 1993; Kemnitz et al., 2002; Muruthi, 1989). Those individuals that tolerated these conditions were able to improve opportunities for their offspring and their fertility. Adult males, unlike females, usually leave their group of birth and disperse into other groups where they reproduce. Therefore, to achieve the advantages of life in a food-enhanced group, most Amboseli males would need to tolerate these altered conditions despite not having grown up in them, perhaps a much greater challenge than that experienced by females, who could adapt to these conditions during ontogeny. In fact, despite the much higher food availability and consequent lower foraging demand experienced by the lodge group, dispersal into this group did not occur over the first 16 years after they moved into close human association. Interestingly, dispersal out

TABLE 6-3 Impact of Foraging Environment on Various Life History Components

Foraging Environment	Offspring Survival to 2 Years	Offspring Growth	Age of Maturation (years)	Reproductive Rate (interbirth interval after surviving offspring)
Food enhanced	0.89	9 g/day	3.72	1.28
Wild	0.70	5 g/day	4.52	1.72
Before move to better habitat (1970s)	0.51		4.69	1.81
After move to better habitat (1990s)	0.70		4.31	1.62

TABLE 6-4 Impact of Ecological and Social Factors on Various Life History Components (Percent change)

	Offspring Survival to 2 Years	Age of Maturation	Reproductive Rate
Food enhanced	+27%	+18%	+26%
Wild-foraging: Improved foraging (1970s-1990s)	+38%	+8%	+15%
Reduced density (fewer adult females)	?		+13%
Improved social status (high ranking)	=	+8%	+20%

of the group by males that matured in the lodge group was reduced in comparison to males from wild-foraging groups; perhaps many males were unprepared or unwilling to face the hardships of a fully wild-foraging lifestyle despite the advantages of access to less closely related mates. As a result, an increasing proportion of potential mates in the lodge group were close maternal and paternal relatives. Although mate avoidance between maternal siblings is strong in many cercopithecines, including baboons, avoidance among paternal siblings is much less so (Alberts, 1999). Consequently, baboons from the lodge group were subject to an increased chance of inbreeding, and behavioral evidence of inbreeding has been associated with reduced offspring survival in wild baboons (Alberts and Altmann, 1995; see also Packer, 1979 for a group in Gombe).

Moving to a Better Wild-Foraging Environment

Between the 1970s and 1990s, the fully wild-foraging study groups moved from their original home range as the habitat degenerated into a richer woodland savannah area to the south and west of the original range, one in which baboon foods and shelter trees were much more abundant (Figure 6-4). The impact of this behavior on the vital rates was similar to that experienced by the lodge group (Table 6-3, rows 3 and 4), and the percentage improvement from the 1970s to the 1990s (Table 6-4, row 2) was again greatest for offspring survival.

In both cases of improved foraging environment, rapid offspring growth rates may be the life history variable mediating the improved survival and fertility that resulted. We were able to examine this possibility indirectly for the food-enhanced contrast; youngsters in the lodge group grew at almost double the rates of those in the wild-foraging groups, 9 versus 5 g per day (growth data were available for only 5 years in the late 1980s, precluding a similar comparison over time in the wild-foraging groups).

Choosing a Social Environment: Fertility, Offspring Survival and Offspring Quality Are Density and Socially Limited

For individuals in the wild-foraging groups, we evaluated social sources of baboon life history variability. In particular we examined the effects of group size as a measure of immediate or experienced density. We also examined the effects of an individual female's social status as study groups changed in size over time. The analyses were performed using a stepwise general linear model, after taking into account the effects of the change in foraging environment. When females were in larger groups (partial r^2 = 0.05; slope, 0.0053; p = 0.0005), and particularly when those groups had more adult females (partial r^2 = 0.08; slope, 0.0212, p = 0.0001), interbirth intervals after the production of a surviving offspring were longer, which lowered fertility for females with surviving offspring (see Figure 6-5). Each additional 10 adult females in a group resulted in an increase of approximately 0.2 years (2.5 months) in interbirth intervals after surviving offspring. In other words, living in small groups enhances reproduction but not offspring survival.

Although we suspected that high density inflicts a slight cost to infant survival, we did not have the power to detect such a cost in the present analyses. In the aggregate, fertility rates do not appear to exhibit density dependence. We postulate a scenario in which in high-density conditions the lower reproductive rates for females with surviving offspring are offset by the higher fertility that occurs when infants die, resulting in no effect on the aggregate fertility measurements used in our matrix models. We do not currently have a clear answer, but the situation highlights the need to look below the surface of overall fertility rates to evaluate density dependence. For baboons in several populations, life in large groups may sometimes entail costs to offspring survival and reproduction (Bulger and Hamilton, 1987; Rhine et al., 1988; Wasser and Starling, 1988).

The impact of large group size on vital rates is probably mediated at least partly through altered hormone levels or indirectly through physiological effects of reduced foraging efficiency from "scramble competition" without direct contest (van Schaik and van Noordwijk, 1988). This is suggested by data from Amboseli (Bronikowski and Altmann, 1996) as well as from other cercopithecine populations (Dunbar, 1996; van Schaik and van Noordwijk, 1988). One theory of primate social diversity and its evolution also assumes that higher rates of direct contest competition will be a source of life history variability in populations such as baboons with clear female dominance hierarchies (van Schaik, 1983, 1989), a mechanism that

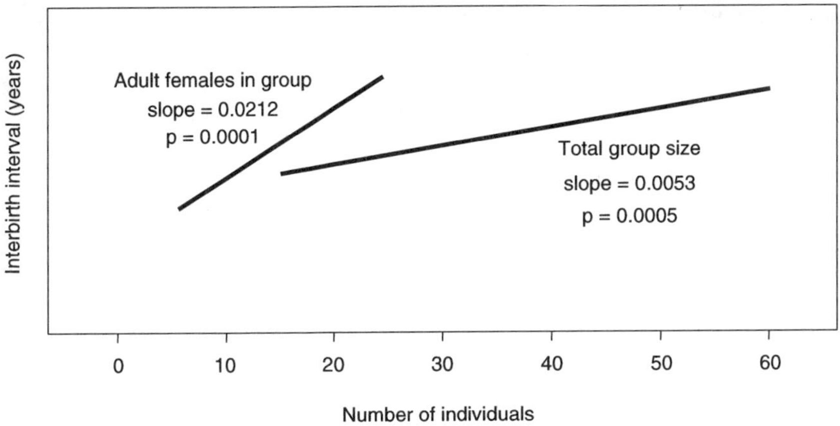

FIGURE 6-5 High density results in lower reproductive rate (longer interbirth intervals following a surviving offspring).
NOTE: Data pooled for all individuals in wild-foraging study groups. Interbirth interval following birth of a surviving offspring is a function of immediate experienced density as measured by group size (total group size and number of adult females in the group) after controlling for change in foraging environment. Although both measures are significant, a change in the number of adult females has a much greater impact (see also Figure 6-6). The range of numbers of adult females and total group sizes depicted here are approximately those observed in wild-foraging Amboseli groups. Interbirth intervals following infant death are excluded from analyses of interbirth intervals in this chapter because baboons, like humans, are not seasonal breeders and, with the loss of a suckling infant, a female rapidly resumes cycling and becomes pregnant in only one or two cycles rather than the usual three to five, resulting in much shorter interbirth intervals.

may occur under some conditions in Mikumi baboons (Rhine et al., 1988; Wasser and Starling, 1988). Future detailed analysis of both behavioral and hormonal variability among individuals may facilitate elucidating selective forces on primate social structure.

Can nonhuman females control group size? In species that exhibit female dispersal in addition to, or rarely instead of, male dispersal, females can control group size as males generally do, through dispersal, and the same is the case for fission-fusion societies (e.g., Wrangham, 1980; Dunbar, 1988). For species exhibiting matrilocality, those in which females remain for life in their group of birth, density may not at first seem to be a variable that females can control. However, control is possible through the rare occurrences of fission (van Schaik, 1996). Although fission of baboon or macaque groups has been reported primarily for groups that have experienced very rapid growth in group size through food enhancement, data on fission of wild-foraging groups are also slowly accumulating (e.g., Nash, 1976; Ron et al., 1994). Amboseli females in fully wild-foraging groups have engaged in such fission events three times in the past three decades (Figure 6-4), resulting in a return to smaller groups and higher reproductive rates.

The costs of group living may not impact all adults equally, particularly in species with a social structure that is relatively hierarchical rather than egalitarian, including most cercopithecines (e.g., Wrangham, 1980; van Schaik, 1983). In baboon groups, inequality is evident in agonistic dominance hierarchies, a pervasive feature of baboon life (e.g., Hausfater, 1975; Altmann et al., 1988) and is predictive of access to various ecological and social resources (Barton, 1993; Barton and Whiten, 1993; Post et al., 1980; Silk, 1987, review for other primates). Adult female rank is very stable throughout adulthood in baboons and macaques, and daughters assume their family's rank prior to adolescence (Hausfater et al., 1982; Pereira and Fairbanks, 1993; Walters, 1980). Despite widespread, though not ubiquitous (e.g., Watts, 1996), findings of dominance effects on foraging in a number of primate species, and despite long-postulated fitness consequences of dominance status, adequate data for rigorous tests remain scarce (van Schaik, 1983, and sequelae; Sterck et al., 1997).

In Amboseli, after taking into account effects of changing environment and group size, rank affects female reproductive rate (partial $r^2 = 0.07$, slope = 0.013, $p = 0.0037$) and age of maturation (partial $r^2 = 0.08$, slope = 0.02, $p = 0.0025$; see Figure 6-6). As with the impact of home range quality, these rank effects may be mediated by differences in offspring growth rate. Offspring of high-ranking females grew more rapidly, and rapid growth was predictive of early maturity. A 10-rank difference in dominance status was associated with a 0.2-year (2.5-month) difference in age of menarche and a 0.13-year (1.5-month) difference in interbirth interval. Busse (1982) reported a similar rank-associated difference in interbirth interval in chacma baboons in Botswana, and rank impacted a number of fitness components in anubis baboons in Gombe, Tanzania (Packer et al., 1995), and under some conditions in Mikumi baboons (Rhine et al., 1988; Wasser and Starling, 1988). Thus, through attainment and maintenance of high status, baboon females accrue fitness benefits from both enhanced fertility and offspring quality. Although the relative status of females in a group is ordinarily transmitted with great fidelity between generations (see Figure 6-7), a low-ranking female can reduce the number of others who dominate her or her daughters by participating in a group fission and thereby escape the costs of low status.

Male fertility is also density dependent in Amboseli and elsewhere (Alberts and Altmann, 1995; Alberts et al., in press; Altmann, 2000). Male mating opportunities are related to the number of females and the number

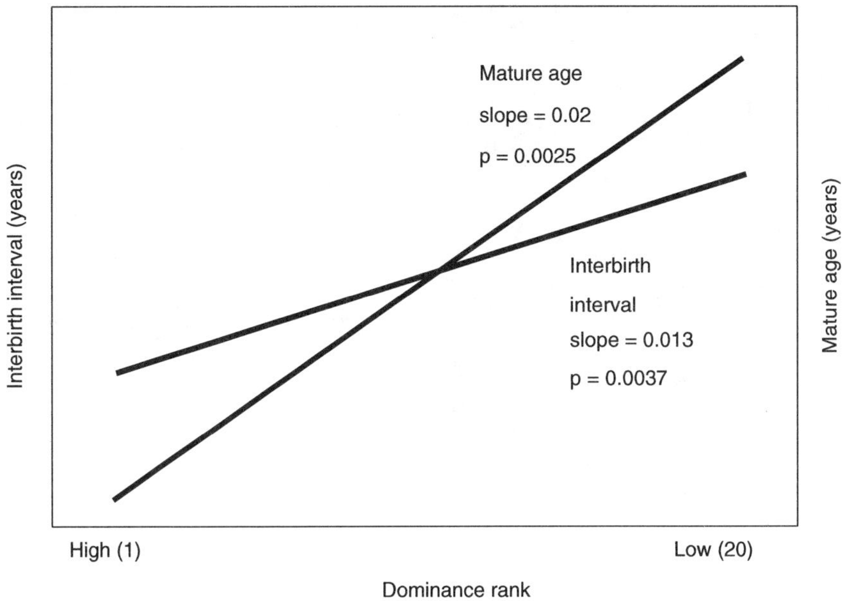

FIGURE 6-6 Age of reproductive maturity and reproductive rate (measured as in Figure 6-5) are functions of social status.
NOTE: High-ranking females experience higher reproductive rates and their offspring mature at younger ages than do low-ranking females (after controlling for changes in foraging environment and group size).

of other adult males in the group. As a consequence, adult males disperse among groups. That is, the costs entailed by living with many other adult males are often avoided or at least mitigated by dispersal to groups with more favorable demographic makeup (Alberts and Altmann, 1995; Altmann, 2000). The relationship between dominance status and mating success in male cercopithecines has a long, controversial, and yet well-documented history. Across species, among baboon populations, and within a single population over time (Amboseli), the relationship accounts for approximately 50 percent of the variance in male mating success but is highly variable (Alberts et al., in press). In most species and populations, male dominance status is strongly negatively associated with age (Alberts et al., in press; Packer et al., 2000). Males who stay in a large group or a group in which they are not of high rank sometimes use coalitions and other social means of enhancing fertility (Alberts et al., in press; Noë and Sluijter, 1990, 1995; Packer, 1977). Some older males who had previously been top-ranking and the father of many offspring also stay in groups in which

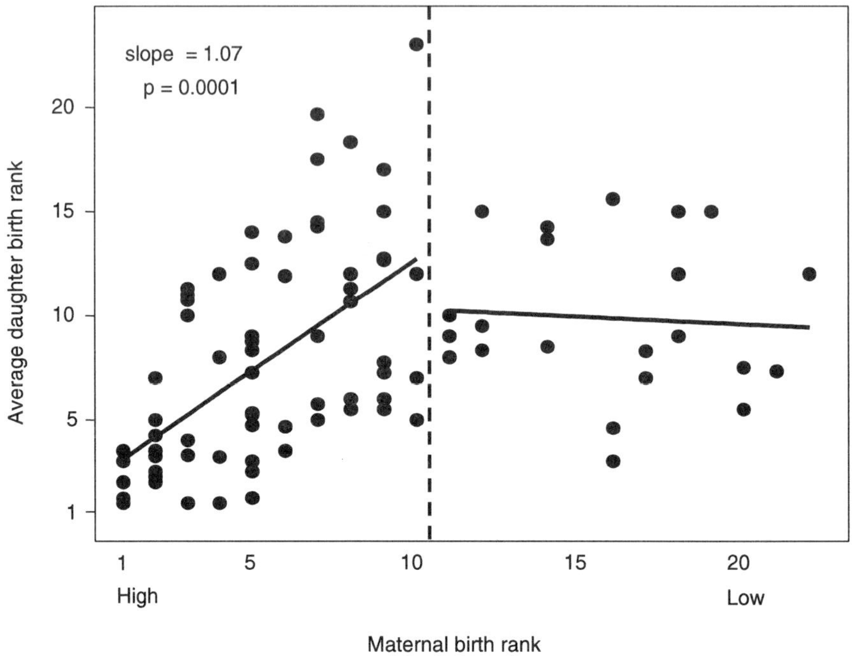

FIGURE 6-7 Daughters' social status as predicted by that of their mothers.
NOTE: For maternal birth ranks 1 through 10 (left side of the figure), this effect is clear and strong (double that expected for a completely heritable trait). No effect occurs beyond rank 10 because group fission occurs beyond this size; females of different matrilines retain the predicted rank relative to each other in the fission products, but at the time of fission the new smaller groups have had 10 or fewer adult females in the wild-foraging groups (three fission events).

their fertility is low. They often provide care and protection for their likely offspring and are thought to reduce the likelihood of infanticide by other males (most recently reviewed in van Schaik and Janson, 2000, and Palombit, 2003), potentially gaining a few matings through female choice rather than dominance status (e.g., Strum, 1982; Smuts, 1985) but also potentially choosing enhancement of offspring survival over greater mating opportunities.

In summary, by altering their home range and their social environments through dispersal (males) or group fission (females), both males and females use behavior to change their physical and social environments. In the process, they often mitigate the effects of low social status, in ways that enhance fitness and sometimes in ways that particularly enhance offspring survival and quality (see Figure 6-8).

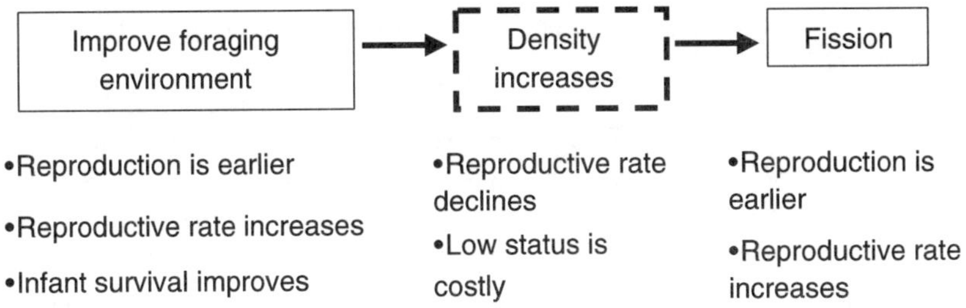

FIGURE 6-8 Overview of behaviors affecting fertility and offspring survival by fully wild-foraging baboons in Amboseli over three decades.
NOTE: The baboons shifted home range when the habitat in their previous range degenerated. Offspring then experienced higher rates of survival and matured at younger ages, and females reproduced more often if their offspring survived. As a result, immediate experienced density (group size and number of adult females per group) increased and reproductive rate then declined as a result of socially constrained reproduction. Group fission followed, removing the density and social constraints.

Covariance of Life History Components

We started with elasticity analyses that assumed independence among life history components. Violations of this assumption may sometimes be significant, and future analyses will need to explore the dependences. From a broad evolutionary perspective, strong linkages among life history variables in the form of life-history "invariants," are central to Charnov's comparative (interspecific) approach to the evolution of life histories (e.g. Charnov and Berrigan, 1993; Charnov, 2001, applications to human evolution in Hawkes, 2002, and references therein). Some of the same correlations may pertain at the level of intraspecific variability as well. However, life history correlations are usually weaker or even in the opposite direction in populations or species than at higher taxonomic levels (see Harvey and Clutton-Brock, 1985; Emerson and Arnold, 1989; Kozlowski and Weiner, 1997; Worthman, this volume). Within a population, some life-history components may be positively correlated because of shared underlying processes (discussed with particular focus on humans in Hrdy, 1999, and Ellison, 2001, and references in both). Under those conditions, behavioral changes will result in several rates increasing or decreasing together. This was seen for infant survival and early maturity in the Amboseli analyses. In other instances, individuals face trade-offs. For instance, producing another infant may inflict higher mortality risk on the mother herself or on her current infant (e.g., Altmann et al., 1988, for baboons). For the Amboseli baboons, we find that these trade-offs seem to be ecologically contingent;

they are evident only in the most stringent ecological habitats or years (Altmann et al., 1988).

Not only might vital rates be correlated within individuals, but the actions of one individual can affect reproduction and offspring survival of another. The most obvious instance is the effect of either parent's behavior on the successful reproduction of the other, particularly in socially monogamous or polyandrous species. The phenomenon is more general, however, as in the case of alloparental care by siblings, grandparents, or other, perhaps more distant, relatives in which one individual may enhance the reproduction of another at a cost to its own reproduction. Enhanced fitness through the actions of others has been postulated for the evolution of alloparental care among some primate species and more specifically as an explanation for humans having "faster" reproductive rates than expected for their body size and otherwise slow life history components (see particularly Hrdy, 1999; Ross and McLarnon, 2000; Hawkes, 2002, and references therein). Covariance and other constraints, within and among individuals, are even more complicated for males. If males cannot appreciably affect total offspring production—that is, if offspring production is determined solely or even primarily by females—increased paternity in one age class will be offset by decreased paternity at other ages, and realistic perturbation analyses for males will need to take this trade-off into account.

The analyses presented here provide clear evidence of behavior that enhances fertility, offspring survival, and offspring quality. Changes in reproductive rates were most pervasive but not of greatest magnitude. Changes in foraging environment affected each parameter but most greatly affected offspring survival. In addition, daughters of low-status females matured later. The matrix model perturbation results raised the possibility that female baboons faced with alternatives might benefit from biasing decisions in favor of offspring survival and quality rather than enhanced fertility. The extent to which baboons are actually faced with such behavioral and life history trade-offs and behave as predicted is not yet clear. Both the simple models themselves and departures from their assumptions, such as population substructure, covariance, and stochastic variability, serve to guide future models and empirical investigations. Furthermore, that the social and environmental factors to which the baboons respond covary and feed back on each other is obvious (Figure 6-8) and is of necessity a topic of future theoretical and empirical investigation. Natural populations of nonhuman primates are relatively small and therefore present challenges to investigations of complexity and change over time, challenges that compound those already inherent in study of species with slow life histories.

CONCLUSIONS

Over a three-decade period, encompassing at least part of the lives of six generations of baboons and just surpassing the full lifetime of the longest living of the animals, individuals experienced great diversity of environmental and social conditions. These included normal wet and dry seasons; years of abundance and others of drought; many close relatives for some individuals or at certain times and few for others; habitat degeneration in the original home area and availability of not-too-distant areas with rich, new opportunities; groups with many competitors or with few. Groups of individuals, and also individuals acting somewhat independently, altered the physical and social conditions in which they lived and thereby considerably changed, through their own behavior, their own reproductive lives and the opportunities provided to their offspring.

Environmental variability has been proposed as the critical environmental context of human evolution (e.g., Potts, 1998). We suggest that adaptation to variable and changing environments is likely to have been an important feature of primate evolution more broadly. Success at responding to environments that change on various temporal and spatial scales and with varying degrees of predictability may be a recurrent theme for the most enduring and widespread primate lineages that we see today and for those likely to persist into the future. Because differences in survival of immature young will have the greatest impact on population growth and individual fitness for species with life histories characteristic of human and nonhuman primates, understanding fertility, parental behavior, offspring behavior, and the mechanisms producing variability in each must of necessity hold a central place in understanding primate adaptation and human origins.

For nonhuman primates as for humans, pregnancy, parturition, and offspring rearing occur within a complex ecological and social context. Few would question that the context of human fertility and parental care behaviors is highly variable and that humans both adjust their behavior to context and are often the agents of altering that context (e.g. Hrdy, 1999; Ellison, 2001; Worthman this volume; and references in each of these). That such variability and agency may also be significant in the lives and evolutionary history of our nonhuman primate relatives has not received comparable status. The opportunity to begin to do so offers considerable potential both for understanding primate behavioral ecology and evolution and for providing a window into human origins and diversity.

Together, the present analyses provide just one piece in beginning to elucidate the conditions, extent, mechanisms, and individual variability in richness of behavioral complexity related to fertility and offspring care in natural primate societies. Future research will benefit from the use of more complex matrix demography models—for example, ones that incorporate temporal heterogeneity and covariance among life history components (Caswell, 2001). Studies of physiological mechanisms, ontogenetic effects, the effect of life history trade-offs on observed behavior (see above), and heritable differences in fertility and parental behaviors will also be essential to the agenda of elucidating ecological and evolutionary perspectives on fertility and parental care behaviors in nonhuman primates. The origin of both an absolutely and a relatively long period between birth and maturation in humans is seen among other large anthropoids. That this period of immaturity historically held and currently holds great opportunities for evolution is unsurprising. Increased links between studies of human and nonhuman primates, and of mechanisms and behavioral ecology, are essential to enhancing the research agenda of each.

ACKNOWLEDGMENTS

We thank the Office of the President of the Republic of Kenya and the Kenya Wildlife Service for permission to work in Amboseli over the years. We also thank the Institute of Primate Research of the National Museums of Kenya for institutional sponsorship in Kenya and the wardens and staff of Amboseli National Park and the local communities of the Amboseli/Longido region for cooperation and hospitality. Particular appreciation goes to the Amboseli fieldworkers who contributed to the data over the years, especially R.S. Mututua, S.N. Sayialel, J.K. Warutere, P.M. Muruthi, and A. Samuels; to K.O. Pinc for database programming in the creation of BABASE and to the series of assistants who organized BABASE entry and extraction of BABASE data—D. Shimizu, S.L. Combes, A. Mosser, and J.M. Zayas. S.A. Altmann, R.A. Bulatao, K. Hawkes, H. Kaplan, J.W. Lynch, K. Wachter, and an anonymous reviewer provided valuable comments on the manuscript. We gratefully acknowledge financial support from the National Science Foundation (IBN-9985910 and its predecessors) and the Chicago Zoological Society.

REFERENCES

Alberts, S.C.
1999 Paternal kin discrimination in wild baboons. *Proceedings of the Royal Society of London-Biological Sciences* 266:1501-1506.

Alberts, S.C., and J. Altmann
1995 Balancing costs and opportunities: Dispersal in male baboons. *American Naturalist* 145:279-306.

2003 Matrix models for primate life history analysis. In *Primate Life History and Socioecology*. P. Kappeler and M.E. Pereira, eds. Chicago: University of Chicago Press.

Alberts, S.C., H.E. Watts, and J. Altmann
In press Queuing and queue-jumping: Long term patterns of reproductive skew among male savannah baboons. *Animal Behaviour*. Available online at <*http://www.duke.edu/~alberts/AlbertsLab/Queuing.pdf*>

Altmann, J.
2000 Predicting male distribution among primate groups: Models of outcome and process. Pp. 236-247 in *Primate Males*. P. Kappler, ed. Cambridge: Cambridge University Press.

Altmann, J., and P. Muruthi
1988 Differences in daily life between semi-provisioned and wild-feeding baboons. *American Journal of Primatology* 15:213-222.

Altmann, J., S.A. Altmann, G. Hausfater, and S.A. McCuskey
1977 Life history of yellow baboons: Physical development, reproductive parameters and infant mortality. *Primates* 18:315-330.

Altmann, J., G. Hausfater, and S. Altmann
1988 Determinants of reproductive success in savannah baboons (*Papio cynocephalus*). Pp. 403-418 in *Reproductive Success*. T.H. Clutton-Brock, ed. Chicago: University of Chicago Press.

Altmann, J., D. Schoeller, S.A. Altmann, P. Muruthi, and R.M. Sapolsky
1993 Body size and fatness of free-living baboons reflect food availability and activity levels. *American Journal of Primatology* 30:149-161.

Altmann, J., S.C. Alberts, S.A. Haines, J. Dubach, P. Muruthi, T. Coote, E. Geffen, D.J. Cheesman, R.S. Mututua, S.N. Saiyalel, R.K. Wayne, R.C. Lacy, and M.W. Bruford
1996 Behavior predicts genetic structure in a wild primate group. *Proceedings of the National Academy of Sciences* 93:5797-5801.

Barton, R.A.
1993 Sociospatial mechanisms of feeding competition in female olive baboons, *Papio anubis*. *Animal Behaviour* 46:791-802.

Barton, R.A., and A. Whiten
1993 Feeding competition among female olive baboons, *Papio anubis*. *Animal Behaviour* 46:777-789.

Benton, T.G., and A. Grant
1999 Elasticity analysis as an important tool in evolutionary and population ecology. *Trends in Ecology and Evolution* 14:467-471.

Blurton-Jones, N., K. Hawkes, and J.F. O'Connell
1999 Some current ideas about the evolution of the human life history. Pp. 140-166 in *Comparative Primate Socioecology*. P.C. Lee, ed. Cambridge: Cambridge University Press.

Boyce, M.S.
1988 Where do we go from here? Pp. 351-361 in *Evolution of Life Histories of Mammals: Theory and Pattern*, M.S. Boyce, ed. New Haven, CT: Yale University Press.

Bronikowski, A., and J. Altmann
1996 Foraging in a variable environment: Weather patterns and the behavioral ecology of baboons. *Behavioral Ecology and Sociobiology* 39:11-25.

Bronikowski, A.M., S.C. Alberts, J. Altmann, C. Packer, K.D. Carey, and M. Tatar
2002 The aging baboon: Comparative demography in a nonhuman primate. *Proceedings of the National Academy of Sciences* 99:9591-9595.

Bulger, J., and W.J. Hamilton, III
1987 Rank and density correlates of inclusive fitness measures in a natural chacma baboon troop. *International Journal of Primatology* 8:635-650.
Busse, C.D.
1982 Social dominance and offspring mortality among female chacma baboons. *International Journal of Primatology* 3:267.
Caswell, H.
2001 *Matrix Population Models*. Sunderland, MA: Sinauer Associates.
Charnov, E.L.
1993 *Life History Invariants*. Oxford: Oxford University Press.
2001 Evolution of mammal life histories. *Evolutionary Ecology Research* 3:521-535.
Charnov, E. L., and D. Berrigan
1993 Why do female primates have such long lifespans and so few babies? or life in the slow lane. *Evolutionary Anthropology* 1:191-194.
Cheney, D.L., and R.M. Seyfarth
1977 Behavior of adult and immature male baboons during intergroup encounters. *Nature* 269:404-406.
Crooks, K.R., M.A. Sanjayan, and D.F. Doak
1997 New insights on cheetah conservation through demographic modeling. *Conservation Biology* 12:889-895.
Dunbar, R.I.M.
1988 *Primate Social Systems*. New York: Cornell University Press.
1996 Determinants of group size in primates: A general model. *Proceedings of the British Academy* 88:33-57.
Ellison, P.T.
2001 *On Fertile Ground*. Cambridge, MA: Harvard University Press.
Emerson, S., and Arnold, S.
1989 Intra- and interspecific relationships between morphology, performance and fitness. Pp. 295-314 in *Complex Organismal Functions: Integration and Evolution in Vertebrates*. D.B. Wake and G. Roth, eds. New York: S. Bernhard.
Fa, J.E., and C.H. Southwick
1988 *Monographs in Primatology: Ecology and Behavior of Food-Enhanced Primate Groups*. New York: Alan R. Liss.
Hahn, N.E., D. Proulx, P.M. Muruthi, S.C. Alberts, and J. Altmann
2003 Gastrointestinal parasites in free-ranging Kenyan baboons (*Papio cynocephalus* and *Papio*). *International Journal of Primatology* 24(2): April.
Harvey, P.H., and T.H. Clutton-Brock
1985 Life history variation in primates. *Evolution* 39:559-581.
Harvey, P.H., and A. Purvis
1999 Understanding the ecological and evolutionary reasons for life history variation: Mammals as a case study. Pp. 232-248 in *Advanced Ecological Theory: Principles and Applications*. J. McGlade, ed. London: Blackwell Science.
Hausfater, G.
1975 *Dominance and Reproduction in Baboons (Papio cynocephalus): A Quantitative Analysis*. Basel: S. Karger.
Hausfater, G., S. Altmann, and J. Altmann
1982 Long-term consistency of dominance relations among female baboons (*Papio cynocephalus*). *Science* 217:752-755.
Hawkes, K.
2002 Grandmothers and the evolution of human longevity. Paper presented at the symposium Strategies for Reproductive Success, Human Biology Association, 13 April.

Hawkes, K., J.F. O'Connell, and N.G. Blurton Jones

2003 The evolution of human life histories: Primate tradeoffs, grandmothering socioecology, and the fossil record. In *Primate Life Histories and Socioecology*. P. Kappeler and M.E. Pereria, eds. Chicago: University of Chicago Press.

Heppel, S., J.R. Walters, and L.B. Crowder

1994 Evaluating management alternatives for red-cockaded woodpeckers: A modeling approach. *Journal of Wildlife Management* 58:479-487.

Heppel, S., C. Pfister, and H. deKroon, eds.

2000 Elasticity analysis in population biology: Methods and applications. *Ecology* 81:605-708.

Hrdy, S. B.

1999 *Mother Nature: A History of Mothers, Infants, and Natural Selection*. New York: Pantheon.

Kappeler, P.M., and M.E. Pereira

2003 *Primate Life Histories and Socioecology*. Chicago: University of Chicago Press.

Kemnitz, J.W., R.M. Sapolsky, J. Altmann, P.M. Muruthi, G.E. Mott, and M.L. Stefanick

2002 Effects of food availability on serum insulin and lipid concentrations in free-ranging baboons. *American Journal of Primatology* 57:13-19.

Kozlowski, J., and J. Weiner

1997 Interspecific allometries are by-products of body size optimization. *American Naturalist* 149:352-380.

Lande, R.

1979 Quantitative genetic analysis of multivariate evolution, applied to brain:body size allometry. *Evolution* 33:402-416.

1982a Elements of a quantitative genetic model of life history evolution. Pp. 21-29 in *Evolution and Genetics of Life Histories*. H. Dingle and J. P. Hegmann, eds. New York: Springer-Verlag.

1982b A quantitative genetic theory of life history evolution. *Ecology* 63:607-615.

Lee, P.C.

1999 *Comparative Primate Socioecology*. Cambridge: Cambridge University Press.

Lee, P.C., P. Majluf, and I.J. Gordon

1991 Growth, weaning and maternal investment from a comparative perspective. *Journal of Zoology of London* 225:99-114.

McDonald, D.B.

1993 Demographic consequences of sexual selection in the long-tailed manakin. *Behavioral Ecology* 4:297-309.

McDonald, D.B., and H. Caswell

1993 Matrix methods for avian demography. Pp. 139-185 in *Current Ornithology*. D.M. Power, ed. New York: Plenum Press.

Mills, L.S., D.F. Doak, and M.J. Wisdom

1999 Reliability of conservation actions based on elasticity analysis of matrix models. *Conservation Biology* 13:815-829.

Muruthi, P.

1989 Food intake and energy expenditure in savannah baboons. MSc. thesis, University of Nairobi.

Muruthi, P., J. Altmann, and S. Altmann

1991 Resource base, parity, and reproductive condition affect females' feeding time and nutrient intake within and between groups of a baboon population. *Oecologia* 87:467-472.

Nash, L.
1976 Fission in free ranging baboons in the Gombe Stream National Park, Tanzania. *American Journal of Physical Anthropology* 44:63-78.

Noë, R., and A.A. Sluijter
1990 Reproductive tactics of male savanna baboons. *Behaviour* 113:117-170.
1995 Which adult male savanna baboons form coalitions? *International Journal of Primatology* 16:77-105.

Packer, C.
1977 Reciprocal altruism in *Papio anubis*. *Nature* 265:441-443.
1979 Inter-troop transfer and inbreeding avoidance in *Papio anubis*. *Animal Behavior* 27:1-36.

Packer, C., D.A. Collins, A. Sindimwo, and J. Goodall
1995 Reproductive constraints on aggressive competition in female baboons. *Nature* 373:60-63.

Packer, C., D.A. Collins, and L.E. Eberly
2000 Problems with primate sex ratios. *Philosophical Transactions of the Royal Society of London Series B-Biological Sciences* 355:1627-1635.

Palombit, R.A.
2003 Male infanticide in savanna baboons: Adaptive significance and intraspecific variation. In *Sexual Selection and Reproductive Competition in Primates: New Perspectives and Directions*. C.B. Jones, ed. Special Topics in Primatology III American Society of Primatology (in press).

Pereira, M.E., and L.A. Fairbanks
1993 *Juvenile Primates: Life History, Development and Behavior*. Oxford: Oxford University Press.

Pfister, C.A.
1998 Patterns of variance in stage-structured populations: Evolutionary predictions and ecological implications. *Proceedings of the National Academy of Sciences* 95:213-218.

Post, D.G., G. Hausfater, and S.A. McCuskey
1980 Feeding behavior of yellow baboons (*Papio cynocephalus*): Relationship to age, gender and dominance rank. *Folia Primatologia* 34:170-195.

Potts, R.
1998 Environmental hypotheses of hominin evolution. *Yearbook of Physical Anthropology* 41:93-136.

Rhine, R.J., S.K. Wasser, and G.W. Norton
1988 Eight-year study of social and ecological correlates of mortality among immature baboons of Mikumi National Park, Tanzania. *American Journal of Primatology* 16:199-212.

Rhine, R.J., G.W. Norton, and S.K. Wasser
2000 Lifetime reproductive success, longevity, and reproductive life history of female yellow baboons (*Papio cynocephalus*) of Mikumi National Park, Tanzania. *American Journal of Primatology* 51:229-241.

Ron, T., S.P. Henzi, and U. Motro
1994 A new model of fission in primate troops. *Animal Behaviour* 47:223-226.

Ross, C., and A. MacLarnon
2000 The evolution of non-maternal care in anthropoid primates: A test of the hypotheses. *Folio Primatologica* 71:93-113.

Shopland, J.M., and J. Altmann
1987 Fatal intragroup kidnapping in yellow baboons. *American Journal of Primatology* 13:61-65.

Silk, J.B.
1987 Social behavior in evolutionary perspective. Pp. 318-329 in *Primate Societies.* B.B. Smuts, D.L. Cheney, R.M. Seyfarth, R.W. Wrangham, and T.T. Struhsaker, eds. Chicago: University of Chicago Press.

Smuts, B.B.
1985 *Sex and Friendship in Baboons.* New York: Aldine.

Strum, S.C.
1982 Agonistic dominance in male baboons: An alternative view. *International Journal of Primatology* 3:175-202.

Stearns, S.C.
1992 *The Evolution of Life Histories.* Oxford: Oxford University Press.

Stearns, S.C., and J.C. Koella
1986 The evolution of phenotypic plasticity in life-history traits: Predictions of reaction norms for age and size at maturity. *Evolution* 40:893-913.

Sterck, E.H.M., D.P. Watts, and C.P. van Schaik
1997 The evolution of female social relationships in nonhuman primates. *Behavioral Ecology and Sociobiology* 41:291-309.

van Schaik, C.P.
1983 Why are diurnal primates living in groups? *Behaviour* 87:120-144.
1989 The ecology of social relationships amongst female primates. Pp. 195-218 in *Comparative Socioecology.* V. Standen and R.A. Foley, eds. Oxford: Blackwell.
1996 Social evolution in primates: The role of ecological factors and male behaviour. *Proceedings of the British Academy* 88:9-31.

van Schaik, C.P. and M.A. van Noordwijk
1988 Scramble and contest in feeding competition among female long-tailed macaques (*Macaca fascicularis*). *Behaviour* 105:77-98.

van Schaik, C.P., and C.H. Janson
2000 *Infanticide by Males and Its Implications.* Cambridge: Cambridge University Press.

Walters, J.
1980 Interventions and the development of dominance relationships in female baboons. *Folia Primatologica* 34:61-89.

Wasser, S.K., and A.K. Starling
1988 Proximate and ultimate causes of reproductive suppression among female yellow baboons at Mikumi National Park, Tanzania. *American Journal of Primatology* 16:97-121.

Watts, D.P.
1996 Comparative socio-ecology of gorillas. Pp. 16-28 in *Great Ape Societies.* W.C. McGrew, L.F. Marchant, and T. Nishida, eds. Cambridge: Cambridge University Press.

Wrangham, R.W.
1980 An ecological model of female bonded primate groups. *Behaviour* 75:262-300.

7

An Evolutionary and Ecological Analysis of Human Fertility, Mating Patterns, and Parental Investment

Hillard S. Kaplan and Jane B. Lancaster

This chapter considers the evolutionary biology of human fertility, parental investment, and mating and is designed to provide a broad overview of the topic. It focuses on three themes. The first is the timing of life events, including development, reproduction, and aging. Second is the regulation of reproductive rates and its relationship to parental investment. Sexual dimorphism and its relationship to mating systems together are the third theme. Each of these themes is addressed from two perspectives: first, in a comparative cross-species context, and second, in terms of variation within and among human groups. Our primary goal is to introduce a new ecological framework for understanding variations in each of those domains and then to apply the framework to understanding both the special characteristics of our species in a comparative perspective and variations within and among human groups. A secondary goal is to discuss how evolutionary biology can be integrated with more traditional approaches to human demography and the new research questions such integration would generate.

The first section of this chapter presents an introduction to life history theory and current thinking in evolutionary biology with respect to the three themes. Since the fitness consequences of alternative fertility and parental investment regimes depend on ecology and individual condition, both specialization and flexibility in life histories are considered. Building on this foundation, an ecological framework for understanding variation in each of those domains is then introduced. The second section discusses humans in a comparative context, with a particular emphasis on the hunter-and gatherer lifestyle because of its relevance to the vast majority of human evolutionary history. The third section applies the framework developed in the first two parts to understanding major historical trends in human fertility, parental investment, and mating regimes. The transition from hunting and gathering to farming and pastoralism is considered first. Land- and power-based stratified societies are then discussed, followed by an analysis of wage-based competitive labor markets and demographic transition. The chapter concludes with a discussion of the new research questions and approaches to research design suggested by this framework.

THE THEORETICAL FRAMEWORK

Fundamental Trade-Offs in Life History Theory

Natural selection acts on variability in the traits of individual organisms within populations. Traits (and the genes that code for them) increase in frequency relative to other traits when their average effects on the individuals possessing those traits act to maximize their long-term production of descendents through time.[1] Fertility is the most direct contributor to an organism's fitness (i.e., the number of descendents it produces). In fact, all other fitness components, such as mortality, only affect fitness through their effects on fertility (e.g., mortality rates affect fitness by affecting the probability of living to the next reproductive event). All else constant, any increase in fertility increases an organism's fitness. However, there are two trade-offs affecting natural selection on fertility.

The first is the trade-off between present and future reproduction. An organism can increase its energy capture rates in the future by growing and thus increasing its future fertility. For this reason, organisms typically have a juvenile phase in which fertility is zero until they reach a size at which some allocation to reproduction increases fitness more than growth. Similarly, among organisms that engage in repeated bouts of reproduction (humans included), some energy during the reproductive phase is diverted away from reproduction and allocated to maintenance so that it can live to reproduce again. The general expectation is that natural selection on age of first reproduction and on the adult reproductive rate will tend to maximize total allocations of energy to reproduction over the life course.

[1]Selection acts on the "inclusive fitness" of genes coding for traits. Inclusive fitness includes effects on both the reproductive success of the individual bearing the gene and other individuals, related by common descent, who also bear the gene. For example, selection on genes affecting alarm calls in response to predators depends both on their effects on the reproductive fitness of the caller (who may risk a greater threat of predation) and on relatives bearing those genes (whose lives may be saved by the call).

The second trade-off is between quantity and quality of offspring, where quality is a function of parental investment in offspring and reflects its ability to survive and reproduce. The general expectation is that natural selection on offspring number and investment per offspring will tend to maximize the long-term production of descendents; this may be estimated by the number of offspring that survive to reproduce themselves during an organism's lifetime (Smith and Fretwell, 1974) or if fertility affects the production and survival of grandchildren, by more distant effects.

Sexual reproduction, which most probably evolved as a means of increasing variability among offspring through the sharing of parents' genetic material, complicates the trade-off between quantity and quality of offspring. This is because offspring share roughly equal amounts of their parents' genetic material, yet parents may contribute unequally to their viability. In this sense, offspring may be considered as "public goods," with each parent profiting from the investments of the other and having an incentive to divert resources to the production of additional offspring. This public goods problem tends to create conflicts of interest between the sexes (see Gangestad, this volume, for a treatment of such conflicts).

In fact, an almost universal by-product of sexual reproduction is the divergent evolution of the two sexes. Sex is defined by gamete size, and the sex with the larger gametes is called female. Larger gametes represent greater initial energetic investment in offspring. With increased investment beyond energy in gametes, the divergence between the two sexes is often exaggerated but may also balance or even reverse. For example, females provide all investment to offspring in greater than 95 percent of mammalian species, but males provide similar amounts or more total investments among most altricial birds, male brooding fish, and some insects, such as katydids (see Clutton-Brock and Parker, 1992, for a review).

To the extent that one sex invests more in offspring than the other, the one that does more investing sex is in short supply resulting in *operational sex ratios* greater than unity and competition for mates among members of the sex that does less investing. This public goods problem generates the third major trade-off: that between mating and parental effort. Sexual reproduction involves two components: finding a mate and achieving a mating, on the one hand, and investing in the resulting offspring to increase its viability, on the other.

To the extent that there are gains from specialization in the two components, one sex will evolve to produce many small highly mobile gametes specialized to mating, and another will evolve to produce fewer larger gametes, specialized for energetic investments in offspring. Trivers (1972) recognized that these differences in relative parental investment affect the structure of mating markets and the characteristics of the more and less investing sexes. The more investing sex is selected to be choosy about when and with whom to mate, and the less investing sex is selected to possess characteristics that increase its mating opportunities. This leads to what economists call negative externalities, since male resources are wasted on costly displays or handicaps (Grafen, 1991) or on fighting, rather than in offspring production. The general expectation is that natural selection acts on mating and parenting effort in populations of males and females so that individual fitness tends to maximize in a competitive equilibrium (i.e., it tends to generate distributions of mating and parenting effort among males and females that cannot be "invaded" by alternative distributions).

Ecology and Life History Evolution

Variations across taxa and across conditions in optimal energy allocations and optimal life histories are shaped by ecological factors, such as food supply, mortality hazards, and the effects of body size on both energy capture and mortality hazards (Charnov, 1993; Kozlowski and Weigert, 1987; Werner, 1986). It is generally recognized that there are species-level specializations that result in bundles of life history characteristics, which, in turn, can be arrayed on a fast-slow continuum (Promislow and Harvey, 1990). For example, among mammals, species on the fast end exhibit short gestation times, early reproduction, small body size, large litters, and high mortality rates, with species on the slow end having opposite characteristics.

It is also recognized that many, if not most, organisms are capable of slowing down or speeding up their life histories, depending on environmental conditions such as temperature, rainfall, food availability, density of conspecifics, and mortality hazards. Within-species variation in life history characteristics can operate over several different timescales. For example, there is abundant evidence that allocations to reproduction, as measured by fecundity and fertility, vary over the short term in relationship to food supply and energetic output among plants, birds, and humans (Hurtado and Hill, 1990; Lack, 1968). Extensive research on many bird species has shown that this phenotypic plasticity tracks fitness quite well (Godfray et al., 1991). Birds under variable conditions adjust clutch sizes in ways that tend to maximize the number of surviving young produced during the life course.

The impact of the environment may operate over longer time intervals through developmental effects (Lummaa and Clutton-Brock, 2002). For example, calorie restriction of rats at young ages tends to slow down growth rates and leads to short adult stature, even when food becomes abundant later in the juvenile period (Shanley and Kirkwood, 2000). Some intraspecific variation operates at even longer timescales, mediated through differential selection on genetic variants in different habitats. For example, rates of senescence vary across different populations of grasshoppers, with those at higher altitudes and earlier winters senescing faster than those at lower altitudes as a result of differential selection on genotypes (Tatar et al., 1997).

Similarly, there is a great deal of evidence suggesting that male and female parental investments vary in relation to local ecology over both the short run and the long run (see Clutton-Brock and Parker, 1992 for a review). For example, among katydids, males provide females with a "nuptial gift" (a bolus of condensed food energy) to support offspring production. Experimental manipulation of food density, affecting the foraging time necessary for males to produce the food package, produces shifts in male and female mating effort. When the food supply is low, male inputs into reproduction require more time than female inputs, males are in short supply, and females actively compete for males; as food density increases, this trend is reversed and males compete for access to females (Clutton-Brock, 1991; Gwyne, 1991; Gwyne and Simmons, 1990). This mix of specialization and flexibility is fundamental to understanding human life histories and mating systems. On the one hand, it is generally agreed that the large human brain supports the ability to respond flexibly to environmental variation and to learn culturally. This suggests that humans may be most capable of short-term flexibility in the timing of life events and investment strategies. On the other hand, the commitment to a large brain and the long period of development and exposure to environmental information necessary to make it fully functional place important constraints on the flexibility of the human life course and require specializations for a slow life history. In fact, consideration of brain- and learning-intensive human adaptation reveals shortcomings in existing biological theory and inspires the development of a more general approach to life history evolution, which is the focus next.

An Evolutionary Economic Framework

A general explanatory framework for understanding our species must be able to account for both its distinctive features when compared to other species and the enormous range of variation exhibited by humans under different conditions, in different societies, and at different points in time. To account for these evolutionary trends, we have expanded existing models of life history evolution by explicitly modeling the three trade-offs discussed above using capital investment theory (Becker, 1975; Kaplan, 1996; Kaplan and Robson, 2002; Robson and Kaplan, 2003). The processes of growth, development, and maintenance are treated as investments in stocks of somatic or *embodied capital*. In a physical sense, embodied capital is organized somatic tissue—muscles, digestive organs, brains, and so forth. In a functional sense, embodied capital includes strength, speed, immune function, skill, knowledge, and other abilities. Since such stocks tend to depreciate with time, allocations to maintenance can also be seen as investments in embodied capital. Thus, the present-future reproductive trade-off can be understood in terms of optimal investments in own embodied capital versus reproduction, and the quantity-quality and mating-parenting trade-offs can be understood in terms of investments in the embodied capital of offspring versus their number.

The central thesis of this chapter is that there are four major factors affecting the timing of reproduction in the life course, reproductive rates, and parental investment for each sex: (1) the important resources consumed and utilized in reproduction and the production process by which those resources are obtained; (2) risks of mortality and the "technology" of mortality reduction; (3) the extent of complementarity between the sexes in the production of offspring; (4) the degree of variation in resource production and capital holdings among individuals and within individuals over time.

With respect to the first factor, the relative impacts of mass-based, brain-based, and extrasomatic physical capital on resource production are critical determinants (see Figure 7-1). What are the marginal effects of an increase in body size on acquisition and turnover rates for energy and other critical resources? What are the marginal effects of increases in brain size, brain complexity, knowledge, and skill on resource production? How does physical capital, such as land or a breeding territory, affect production? How do body mass, brain-based abilities, and extrasomatic physical capital combine in resource production? The general expectation is that, since investments in each of those forms of capital trade off against each other and against allocations to reproduction, natural selection will optimize those investments so as to maximize descendent production.

The brain is a special form of embodied capital. On the one hand, neural tissue monitors the organism's internal and external environment and induces physiological and behavioral responses to stimuli (Jerison, 1973; 1976). On the other hand, the brain has the capacity to transform present experiences into future performance. This is particularly true of the cerebral cortex, which specializes in the storage, retrieval, and processing of experiences. To the extent that capital investments in the brain generate rewards that are realized over time (e.g., an increased reproductive rate during adulthood), the payoffs to those investments depend on mortality rates, since they affect the length of time over which the return will be realized. Dynamic models of this process show that investments in embodied capital coevolve with investments affecting mortality and longevity (Kaplan and Robson, 2002; Robson and Kaplan, 2003). The longer the time spent growing and learning prior to reproducing, the more natural

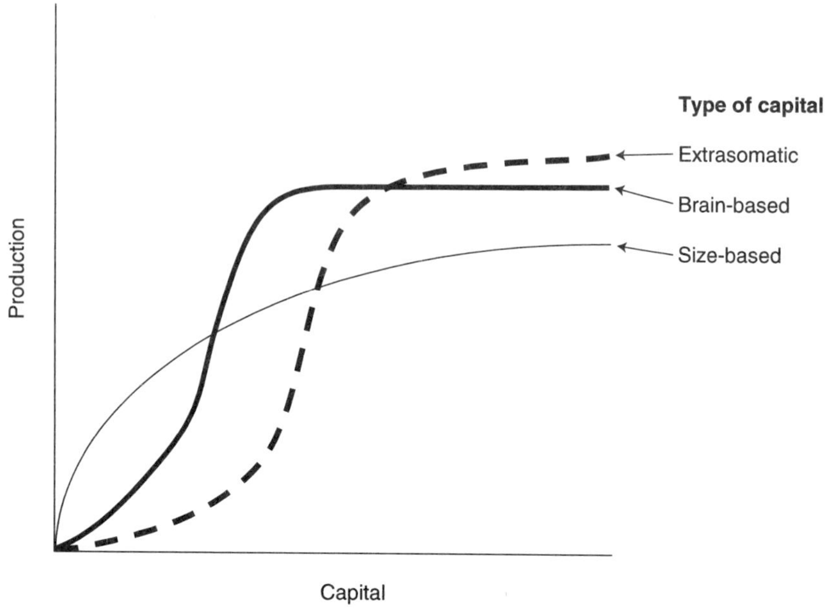

FIGURE 7-1 Production as a function of the capital stock.
NOTE: The relationship between production and each form of capital varies with ecology and the resources produced. Capital may be size-based, brain-based, or extrasomatic. More or less initial investment may be required before returns increase, and with further increases in investment, returns may diminish rapidly or slowly.

selection favors investments in staying alive to reap the benefits of those investments. Similarly, any investments that produce increased energy capture rates later in life, such as learning, select for additional investments to reach those older ages.

In addition to the production of energy, organisms can allocate energy and/or invest in forms of capital that reduce risks of mortality. While most biological models treat mortality as essentially exogenous, observed mortality is best understood in terms of an interaction between exogenous risks (environmental assaults) and endogenous responses designed to reduce mortality in the face of those risks. The technology of mortality reduction (the immune system, the ability to run, protective coverings such as shells, defensive weapons) also affects the likelihood of dying from environmental assaults. Models of embodied capital also show that ecological features or investments that increase the probability of survival to older ages also produce selection for greater investments in income-related embodied capi-

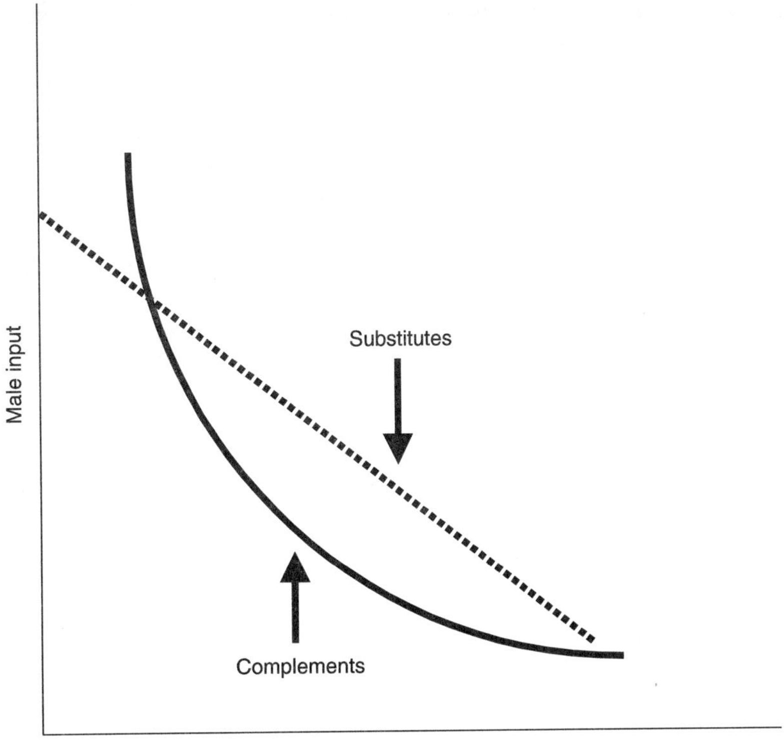

FIGURE 7-2 Offspring viability isoclines (indifference curves) as a function of male and female inputs.

tal. These coevolutionary effects appear to have been particularly important in human life history evolution.

With respect to the third factor, complementarity, each parent in sexually reproducing species contributes approximately half the offspring's genes and some amount of parental investment. The fitness of offspring is likely to be some function of the genetic material and the investments received from each parent. Each of these inputs may act as substitutes or complements, as illustrated in Figure 7-2. Stated simply, *complementarity* occurs when the value of male investment in offspring depends *positively* on the amount given by females and vice versa (with fitness held constant).[2] In

[2]Technically, complementarity occurs when marginal rates of substitution along fitness isoclines or indifference curves change as the ratio of the two inputs changes, making those curves convex to the origin.

contrast, male and female inputs are substitutes when the relative values of the two inputs are independent of the amount provided by the other sex (again holding fitness constant). Thus, there are four axes of potential complementarity (e.g., between mother's and father's genes, between mother's and father's investment, and between each parent's genes and their own and the other parent's investments). Gains from specialization in parenting and/or mating effort and complementarity between genes and investment are forces favoring sexual dimorphism, with females typically specializing in parenting effort and males specializing in mating effort.

Complementarity between the investments of each sex is the force favoring decreased sexual dimorphism and increased male parental investment. This kind of complementarity can occur when both direct care and resources are important to offspring viability and when the provisioning of each conflicts with, or is incompatible with, the provisioning of the other. For example, protection and feeding of nestlings are incompatible among many flying bird species. Protection of the young by one parent complements provisioning by the other parent, since food is only valuable to offspring that have not been preyed on. This ecology favors biparental investment and taking turns in feeding and nest protection by males and females. Among grazing mammals, however, offspring follow their mothers, who are able to nurse and protect them simultaneously. Investments by males in this case are less complementary and would only substitute for the investments of females.

Mate choice criteria and mating "market" characteristics are expected to result from the variance among and within individuals over time with respect to the resources critical for reproduction. When females provide all the parental investment in response to the conditions discussed above, they are expected to exercise choice among males in terms of their genetic quality, and males are expected to compete with other males for access to fecund females, either through physical competition or appeals to female choice.

As support from males increases in value with a resultant increase in their contribution to reproduction, we expect female choice to respond to *variation* in male offers of investment and in their ability to acquire resources utilized in reproduction. Males, in turn, as their investments in offspring increase, are expected to exert choice with respect to variation in female quality and to compete with other males for access to the resources utilized in reproduction. Ecological variability affecting the variance among males and females in resource access or access to mates is expected to exert a significant influence on mating market dynamics and in male and female investments in parenting and mating effort. Intertemporal variation in productivity within individuals is also likely to affect their mate value because it increases the likelihood of shortfalls.

Our proposal is that human evolution has resulted in a specialized life history that is due to a particular constellation of the factors discussed above. This constellation derives from the hunter-gatherer way of life, which characterized the vast majority of human evolutionary history. While, as discussed in the next section, there are some universal features associated with this way of life, there is significant ecological variability across habitats. We also propose that as a result of exposure to such variation, human psychology and physiology have evolved to respond in systematic ways to variations in the four factors discussed above. Finally, the domestication of plants and animals and subsequent economic transformations produced new socioecological conditions to which people responded in radical shifts in parenting and mating practices.

HUMAN LIFE HISTORIES IN A COMPARATIVE CONTEXT

Relative to other mammalian orders, the primate order is slow growing, slow reproducing, long lived, and large brained. Humans are at the extreme of the primate continuum. Compared to other primates, there are at least four distinctive characteristics of human life histories: (1) an exceptionally long life span, (2) an extended period of juvenile dependence, resulting in families with multiple dependent children of different ages, (3) multigenerational resource flows and support of reproduction by older postreproductive individuals, and (4) male support of reproduction through the provisioning of females and their offspring. The brain and its attendant functional abilities are also extreme among humans.

Our theory (Kaplan et al., 2000; Kaplan and Robson, 2002; Robson andd Kaplan, 2003) is that these extreme values with respect to brain size and longevity are coevolved responses to an equally extreme commitment to learning-intensive foraging strategies and a dietary shift toward high-quality, nutrient-dense, difficult-to-acquire food resources. The following logic underlies our proposal. First, high levels of knowledge, skill, coordination, and strength are required to exploit the suite of high-quality, difficult-to-acquire resources that humans consume. The attainment of those abilities requires time and a significant commitment to development. This extended learning phase during which productivity is low is compensated for by higher productivity during the adult period, with an intergenerational flow of food from old to young. Since productivity increases with age, the time investment in skill acquisition and knowledge leads to selection for lowered mortality rates and greater longevity because the returns on the investments in development occur at older ages.

Second, the feeding niche specializing on large valuable food packages, and particularly hunting, promotes cooperation between men and women and high levels of male parental investment, because it favors sex-specific specialization in embodied capital investments and generates a complementarity between male and female inputs. The economic and reproductive cooperation between men and women facilitates provisioning of juveniles, which both bankrolls their embodied capital investments and acts to lower mortality during the juvenile and early adult periods. Cooperation between males and females also allows women to allocate more time to child care and improves nutritional status, increasing both survival and reproductive rates. The nutritional dependence of multiple young of different ages favors sequential mating with the same individual, since it reduces conflicts between men and women over the allocation of food. Finally, large packages also appear to promote interfamilial food sharing. Food sharing assists recovery in times of illness and reduces the risk of food shortfalls due to both the vagaries of foraging luck and the variance in family size due to stochastic mortality and fertility. These buffers against mortality also favor a longer juvenile period and higher investment in other mechanisms to increase life span.

Thus, we propose that the long human life span, lengthening of the juvenile period, increased brain capacities for information processing and storage, intergenerational resource flows, and cooperative biparental investment in offspring coevolved in response to this dietary shift and the new production processes it entailed.

It is not yet possible to know many vital statistics and behavioral characteristics from paleontological and archeological remains. It must be recognized that modern hunter-gatherers are not living replicas of our Stone Age past, and global socioeconomic forces affect them all. Furthermore, many foragers today live in marginalized habitats that underreward male hunting efforts. Yet despite the variable historical, ecological, and political conditions affecting them, there is remarkable similarity among foraging peoples, and even the variation often makes adaptive sense. Comparisons between foraging peoples and other modern primates are an important source of information about the life histories of our ancestors and the selection pressures acting on them, the subject of the next sections.

Mortality and Production

The age-specific mortality profile among chimpanzees is relatively V-shaped, decreasing rapidly after infancy to its lowest point (about 3 percent per year) at about age 13, the age of first reproduction for females, and increasing sharply thereafter. In contrast, mortality among human foragers decreases to a much lower point (about 0.5 percent per year) and remains low with no increase between about 15 and 40 years of age. Mortality then increases slowly, until there is a very rapid rise in the 60s and 70s. The pattern is much more block U-shaped. The strong similarities in the mortal-

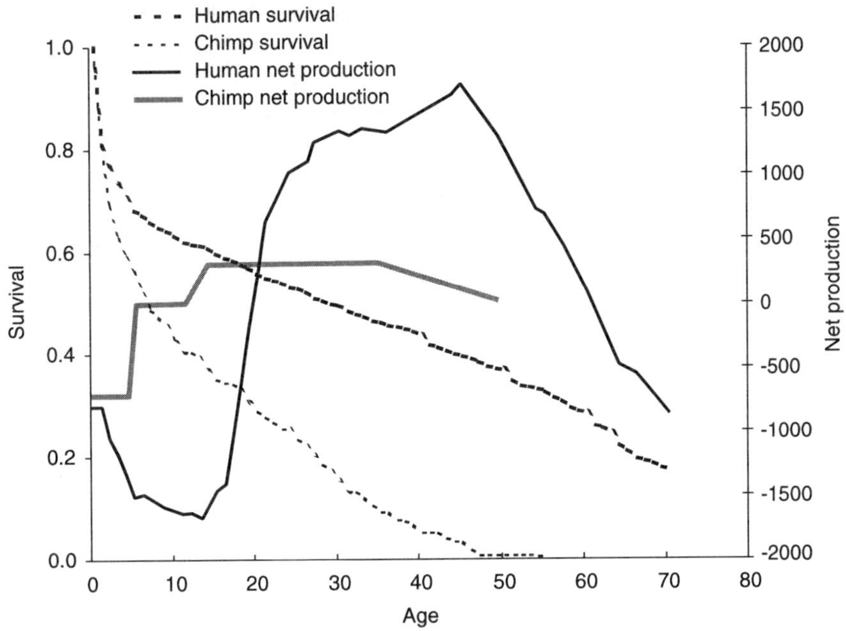

FIGURE 7-3 Net food production and survival: Human foragers and chimpanzees.

ity profiles of the foraging populations suggest that this pattern is an evolved life history characteristic of our species.

Figure 7-3 illustrates the differences between human foragers and wild-living chimpanzees. As a result of these differences in mortality pattern, hunter-gatherer children experience higher survival (60 vs. 35 percent) to age of first reproduction, at about ages 13 and 19 for chimpanzees and foragers, respectively. Chimpanzees have a much shorter adult life span than humans as well. At first reproduction, chimpanzee life expectancy is an additional 15 years, compared to 38 more years among human foragers. Importantly, women spend more than a third of their adult life in a postreproductive phase, whereas very few chimpanzee females survive to reach that phase. Fewer than 10 percent of chimpanzees survive to age 40, but more than 15 percent of hunter-gatherers survive to age 70.

Age profiles of net food production (food produced minus food consumed) also differ dramatically. Among chimpanzees, net production before age 5 is negative, representing complete, and then partial dependence on mother's milk. The second phase is independent juvenile growth, lasting until adulthood, during which net production is zero. The third phase is reproductive, during which females produce a surplus of calories that they allocate to nursing. Humans, in contrast, produce less than they consume for some 15 to 22 years, depending on the group. These same patterns appear to hold true even among subsistence agriculturalists (Kramer, 2002). Net production becomes increasingly negative until about age 14 and then begins to climb. Net production in adult humans is much higher than in chimpanzees and peaks at about 35 to 45 years of age. This peak is about five times as high as the chimpanzee peak. The human age profile of production could not exist if humans had the same mortality profile as chimpanzees (Kaplan and Robson, 2002; Robson and Kaplan, 2003). Only 30 percent of chimpanzees ever born reach the age when humans produce what they consume on average, and less than 10 percent reach the age when human production peaks.

Role of Men in Human Reproduction

Unlike most other mammals, men in foraging societies provide the majority of the energy necessary to support reproduction. After subtracting their own consumption from total production, women supply an average of 3 percent of the calories to offspring, with men providing the remaining 97 percent among the 10 foraging societies for which quantitative data on adult food production are available (Kaplan et al., 2001a). Hunting, as opposed to gathering of animal protein in small packets, is largely incompatible with the evolved commitment among primate females toward intensive mothering, carrying of infants, and lactation on demand in service of high infant survival rates. First, it is often risky, involving rapid travel and encounters with dangerous prey. Second, it is often most efficiently practiced over relatively long periods of time rather than in short stretches, due to search and travel costs. Third, it is extremely skill intensive, with improvements in return rate occurring over two decades of daily hunting. The first two qualities make hunting a high-cost activity for pregnant and lactating females. The third quality, in interaction with the first and second, generates life course effects such that gathering is a better option for females, *even when they are not lactating*, and hunting is a better option for males (Kaplan et al., 2001b). Since women spend about 75 percent of their time either nursing or more than 3 months' pregnant during their reproductive lives, it would not pay to hunt; therefore they never get enough practice to make it worthwhile, even when they are not nursing or pregnant or are postreproductive.

The fact that humans are unique in raising multiple dependent offspring of different ages also reduces the payoffs to defection and increases the benefits for men and women to link their economic and reproductive lives over the long run. Men and women who divorce and remarry during the time they are raising offspring will face conflicts of interest with new spouses over the division of resources. If they marry someone with children from previous marriages, they may disagree with their new spouses over the allocation of food and care to their joint children, relative to children from the previous marriage. Those conflicts increase the benefits of spouses staying together and having all or most of their children together.

Human females evidence physiological and behavioral adaptations that are consistent with an evolutionary history involving extensive male parental investment. They both decrease metabolic rates and store fat during pregnancy, suggesting that they lower work effort and are being provisioned (Ellison, 2001a; Lawrence and Whitehead, 1988; Pike, 1999; Poppitt et al., 1993). During lactation, women in foraging societies decrease work effort and focus on high-quality care (Hurtado et al., 1985; Lancaster et al., 2000). In contrast, nonhuman primate females do not store appreciable fat, and they increase work effort during lactation; as a result, they have increased risk of mortality (Lancaster et al., 2000). The human specialization could not have evolved if women did not depend on men for most of their food provisioning throughout human history.

Extensive cooperation among human men and women would only make sense if the reproductive performance of spouses were linked. When women reach menopause in their late 40s, men have the option to continue reproducing with younger women but generally do not do so. Among the Ache, for example, 83 percent of all last births to women also represent a last birth for the fathers of these children (Kaplan et al., 2001b).

The importance of male provisioning interacts with free access to the means of production, resulting in relatively low levels of polygyny. Although there are often territorial boundaries and disputes among neighboring groups, there is generally open access to foraging sites. Production is therefore determined by work effort and ability and is less variable as a result (although differences due to ability can be significant). The comparatively low variance in adult men's food production, coupled with the importance of male provisioning, may be why monogamy is the predominant marriage form among foragers. Figure 7-4 (using cross-cultural data from Binford, 2001) shows that the modal percentage of marriages that are polygynous among foragers is about 3 percent, with the major outliers coming from Australia (see below).

Flexibility in Fertility, Parenting, and Mating

Traditionally, demographers have attempted to understand the onset and termination of reproduction and birth intervals in natural fertility regimes in terms of proximate determinants (Bongaarts and Porter, 1983; Wood, 1994). For the most part, those determinants are treated as givens, and there has been little consideration of the causal processes shaping them.

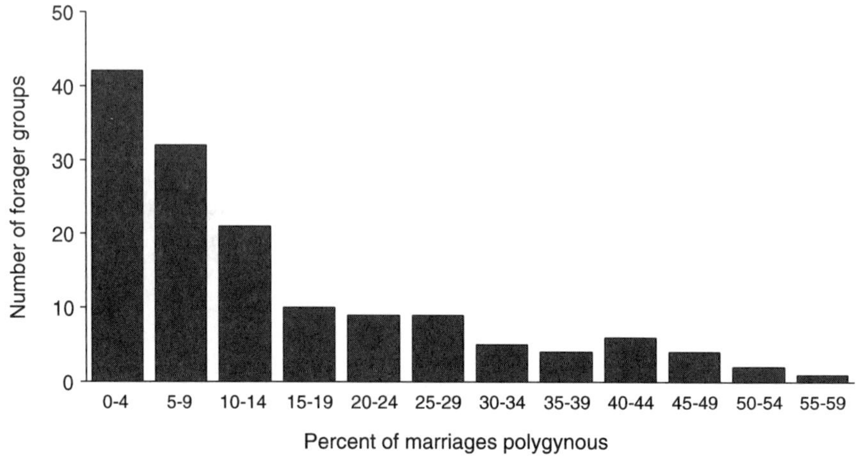

FIGURE 7-4 Frequency distribution of percentage of marriages that are polygynous among foragers.

In contrast, evolutionary demographers approach those determinants in terms of design and ask *why* the physiological, psychological, and cultural processes that regulate fecundity take the forms they do. The three trade-offs discussed above (current vs. future reproduction, quantity vs. quality of offspring, and mating vs. parenting effort) have organized research into those design features.

There is mounting evidence that human reproductive physiology is particularly specialized toward the production of high-quality, large-brained offspring. Two implications of this specialization are rigid control over embryo quality and a series of adaptations on the part of both mother and offspring designed to ensure an adequate energy supply to the nutrient-hungry, fast-growing brain. Given the massive investment in human offspring, this system ensures that investment is quickly terminated in an offspring of poor genetic quality. Fetal growth is more rapid in humans than in gorillas and chimpanzees, and both mother and offspring store exceptional amounts of fat (Kuzawa, 1998), probably to support an equally exceptional rate of extensive brain growth during the first five years of life (Ellison, 2001a, 2001b).

The physiological regulation of ovulation, fertilization, implantation, and maintenance of a pregnancy is highly responsive to energy stores in the form of fat, energy balance (calories consumed minus calories expended), and energy flux (rate of energy turnover per unit of time). Low body fat, weight loss due to negative energy balance, and extreme energy flux (either very low intake and very low expenditure, or very high intake and very high expenditure) each lower monthly probabilities of conceiving a child that will survive to birth. Seasonal variations in workloads and diet have been shown to affect female fecundity and fertility (Bailey et al., 1992; Hurtado and Hill, 1990; Prentice and Whitehead, 1987). Variation across groups in both age of menarche and fecundity has been linked to differences in food intake and workloads.

Behavior and the underlying psychological processes that govern parental investment affect fertility indirectly via maternal physiology. One route is through breast-feeding. Patterns of breast-feeding and solid food supplementation vary both cross-culturally and among mother-infant pairs (McDade, 2001; Sellen and Smay, 2001).

The second route is due to the additional energetic constraints involved in provisioning children. One fundamental trade-off with respect to activity profiles is between present and future production (Bird and Bliege Bird, 2002; Bliege Bird and Bird, 2002; Bock, 2002; Kaplan, 1996; Kramer, 2002). If children engage in easy-to-perform foraging activities, such as fruit collection, this will provide immediate caloric benefits and lower the parental subsidy required. However, time allocation to those activities detracts from time spent learning more difficult activities, such as hunting and extractive foraging. During the learning phase, those activities produce very little food but generate high rates of production in the future. Another fundamental trade-off is between production and mortality risks, since foraging exposes people to predation, accidents, and getting lost. This suggests that parental psychology should be responsive to age-specific mortality rates and how they are affected by alternative activity profiles and on their short- and long-term consequences for production/productivity.

There is a growing body of evidence to support the view that people in foraging societies are sensitive to these trade-offs and adjust their behavior accordingly. A seminal series of papers by Blurton Jones and colleagues (1994a, 1994b; Hawkes et al., 1995) shows that !Kung hunter-gatherer parents consciously assess foraging risks to children and that differences between !Kung and Hadza children's productivity are due to features of the local ecology related to ease of resource extraction and dangers associated with productive tasks. A study of foragers/agropastoralists in Botswana showed that the age profiles of children's activity budgets reflected immediate skill and strength requirements as well as opportunities to learn (Bock, 1995). In all foraging societies for which data are available, people are aware of the many years of learning required to become a competent hunter, and young men are provisioned while they learn those skills (Kaplan et al., 2000).

These time allocation decisions affect fertility through maternal energetics. The connection between psychology and fertility is indirect in that psychology adjusts parental investment (through productive behavior, wealth flows, and breast-feeding) and reproductive physiology translates parental investment decisions into fertility. The key to this system is that maximizing lifetime-expected resource production through optimal allocation of activities and wealth flows will tend also to maximize fitness when all wealth is in the form of food and extra food translates into higher fertility.

There have been several empirical applications of optimality models, designed to determine whether the onset and termination of reproduction and the size of interbirth intervals actually maximize fitness. The results of those analyses have been mixed. Blurton Jones et al. (1989) analyzed the relationship of the birth interval following a child who survived until the birth of its next sibling to the survival of either member of the sibling pair among the !Kung (Jo'hansi) in order to determine whether the observed mean interval of 48 months maximized the total number of surviving offspring. This analysis showed that 48-month birth intervals were, in fact, optimal (see Harpending, 1994; Pennington, 2001, for a critique).

In contrast, similar analyses among the Ache showed that observed birth intervals were longer than optimal (Hill and Hurtado, 1996). Phenotypic covariation, however, poses a major problem in those analyses. If healthier women have shorter birth intervals than less healthy women because they have larger effective energy resources, the estimated effect of birth intervals on offspring survival would be downwardly biased. In fact, studies examining natural variation among nonhuman organisms often show a positive, rather than a negative, relationship between fertility rate and offspring survival for the same reason (Partridge and Harvey, 1985). When fertility rate is experimentally manipulated among those same organisms, the relationship is reversed, as would be expected by a quantity-quality trade-off. Consistent with the self-selection hypothesis, Gambian women who had higher hemoglobin levels following the birth of a child exhibited both shorter interbirth intervals and higher child survival (Sear et al., 2001). Thus, it may be that women's physiology tracks its own condition in such a way as to maximize their individual fitness.

Hill and Hurtado (1996) also examined age of first reproduction and menopause to test optimality models. They found that women began reproducing at the optimal weight to maximize their lifetime fitness. However, they did not find support for the proposition that menopause maximizes fitness, as expected by the "grandmother hypothesis" (Williams, 1957). The effects of grandmothers on the fertility of their children and on the survival of their grandchildren were not large enough to overcome the fitness costs of reproductive cessation. In a parallel "contrary-to-prediction" analysis, Rogers (1993) found that the expected reproductive success of older women would have to be implausibly low to favor menopause. However, as Hill and Hurtado (1991, 1996) point out, self-selection also complicates this analysis. Grandmother's death is used to assess the impacts

TABLE 7-1 Regressions for Percent of Families That Are Polygynous Among Foragers

Parameter	*B*	Standard Error	*t*	Significance
Intercept	6.004	2.294	2.618	.010
Group size	0.294	.110	2.676	.008
% of diet from gathering	0.137	.044	3.089	.002

NOTE: $N = 145$, $R^2 = .10$.
SOURCE: Binford (2001).

of older women on the fitness of their children and grandchildren, but in kin-based societies other relatives probably compensate for the death of a kinswoman, producing another downward bias in effect estimation.

Finally, there is evidence that mating behavior responds to ecological variability in subsistence ecology, associated with complementarity and variance in access. Using the same cross-cultural data set as in Figure 7-4, a regression of the percentage of marriages that are polygynous on the percentage of the diet derived from gathered foods and the size of mobile foraging groups suggests that increased reliance on female contributions is associated with higher levels of polygyny (see Table 7-1). The one exceptional area, where polygyny is much greater than average, is Australia. There high rates of polygyny are found in the northern territories and Queensland, with the most extreme case being the Tiwi (51 percent of marriages being polygynous). In a sense they are the exception that proves the rule because, according to ethnographic sources (Goodale, 1971; Hart and Pilling, 1960), Tiwi women are actively involved in hunting and fishing. In that coastal environment there are small game and fishing opportunities that are more like gathering than hunting (e.g., catching small, sleeping animals) and women can be more economically self-sufficient.

The next section treats major historical trends in reproduction, parenting, and mating practices associated with the domestication of plants and animals.

REPRODUCTIVE BEHAVIOR SINCE THE DOMESTICATION OF PLANTS AND ANIMALS

Sedentism and Tribal Horticulture

The Socioecological Context

Village sedentism and the domestication of plants had a profound, yet limited, impact on human socioecology. Subsistence based on horticulture rests on land-extensive, slash-and-burn agriculture on prime resource patches, access to which was maintained by the social group and defended by males against outsiders. Within the group, access is on the basis of a usufruct system of land tenure that gives all group members direct rights to the means of production and reproduction (Boserup, 1970; Goody, 1976). People live in small villages, larger than hunter-gatherer bands but similarly scaled in terms of face-to-face, kinship-laden interactions.

There is evidence that sedentism brings a reduction in child mortality compared to hunter-gatherers, as well as higher female fertility, although it is unclear whether the strongest effects are in reduced birth spacing or higher rates of child survival (Bentley et al., 2001). The potential of deaths from chronic intergroup warfare and raiding increases, particularly affecting males in which the percentage mobilized often reaches 35 to 40 percent and male deaths from 10 to nearly 60 percent (Keeley, 1996). Complementarity in the male and female division of labor is complex because of its link to local ecology. Garden production by women using the dibble and hoe provides the carbohydrate and caloric base of the diet and is easily combined with child care (Boserup, 1970; Goody, 1976). Males contribute their labor in clearing fields, in animal protein through hunting and fishing, and in protection of the village resource base through defense.

The relative contribution and imperative of male help vary by ecological context. For example, female gardening of high-protein crops on riverine alluvial soils, such as millet and sorghum in much of village Africa (Colson, 1960; Lancaster, 1981), is very different from subsistence based on manioc in the thin soils of South America. There male hunting is critical to balanced macronutrients in the diet and frequent clearing is necessary. Similarly, the critical need for defense of the village resource base is supplied by males as an umbrella benefit rather than to specific wives. More recently, the benefit of such defense was much reduced under colonial suppression of warfare and raiding. However, since neither males nor females produce beyond subsistence needs and the means of production are held in common through usufruct, there is little opportunity for major variance in resource holding. However, variance in male reproductive success does arise on the basis of their success in raiding, which brings certain males both high status and more wives (Chagnon, 1979).

Mating Patterns, Parental Investment, and Reproduction

Reproduction in horticultural societies is associated with near-universal marriage for both sexes, with reproduction beginning at sexual maturity for women and extending through the entire period of fecundity. Reproduction for men is somewhat delayed due to the need to access wives through either bride service (local group) or bride capture (outside group), the first being a personal cost in labor contributed to the bride's family and the second a personal cost in terms of risk. However, polygyny extends the male reproductive period as new and younger wives are added through time.

The high frequency of polygynous marriages associated with horticulture may be because each wife is essentially able to support herself and her children through her own labor (Lancaster and Kaplan, 1992; Murdock, 1967). Males do not have to ponder whether they can afford additional wives and children, only how they can get and keep them. As White and Burton (1988) found, polygyny is most associated with fraternal interest groups, warfare for the capture of women, absence of constraints on expansion into new lands, especially for horticulturalists, environmental quality, and homogeneity. The practice of widow inheritance by husband's kin also increases the frequency of polygyny (Kirwin, 1979). The form, sororal polygyny, is at its highest frequency due to the ease of sisters forming collaborative horticultural work groups (Irons, 1979b).

Parental investment in horticultural societies focuses on raising healthy children without concern for their marriage market endowments or inheritance of resources. Birth into a social group provides all the inheritance a child would need to access the means of production and reproduction. Such concepts as bastardy or disinheritance do not play a formal role in family dynamics. Child labor is valuable to families since horticulture provides a number of relatively low-skilled tasks that older children can perform. In fact, Kramer (2002) demonstrated that among Maya horticulturalists older children contribute at the level of "helpers-at-the-nest," significantly increasing their parents' fertility and without whose help their parents could not add further offspring to the family.

Variance in reproductive success is relatively low for women because marriage is universal, and female fertility and fecundity depend on their own productivity and work effort (Ellison, 2001a; Jasienska, 2000; Prentice and Whitehead, 1987). Greater variance among men was possible on the basis of raiding and bride capture, but the social system itself is not stratified and individual men cannot amass or control access to resources relative to other men or pass them on to their sons.

Extrasomatic Wealth and Tribal Pastoralism

The Socioecological Context

The domestication of animals, particularly large herd animals such as cattle, camels, and horses, proved to have a profound effect on human social and reproductive patterns. Large domesticated livestock have intrinsic qualities that affected human social relationships, marriage patterns, and investment in children. For the first time in human history, men could control a form of extrasomatic wealth that could be held by individuals, thus increasing the variance in male quality based on the resources each could control.

Second, herds are the basis of the domestic economy through their products of meat, milk, and hides. There are advantages to dependence on such a resource supply: (1) improvements in diets rich in animal protein, (2) stability of diets since animals are stored hedges against fluctuations in annual or seasonal climatic effects, and (3) flexibility due to the divisibility of herds into smaller units that can be moved about the landscape on the basis of the richness and concentration of local resources. This improvement in diet may result in higher fertility and survivorship of women and children compared to foraging and horticulture but also higher mortality for males due to endemic conflict. Generally, however, pastoralists show a wide range in fertility levels due to the many different kinds of pastoralism with respect to agricultural supplementation, disease risk, mobility, and so forth (Borgerhoff Mulder, 1992; Sellen and Mace, 1997). Large-animal herding demands a high degree of complementarity between female processing and child care and male risk taking in herd management and defense. The products of herds require intensive processing of meat, milk and hides, labor provided by women. In contrast, the very existence of extrasomatic wealth in large stock in such a readily divisible and moveable form (as opposed to agricultural land) puts a high premium on males as defenders and raiders. We find the warrior complex full blown, with chronic internal warfare, blood feuds, the social segregation of a male warrior age class, fraternal interest groups, a geographic flow of women from subordinate to dominant groups through bride capture, and expansionist segmentary lineages based on the male line (DiVale and Harris, 1976; Low, 2000; White and Burton, 1988). Men with strong social alliances are more likely to find at least some of their wives from within their own social groups, whereas men from small or subordinate lineages are willing to take more risks in lieu of performing bride service (Chagnon, 1988, 2000; Lancaster, 1981).

The original distinction made by Orians (1969) between resource defense polygyny and harem defense polygyny is relevant here. The chronic warfare of pastoralists (Keeley, 1996; Manson and Wrangham, 1991; White and Burton, 1988) can be understood as resource defense polygyny, as opposed to the harem defense polygyny described earlier for horticultural societies. Both types of societies raid to capture women, but pastoralists also raid to capture resources that can be used to acquire and maintain new wives and their children. In a study of 75 traditional societies, the principal cause of warfare was either women (45 percent of cases) or material resources for obtaining a bride (39 percent of the cases), particularly in pastoral societies where bride wealth must be paid (Manson and Wrangham, 1991).

Mating Patterns, Parental Investment, and Reproduction

Resource defense polygyny means that males will compete to control the resources that females must have for successful reproduction. A male's ability to successfully control more resources translates directly into more wives and children (Borgerhoff Mulder, 1989, 1991, 1995). One extraordinary result of extrasomatic wealth, particularly readily partible wealth, is the institution of a new pawn on the marriage market table—bride wealth. Women and their families come to marriage negotiations with their traditional offers (youth, health, fecundity, and female labor). Men, however, now have to come up with a significant payment of resources in the form of bride wealth as a preferred substitute for bride service.

Bride wealth among pastoralists consists of horses, cattle, or camels, with sheep or goats as supplements or lower-valued substitutes. Among African pastoralists the close male kin of the groom helps him with his first bride wealth payment, but the acquisition of subsequent wives is his own responsibility. Livestock used for bride wealth has interesting attributes: (1) it creates conflicts of interest between fathers and sons and among brothers for its use to obtain a bride (Borgerhoff Mulder, 1988), (2) men from poor families will be more willing to take risks to obtain bride wealth or brides though capture (see Dunbar's 1991 discussion of war chiefs and peace chiefs among the Cheyenne), and (3) livestock can be inherited.

Investment in children takes a novel form under a pastoralist system. The payment of bride wealth improves health and survivorship among young girls because their marriages bring in resources that can be used by their fathers and brothers to acquire more wives (Borgerhoff Mulder, 1998). Sub-Saharan Africa is notable for the fact that despite the patrilineal bias in so many societies, neither a survival nor a nutritional advantage is found for boys over girls (Svedberg, 1990). Furthermore, among the Kipsigis, who are agropastoralists, early-maturing (and presumably better fed and healthier) women have higher lifetime reproductive success than late-maturing women, command higher bride wealth, and hence constitute a higher return on parental investment in their upbringing (Borgerhoff Mulder, 1989). They also represent a better investment for a husband's bride wealth payment because of a higher return in fertility.

Furthermore, children are able to provide child care of younger siblings as well as low-skilled labor in stock care and the processing of animal products, so they are able to substantially but not completely offset the costs of their rearing (Bock, 1995, 2002). However, this is countered by the fact that the parents of sons now have a new cost to meet, the balloon payment (bride wealth) needed at the end of their sons' development and perhaps equal to the summed previous investment to establish sons on the marriage market. The flow of stock through families that are both bride wealth receivers and givers helps maintain the system at the same time that it creates problems for families with unfavorable ratios of sons to daughters (Borgerhoff Mulder, 1998).

Finally and most significantly, there is suggestive evidence that for the first time humans began to reproduce at levels that may not maximize the number of descendents with the appearance of extrasomatic wealth and its inheritance. Men appear to marry fewer wives than they could afford in the interests of providing each child with a greater endowment. In other words, male pastoralists may pit quality against quantity of children to preserve a lineage status and resource base rather than simply maximizing the number of descendents (Borgerhoff Mulder, 2000; Mace, 2000).

Social Stratification in the PreModern Era: States and Despotism

The Socioecological Context

The rise of civilizations, beginning about 6,000 years ago in Mesopotamia and occurring at different times and places (e.g., Egypt in the Near East, the Aztec and Inca in the Americas, and India and China in Asia) marked a critical shift in how humans organized themselves in social systems and in relation to the environment (Betzig, 1993; Goody, 1976). These civilizations appear to have developed independently in response to local conditions without being the products of either conquest or diffusion. Despite this historical independence, they evidence significant similarities: (1) the presence of large stratified social groupings settled on particularly large and productive resource patches and (2) the appearance of social despots, men who use coercive political power to defend their wealth and reproduction and warfare to acquire more resource patches and slaves (Betzig, 1986). These two major effects flow from the nature of the resource patches.

The patches on which the first civilizations were settled had special qualities: (1) they were highly productive but set in environments where there was a rapid falloff to unproductive lands such as desert or forest and (2) these productive patches could not be intensively utilized without complex political organization as in regional irrigation systems. Political control and organization rested on the power of men. Although female nonhuman primates often form alliances with their female kin to protect and control access to the resources necessary for their reproduction (Isbell, 1991; Sterck et al., 1997), the reproductive benefits of resources are much greater for men than for women because of their impacts on polygyny. The end result of these environmental conditions associated with early social stratification was that men competed for control of the resources necessary for reproduction and formed despotic hierarchies involving social alliances and stratification, with low-status men "agreeing" to live under political despotism because they could not readily move to another resource base.

The increased reliability of food resources, the costs of warfare, and the concentrations of large populations into small urban areas each had impacts on mortality and morbidity. A cross-cultural analysis of fertility and mode of subsistence found that, for a 10 percent increase in dependence on agriculture between "sister" cultures, there is a fertility increase of approximately 0.2 live births per woman (Sellen and Mace, 1997). Bentley et al. (2001), in reviewing the cross-cultural and archeological evidence, suggested a series of multidirectional effects: higher fertility due to more consistent food supply and earlier maturation; increased infectious diseases with regular visitations as well as endemic diseases, such as malaria and tuberculosis, due to long-distance trade and large urban populations; and a shift in peak mortality from infancy to middle childhood. Furthermore, warfare continues to reduce the numbers of young men in the mate pool.

With social stratification comes a complex division of labor with specialists in war, farming, crafts for the production of goods and services, and war captives and slaves for the hardest manual labor, as well as long-distance trade in luxury goods and slaves. The introduction of the plow in Eurasia and the need for food production beyond simple subsistence to service the needs of urban markets led to significant changes in the division of labor (Ember, 1983; Goody, 1976) and extremely high complementarity between male labor and resource acquisition and female labor and child care. There is evidence of increased workloads for women despite the fact that men assume more responsibility for farm labor, because of increased demands for women to process grains or secondary animal products such as milk, hides, and wool (Bentley et al., 2001). They cite evidence that women's physical activity levels as measured by PALs (the multiple of resting basal metabolic rate required for activity) among hunter-gatherers and horticulturalists are very similar, with means of 1.72 and 1.79, respectively, but that with agriculture it increases substantially to 2.31.

Variance in male resource holding was probably the greatest it has ever been in human history (Betzig, 1986, 1992a, 1992b, 1993). The reason for this is that despotic males had enormous political and social control with the ability to eliminate rivals and their entire families through despotic edicts, to wage war to increase personal and state resource bases, to acquire slaves and war captives for labor and reproduction, and to determine political succession for favored sons. This extreme variance in male resource holding inevitably produces political instability due to the creation of too many potential heirs (sons of many wives) and too many males (slaves) without access to the means of reproduction. The great wealth to be gained from domination also motivated expansion and intergroup conflict among would-be despots.

Finally, a notable characteristic of the premodern period in many parts of the world is evidence for a growing rural population resulting from higher fertility and associated growing concerns regarding saturation of the resource environment. This is often associated with urban growth, empire building and colonial expansionism, providing opportunities for migration by noninheriting or low-status children to areas of both higher mortality and risk but also with the potential for the acquisition of employment, land, or wealth and power. It also generated a great deal of concern about keeping the family estate intact and about the management of inheritance.

Mating Patterns, Parental Investment, and Reproduction

Despotic males are an extreme example of resource defense polygyny (Orians, 1969); that is, as individuals they control access to the resource base for reproduction that females require and, with few competitors, polygynous marriages to them become the only family formation strategy option for many women. The mating markets of despotic systems are characterized by historic extremes in male variance in resource holding and power. Table 7-2 presents data on the numbers of wives and children of despots in some of these early civilizations. As Betzig (1993) notes, the extreme sizes of royal harems ranging from 4,000 to 16,000 women in these examples are associated with smaller but still impressive numbers of wives and concubines for the royal supporters. In the case of the Inca, the size of a man's harem was regulated by law and was in direct relationship to his social/political rank. Among the Inca there were nine levels of political rankings with polygyny ceilings for each except the top-most. These harems were exclusive holdings of large numbers of young fecund women with their children, and access to them was restricted to their mate and regulated

TABLE 7-2 The Wives of Despots

Country	Century	Royal Harems	Reign
India	5th B.C.	16,000	Udayama
	15th A.D.	12,000	Deva Raya II
	16th A.D.	4,000-12,000	
China	618-907 A.D.	10,000	
Inca Peru	early 16th A.D.	1,500 per province	
Aztec Mexico	early 16th A.D.	4,000	

SOURCE: Betzig (1993).

with some sophistication to optimize female fertility. Many of these wives and concubines were collected as tribute or war booty, but others, as principal wives, probably represented important political alliances with their male relatives.

There are two clear outcomes of such variance. The first is that many men remain unmated or have only one wife, so male celibacy or at least nonmarital sex is prominent. In the words of Dickemann, polygyny in the context of extreme social stratification is "characterized not only by arbitrary sexual rights of lords and rulers but by large numbers of masculine floaters and promiscuous semi-floaters, beggars, bandits, outlaws, kidnappers, militia, and resentful slaves and serfs." (Dickemann, 1981:427). Nevertheless, these early despotic states lasted for thousands of years. A second outcome of variance in male resource holding and male mating success is that there tends to be universal marriage for women, with only those most severely compromised by health or other personal qualities being unlikely to find a role as secondary wife or minor union. For access to the mating market, men must bring wealth, power, and land in order to be favorably placed or else get wives as high-risk booty in state warfare (Clarke and Low, 2001; Low, 2000).

Women, too, bring their traditional qualities of youth, health, and fecundity along with their labor. However, there is a historic shift in how women and their families approach the mating market that has been richly described in a series of papers on hypergyny, dowry, female infanticide, and paternity confidence (Dickemann, 1979a, 1979b, 1981). The extreme variance in male quality created by despotism and harem polygyny forces the families of women to put down more and more value on the mate market table to access a desirable groom or to move a daughter up in the social hierarchy. These extra payments form an area of female-female competition that includes actual wealth, in the form of dowry, and guarantees of paternity confidence (bridal virginity and wifely chastity; (Gaulin and Boster, 1990). Guarantees of a daughter's virginity and chastity (a prerequisite for a bride destined to produce heirs to a male lineage holding a reproductive estate) are costly, involving female seclusion (special women's quarters, harem guards, chaperones) and female incapacitation (e.g., foot binding and corseting) that bars their daughters from the outside world of productive labor.

Endowment of Children with Access to Reproductive Estates

Parental concern over the ability of their children to access reproductive estates transforms the nature of the marriage market. Parental investment in these systems varies in relation to the power and wealth of the male's family. As is to be expected, under such conditions where male access to and control of resources is the basis of social stratification, patrilineal descent and patrilocal residence are highly favored since males are the principal resource holders (Hartung, 1982). Resource-holding parents commit to a balloon payment, very large and late in the period of parental investment, to launch their children in marriage. This balloon payment takes the form of endowments, promised inheritance, and dowry as anticipatory inheritance for daughters (Dickemann, 1979a, 1979b; Goody, 1973, 1976). For resource-holding families, then, the marriage market formed by stratified social systems proves costly in terms of parental investment and forces a focus on endowments for both sexes at the age of marriage. Poor parents, on the other hand, attempt to balance labor demands with fertility, since in agricultural systems children can be productive at low-skill tasks or child care and thus add to the family economy. They might try to regulate birth spacing to optimize the productivity of already-born children before another mouth to feed is added to the family.

Historic Trends in the Reduction of Claimants to the Family Estate

With population growth and increased saturation of arable lands, parents adopt patterns of restricted and differential inheritance in order to keep the family estate intact and maintain the concentration of wealth or, in the case of the poor, to balance food supply with family size. Boswell (1990) and Hrdy (1994) provide evidence from classical Europe of attempts by parents to limit the burden of excess children through abandonment. However, well-to-do families also practice abandonment in an attempt to limit the number of potential heirs to political succession and inheritance, as evidenced by the placement of secret identifying markers so that a child might be retrieved later should its older same-sex sibling die.

This trend is particularly well documented in premodern Europe. Human evolutionary ecologists in collaboration with historical demographers have provided a unique record of the relationships between fertility, family formation strategies, and the socioecological context during the premodern and early modern periods of European history (see review in Voland, 2000)). Their studies, based on heraldic or parish records of births, marriages, deaths, and inheritance of estates, can be used to directly link reproductive strategies with resource holdings. This time period witnessed developments that had began centuries earlier but occurred without the benefit of quantifiable documentation. Boone, for example, traces the historical process of parental investment among Portuguese elites during the medieval/early modern periods of the 15th and 16th centuries (Boone, 1986, 1988). Saturation and resource stress are evident with a progressive narrowing of the numbers of claimants to an inheritance, first through monogamy and bastardy creating a single bloodline of inheritors (Goody, 1976, 1983), followed by a preference for sons over daughters as inheritors, and finally by birth-order effects with preference for primogeniture within each sex for access to resources and the creation of celibate children to live as priests, nuns, bachelors, and spinsters (Hrdy and Judge, 1993). For the first time in human history, mating and reproduction are no longer universal for women. With survival through childhood and young adulthood still quite problematic, ancillary practices develop in which both sons and daughters would be held in reserve in monasteries and nunneries for inheritance should their older same-sex sibling die before reproduction (Boone, 1986, 1988; Goody, 1976, 1983). Within the scope of these restrictions that limit half-sibling and sibling competition, parents with wealth raise as many children as they can but endow a select number at adulthood.

During most of this historical period there is a strong correlation between wealth, probability of marriage, younger age at marriage, and completed fertility (Voland, 2000). However, restricted inheritance decreases the reproductive benefits of polygyny. The desire to concentrate wealth also limits the reproductive success of noninheriting sons and daughters. This may be another example in which reproductive and parental investment behavior in response to extrasomatic wealth results in outcomes that do not maximize parental fitness. In fact, toward the end of the period, as life expectancy improved and economic structures became saturated, resource holding groups delay marriage into the late 30s and early 40s for men and mid-20s for women (Szreter and Garrett, 2000; Voland, 2000).

Family reconstruction studies document very different reproductive strategies according to class.[3] Generally, wealth brings higher probability of marriage at a younger age, to a younger spouse, and more children. However, as environments become more saturated, local resource competition among siblings differentially affects resource-holding families, as opposed to day laborers, and increases the likelihood of dispersal of later-born children (Clarke and Low, 1992; Towner, 1999, 2001; Voland and Dunbar, 1997). With saturation the benefits to resource holders of having an above-average number of children is offset by more and more intense sibling competition for access to inheritance (Voland, 2000). Parents without resources have no need to manipulate their offspring and are more likely to benefit from opportunistic strategies by their children (Voland and Dunbar, 1995). An extreme form of such parental manipulation of offspring marital

[3]The behaviors of nobility are documented by Boone (1986, 1988) for Portugal; Dickemann (1979a, 1979b, 1981) for Europe, the Middle East, China, and India; for gentry and land-holding peasants as well as day laborers by Voland and colleagues for Germany (Voland, 1990, 2000; Voland and Chasiotis, 1998; Voland and Dunbar, 1995, 1997; Voland et al., 1991, 1997; Voland and Engel, 1990), Low (1990, 1991, 1994) for Sweden; Towner (1999, 2001) for the United States; and Hughes (1986) and Scott and Duncan (1999) for England.

opportunities is polyandry in which a male sibship jointly marries a single woman in order to avoid division of property and labor among competing households of wives and children of brothers (Crook and Crook, 1988; Haddix, 2001). Wet-nursing during this period presents a fascinating example of how differentiation in parental investment strategies develops into extreme forms for both the highest and the lowest status groups of women. Throughout human history there has always existed a conflict between production and reproduction for women, a conflict that in fact troubles female mammals in general. Human women are especially caught in this conflict because they have multiple dependent young of differing ages and needs (Draper, 1992), which means that a true respite never occurs until all children are reared. Cross-culturally women's work is organized by its compatibility with child care (Brown, 1970); however, this compatibility is never complete—only more or less so (Hurtado and Hill, 1990; Lancaster, 1997; Lancaster et al., 2000). During this period of social stratification some women, for the first time, are able to subvert the physiological capacity of lactation of other women to serve their own reproductive ends. Since intense breast-feeding lowers the likelihood of ovulation, wet-nurses, even if paid, are sacrificing their own fecundity to another's (Hrdy, 1994, 1999).

Typically high-status women do not breast-feed their own children but use wet-nurses. This increases the fertility of high-status women, whose main function is to produce heirs, to a nearly annual birth rate (among the highest for any group of women in human history). In contrast, the birth spacing for their wet-nurses is closer to 4 years (Hrdy, 1994). A second group of women also used wet-nurses, especially towards the end of this historic period. These were single women working in urban centers or the wives of poor tradesman who found themselves in positions of servitude or trade where the incompatibility between breast-feeding and work was complete. To great detriment to their infant's survival, these women placed their children with commercial wet-nurses. In these cases the demands of maternal work far outweighed the needs of infant growth, perhaps to further the interests of weaned older children.

Modern Labor Markets

The Ecological Context

Given rural reproductive and survival rates, the restricted inheritance system discussed above produces excess adults without access to land and the means of production. Colonization through conquest was one response by males, especially later-born sons (Boone, 1986; Curtin, 1989) to this situation. Another response by both men and women was to provide services for others and migration to cities in search of employment. This supply of labor and of consumers helped fuel the growth of a mercantile economy that was to gradually supplant the power- and land-based hierarchies of the pre-modern period.

The directional change in the nature of labor markets toward greater wage premiums for skill- and education-based capital over the last two centuries is well documented (e.g., Burck, 1976; Herrnstein and Murray, 1994; Newcomer, 1955; Vinovskis, 1994). The relationship between education and income increased considerably during the second half of the 20th century. For example, in the United States, real wages actually dropped from 1958 to 1990 among men without high school degrees. In 1958, men with a graduate education earned about 2.3 times as much as men with an elementary school education; by 1990 they earned more than 3.5 times as much. Wage differentials among men with some college education, bachelor's degrees, and graduate degrees also increased substantially. For women, wage differentials by education levels increased substantially in the 1980s (Kaplan et al., 2002).

As the extent of the labor and consumer markets grew, along with advances in production technologies, there was a concomitant increase in both private and public investments in education. In a sense, the relationship between embodied capital and production in modern skills-based labor markets is more similar to the foraging way of life than to its agricultural predecessor. Rather than generating wealth through control of land, people invest in learning to increase productivity, and individuals are free to move through the environment in search of economic opportunities.

These increases in educational capital investment and the nature of labor markets were accompanied by improvements in the "technology" of disease prevention and treatment and by increased public and private investments in health and mortality reduction. During the 19th century, there were large changes in the scientific understanding of disease (see Preston and Haines, 1991, for a review). This led to dramatic declines in infant, child, and adult mortality rates that continued for close to a century. As scientific advances enabled reductions in mortality rates, there was strong pressure to increase public investments in health and disease prevention, from protection of the water supply to development of vaccines and public access to medical care. As a result, infant and child mortality rates were reduced dramatically, greatly increasing the probability that investments in children would be realized in terms of productive adulthood. The length of the productive adult life span, especially when time lost to morbidity is taken into account, has also increased significantly. Together, the two shifts in production processes and mortality rates favor increased human capital investment in a way that is reminiscent of the initial dietary shift leading to the hominid specialization discussed above.

This historical process also resulted in much greater labor force participation by women. During the initial demographic transition in the developed world, the breadwinner-homemaker family structure was dominant. With increased demand for labor that requires skill as opposed to strength and with growth in the service sector of the economy, wage-earning opportunities for women increased. At the same time, the payoffs to "home" production decreased with labor-saving devices, such as washing machines and refrigerators, and with smaller family size reducing the number of years spent caring for small children. Over time, therefore, there was a trend from greater to lesser complementarity between men and women.

Although the shift toward an education-based wage structure has been largely monotonic, those changes occurred at different times in the developed and developing worlds, and the details of the supply and demand for labor of different levels of human capital have been both historically and regionally variable. Moreover, both within and among societies, there appears to be a great deal of variation in rates of return on investments in educational capital.

The production of human capital is human-capital intensive (Becker and Barro, 1988). To see this, it is useful to think of an "education production function." In each year of a child's life, the amount he or she learns and the changes in his or her knowledge, reading, writing, logic and mathematical skills will depend on many different inputs, such as time, prior abilities, parents' time, and teacher's time. The value of those inputs, in terms of the educational capital produced, depends on the quality of those inputs. First, consider parents' time. There is significant evidence that the nature of parent-child interaction varies with the educational level of the parents (Hart and Risley, 1995; Hoff-Ginsberg and Tardiff, 1995). For example, Hart and Risley report that, by the age of 3, children heard six million words if their mothers were professionals, 3 million words if their mothers were "working class", and only 1 million words if their mothers were on welfare. By the time children enter the public education system there are clear differences in school-related skills, and those differences are related to socioeconomic status.

Second, the rate at which a child learns may depend on the knowledge and skills he or she already possesses. Much of the education offered in schools is based on the premise that knowledge is cumulative (Cromer, 1993). Basic skills are acquired first, and those skills are used as a foundation for the acquisition of the next set of skills. This implies that the impact of a child's time inputs would depend on the skills already in place. It also means that the net increase in embodied capital at each age is a function of both the quality of inputs and the capital acquired at younger ages.

Moreover, those qualities tend to be correlated across inputs. Children with more educated parents also attend better schools with better teachers and better fellow students. At the other extreme, children in developing nations often come from families in which neither parent has had formal schooling and attend schools with very large class sizes, almost no library resources, and teachers with only a primary education themselves. Under those conditions, much less is learned per year spent in schooling. For example, in a study of a predominantly black school in Cape Town, South Africa, Anderson et al. (2001) found that, on average, it took children 15 years to complete 12 grades of schooling. By that age (20 to 21), only about 10 percent of students passed the final matriculation exam and earned a high school diploma. The variance in those inputs leads to an increasing differentiation in educational capital with age.

This within-population heterogeneity in the costs of embodying capital in children means that environment does not determine diminishing returns to parental investment as it would be in primary production economies but will be frequency dependent. First, consider the highest-skilled jobs in the economy. Those jobs would be filled by individuals with the lowest costs of skill acquisition in decreasing rank order until the point is reached when the next-cheapest worker is more expensive than the product he or she produces. His or her parents would therefore invest less in his or her than would be necessary to obtain the highest-skilled jobs, and he or she would find employment in the next skill tier. That tier would then be occupied by individuals in decreasing rank order, until the next-cheapest worker will not be paid enough to compensate for skill embodiment. This process would continue through to the lowest-skilled jobs in the economy.

Individuals with low levels of human capital are more likely to be unemployed as well as to have a lower income when they are employed. This is especially true in urban areas in the developing world. The massive rural to urban migration over the past 40 years has resulted in very large populations of people with low levels of education competing for a limited number of low- skilled jobs. In many places, male unemployment can be as high as 70 percent. This variability in educational capital, along with its impacts on income variation across individuals and within individuals over time, has profound effects on family formation and reproduction.

Reproduction and Parental Investment

There is considerable evidence that in response to these conditions people in modern societies do not maximize fitness through their fertility decisions (see Kaplan and Lancaster, 2000, for a review). Observed fertility behavior deviates from the predictions of fitness maximization in two ways. First, and most important, observed fertility is lower than would be predicted based on models of fitness maximization. For example, among men in Albuquerque, New Mexico, the number of third-generation descendants (i.e., grandchildren) is highest among those who produced the most (i.e.,

>12) children (Kaplan et al., 1995). This contrasts sharply with the observed modal fertility of two. Mueller (2001) presents similar evidence from several other data sets in Europe and the United States. Higher parental fertility in modern developed societies is associated with lower educational and economic status of offspring (Blake, 1989; Downey, 1995), but the lower earning capacity of children from large families does not decrease their fertility, and so there is no apparent fitness reduction associated with lowered parental investment per child (Kaplan et al., 1995).

The second way in which modern behavior deviates from the predictions of simple budget constraint models of quantity-quality trade-offs is that higher-earning adults produce no more children than their lesser-earning counterparts, even in well-controlled studies. Whereas available data on preindustrial societies consistently exhibit a positive relationship between resources or power and reproductive success (Betzig, 1986; Boone, 1986; Chagnon, 1988; Hughes, 1986; Irons, 1979a; Kaplan and Hill, 1985; Low, 1990; Voland, 1990), studies of postdemographic transition societies either find no relationship or a negative one (Kaplan et al., 1995; Vining, 1986).

There is some evidence that the transition to low fertility begins with a negative association between income and fertility and then proceeds to a phase in which there is no association between the two (Kaplan and Lancaster, 2000; Retherford, 1993; Szreter and Garrett, 2000). Perhaps, the reason why the transition begins with a negative association between wealth and fertility is that the payoffs to investment in oneself and one's offspring were not the same across economic strata. First, infant and child mortality rates are much lower among the wealthy than the poor (Preston and Haines, 1991) in both Europe and America. Second, wealthy parents tend to be more educated and to have greater access to educational resources. Our hypothesis is that, as a result, wealthier parents were able to educate their offspring more efficiently than poorer parents could and had a greater return on investments in both their and their offspring's education.

Public- and private-sector responses to these trends then begin to change the payoffs to such investments among the poorer and less educated sectors of society. Increased public investments in health and schooling decrease mortality rates and increase the efficiency of private investments in children's schooling for all sectors of society. More effective and less costly forms of birth control technologies allow for a significant reduction in birth rates. A more educated populace expands the expertise in firms with respect to both management and the technology of production, further increasing the demand for skilled workers. Ultimately, those interactions produce equal fertility among economic strata. Wealthier, more educated people invest more per child than poorer, less educated people because they are still more efficient at embodying capital in their children, but their higher wealth allows them to have as many children (although more costly) as less wealthy individuals.

Thus, what appears to be a gradual decrease in fertility through time according to national-level statistics may actually be a process in which an increasing proportion of the population exhibits very low fertility.

The effect of education on fertility varied with the total fertility rate during the 20th century. For men and women born early in the century, who reproduced during the Depression and war years, education delayed fertility. There was little effect of education on fertility during the Baby Boom years, when all education groups showed a reduction in age of first reproduction. As education became an increasingly important determinant of wages in the last third of the 20th century and fertility decreased again, the effects of education on fertility were most pronounced (Kaplan et al., 2002).

Virtually all of the effects of education on fertility are due to postponement of marriage and a delay from marriage to reproduction. The delay, coupled with age effects on fecundity due to reproductive physiology, results in lower completed fertility. For example, data from the National Survey of Families and Households show that among women 35 to 44 years of age in 1990, high school dropouts have a mean of 2.77 children, which drops to 2.22 for those with high school degrees, 1.95 for those with bachelor's degrees, and 1.43 for those with graduate degrees (Kaplan et al., 2002).

These shifts in the economy also appear to have had profound effects on mating and marriage. Two opposing forces act on marital stability. The decrease in complementarity associated with women's entry into the labor force (especially when women began to reenter the labor force after short maternity leaves) renders divorce less costly, since women no longer rely solely on males for financial support. This change in the costs of divorce inspired the reform of divorce laws and, ultimately, increases in the divorce rate. On the other hand, the greater importance of education in wage determination increases educational homogamy in the mating market and parental assessments about the level of investment children require. Support for college is another form of balloon payment in the parental investment stream. Divorce has a large negative impact on both the probability that offspring will attend college and the likelihood of paternal financial support for college (Anderson et al., 1999b; Kaplan et al., 2002).

These two opposing forces affect people differentially, on the basis of their education and presumably their expected rate of return on investments in their children's education. The effects of education on divorce when children are young are striking. Figure 7-5 shows the probability that a man will cease to live with a child before the age of 6 as a function of the child's birth cohort and the father's education level among men in Albuquerque, New Mexico. The increase in divorce rates is clearly evident. However, there is an interaction effect between a man's education and the child's birth cohort on the probability of separation between a child and its father. Among children whose father has less than a high school education,

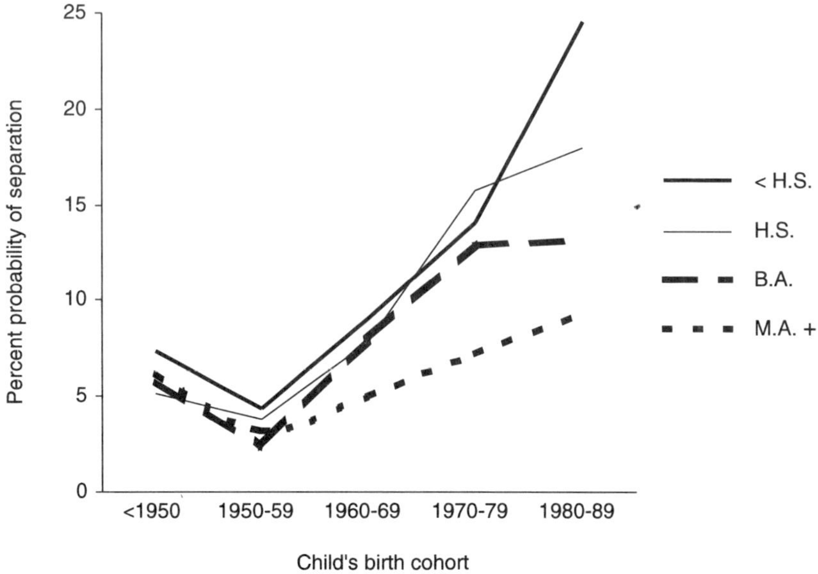

FIGURE 7-5 Father's probability of ceasing to live with his child before the age of 6.
SOURCE: Kaplan et al. (2002). Reprinted with permission of Wiley-Liss, Inc., a subsidiary of John Wiley & Sons, Inc.

the percentage of children who cease to live with him before age 6 rises from about 5 percent for children born before 1960 to 23 percent for children born in the 1980 cohort. Among children whose father has a graduate degree, the percentage of children who cease to live with him before age 6 did not change significantly during this period and remains between 5 and 8 percent.

On the high end of the education continuum, both men and women delay marriage and delay the onset of childbearing after marriage until they are confident about their readiness to have children. After childbearing, their marriages are more stable, and their children are more likely to attend college and receive parental support to do so. The major cost of this strategy is that the delay can result in lower total fertility than desired because of age-related changes in fecundity (Kaplan et al., 2002).

We propose that a third factor comes into play at the low end of the education continuum. It has been pointed out that men who are less educated have higher mortality rates and greater rates of incarceration (Geronimus et al., 1999; Willis, 1987, 1994). This tends to make sex ratios female biased and promotes single parenthood. Additionally, periods of unemployment are likely to be interspersed with periods of employment, making the income stream highly variable. This variability in male income streams may shift female strategies of mate choice and family formation. Rather than relying on a single man to provide resources over the long term, women derive support for themselves and their children from a number of different sources: (1) their own market labor; (2) assistance from female kin and other women (Geronimus, 1996; Geronimus and Korenman, 1992; Stack, 1974); or (3) temporary boyfriends, who are chosen in part because they are currently employed (Lancaster, 1989; Tucker and Mitchell-Kernan, 1995).

This pattern results in a system of serial and simultaneous polygynandry, where both women and men have multiple reproductive relationships (Lancaster, 1989; Lancaster and Kaplan, 1992). It also results in residential sibships composed of half-siblings with different fathers. Since it may be difficult for fathers to control the distribution of resources they provide to ex-partners so that they are preferentially directed toward their genetic offspring, men have less incentive to invest in them (Weiss and Willis, 1985; Willis and Haaga, 1996), placing further pressure on women to garner resources from other sources.

In the United States, many women, especially ethnic minorities, who face a mating market where male unemployment is great, choose to reproduce at younger ages while they are still living with their mothers, so that they can receive maternal or grand-maternal assistance in child rearing (Burton, 1990; Geronimus, 1996). The change in the family structure associated with teen childbearing over the second half of the 20th century was dramatic. For example, in 1960 only 15 percent of births to women under age 20 were to unmarried women; by 1994 the figure had risen to 76 percent (Child-Trends, 1995, 1996). Among ethnic groups with high levels of unemployed males, the proportion of all births to unmarried women has shown an equally dramatic increase; for example, by the late 1990s, more than 70 percent of all births to black and Native American women were nonmarital.

This trend is especially pronounced in the developing world, where male unemployment among migrants to the cities is exceptionally high. For example, Figure 7-6 shows the household living arrangements of the students in the Cape Town study discussed above. Less than a quarter of the students were living with both natural parents, about half were living either with their mother alone or with their mother and step-father, and more than a quarter were living with other relatives. It is interesting to note that the switch to the matrifocal family in South Africa from the traditional patrilineal patrilocal form was noted as early as the 1940s, as soon as there was significant migration to urban areas by women (Burman and Preston-Whyte, 1992; Burman and Reynolds, 1986). The global emergence of the matrifocal family in response to urbanization is another example of convergence among people with very different cultural backgrounds.

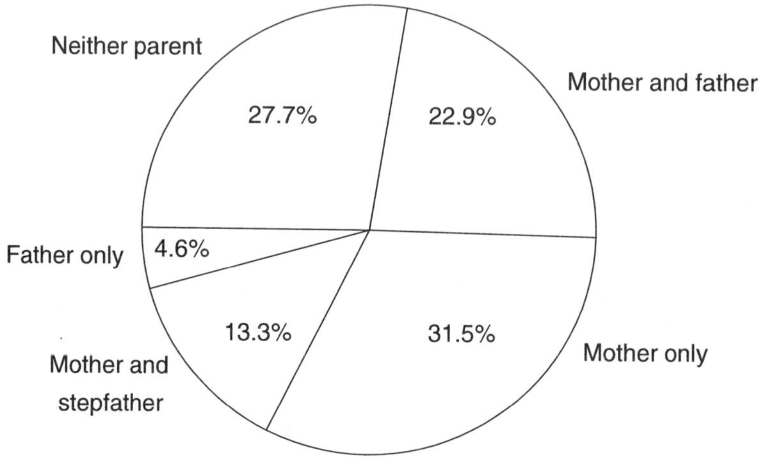

FIGURE 7-6 Living arrangements of I.D. Mkize High School students in Guguletu, South Africa.
SOURCE: Anderson et al. (2001).

Summary

In horticultural societies, access to the resources necessary for production and reproduction are reached through group membership. Groups are centered on productive resource patches that are used extensively and not possessed by individuals except through recognition of usufruct. Production by both males and females is for subsistence, and female labor underwrites much of the cost of supporting themselves and their children. This frees men to take as many wives as they can acquire through bride service or bride capture, creating conditions favoring endemic raiding for women. Parents focus their parental investment on raising as many healthy children as possible without concern for marriage market endowments or inheritance.

Pastoralism creates extrasomatic wealth in the form of highly mobile, easily divisible herds. This quality of livestock produces a reliable source of food but also a constant temptation to neighbors. Endemic warfare and raiding for women and livestock are the focus of the male life course, leading to expanded variance among men in resource holding and fertility based on the number of wives they can pay for or capture. At the same time that males must pay higher costs in bride wealth and in risk to access women, their families begin to help them by contributing a balloon payment at maturity to position them favorably on the mating market. Families of men now take responsibility not only to raise healthy children but also to help sons find mates. Finally, owing to the fact that extrasomatic wealth creates a reproductive estate, families husband that estate for future generations by balancing quality of children (marriage endowments and inheritance) against quantity of children.

Early civilizations and premodern stratified social systems witness a complex of socioecological and reproductive patterns that are different from those of tribal societies. The first is an even stronger correlation between extrasomatic wealth and reproductive success than already found among pastoralists and brings into focus female-female competition in the marriage market. Since extrasomatic wealth has the potential of being controlled by powerful resource holders, social stratification and the ensuing variance among men restructure the mating market. The families of daughters compete for access to quality grooms by offering not only the youth and fertility of their daughters but also their virginity, chastity, and a dowry payment. Families that are resource holders focus on ways to maintain the integrity of the family estate through inheritance, at the same time that they promote both sons and daughters with an advantageous foothold in the marriage market. These families make reproductive decisions with an eye to long-term resource management considerations (Voland, 2000). Families without reproductive estates (laborers) live as reproductive opportunists in the here and now.

Over time, population growth and environmental saturation led to an ever-increasing emphasis on parental limitation of claimants to family reproductive estates through monogamy and bastardy, sex preference, sibling birth-order effects, and delayed or nonreproduction by selected sons and daughters. However, unlike the conditions of the early civilizations, population movement through urbanization, warfare, colonialism, or migration siphons off excess reproduction to less saturated areas.

The existence of extrasomatic wealth may be the critical environmental condition to which the evolved human physiology and psychology do not respond so as to maximize fitness. When there is heritable wealth, such as cattle or land, the breast-feeding/energy balance system may generate higher fertility than parents desire, in terms of their own wealth and the resources they wish to pass on to their children. Adjustments to this situation may involve primarily differential inheritance, such as primogeniture and illegitimacy, but may also include late age of marriage (Coale and Treadway, 1986) or even celibacy (Boone, 1986) and lowered rates of polygyny by wealthy men (Luttbeg et al., 2000). Thus, perhaps we should not be surprised to find deviations from fitness maximization as soon as there are forms of extrasomatic wealth.

The extremely low fertility in modern societies may reflect the extreme importance of extrasomatic wealth and the multiple ways in which it can be used. Changes in the economy and public health increase the rate of wage returns on investments in education, albeit not equally both within and among societies. Moreover, in modern society, people face a tremendous array of consumption goods, including housing, clothing, electronic equipment, and vehicles. The medium of exchange for obtaining those goods is money. Money is highly fungible in that it can be translated into any one of those goods. As diminishing returns to consumption of one good are reached, money can then be allocated to other goods. With all the goods available, there is always some good of which little has been consumed and returns to purchasing some amount of it are still high. The same can be said for investment in offspring's embodied capital, which appears to include not only investments in schooling but also in goods associated with social training and social status, such as hobbies and sports, clothing, and toys. Much of these investments are commitments to favorable placements of children in the mating market. The low fertility exhibited in modern societies may reflect both the payoffs to investments in offspring income and a perceived lack of diminishing returns to other forms of consumption (see Haaga, 2001, for a related discussion).

Changes in male-female complementarity affect people differently, on the basis of returns to investments in education. Those with the highest returns delay marriage and fertility, preferentially mating with one another and having fairly stable reproductive unions. Those with the lowest returns converge on the matrifocal family in response to insecurity in the income flow and the high relative costs of purchasing child care.

CONCLUSIONS

The final aim of this chapter is to discuss the implications of this evolutionary framework for new research and theory building. The above overview examined broad trends in fertility, parental investment, and mating behavior in response to large-scale shifts in socioecology. The utility of the framework, however, will depend on its ability to stimulate productive research designed to explain more fine-grained patterns of variation within and among populations over time.

Perhaps the most fundamental set of questions raised by this analysis concerns how people allocate resources among their own consumption, their children's consumption, investments in their own and their children's human capital, and reproduction. An understanding of the decision-making processes underlying those allocations remains elusive. For example, many men in our focus group discussions conducted in 1991 in Albuquerque, New Mexico, mentioned that the major factor limiting their fertility was the monetary and time costs necessary to raise a child. Several Hispanic men, who had come from large families, observed that when they were growing up it was considered acceptable to have several children share the same bedroom, but today each child needs his or her own room. Very little is known about how individual decisions are made and how social standards evolve regarding investments in children.

The same can be said of allocations to a person's own consumption. We do not know why members of the elite in all societies engage in and institutionalize elaborate displays of consumption (Boone and Kessler, 1999). We also have a very incomplete understanding of the preferences and decision-making processes underlying consumption patterns in modern societies. Given limited budgets, decisions about one's own and one's children's consumption impinge on fertility decisions.

With respect to the second major theme in this chapter, mating systems and parental investment by sex, our understanding is even more incomplete. The factors affecting convergence and divergence between the sexes in each of those allocation decisions have not yet been systematically investigated. Clearly humans exhibit a great deal of flexibility in their family arrangements; the relationships between allocation decisions by sex, mating markets, and socioeconomic conditions are a new frontier for research.

These considerations suggest a "two-pronged" research program. One prong is to understand the mechanisms underlying those allocation processes, and the other is to understand how those mechanisms interact with socioeconomic conditions in generating behavioral and demographic outcomes. Several distinct lines of research may each contribute to such an understanding.

One approach is to examine individual variation in the weights or relative values that people attach to changes in their own and their children's consumption, to relative social standing, to sexual gratification, and to number of children. It would be useful to know if some portion of that variation is associated with additive and nonadditive genetic variation. Rather than simply examining the heritability of fertility per se, a productive direction for genetic mapping and behavioral genetics research may be to examine psychological characteristics hypothesized to be directly or indirectly involved in fertility and mating decisions. For example, it has been suggested that natural selection has resulted in a desire for sexual gratification but not for children per se (Potts, 1997). However, this has not been examined empirically although there is some evidence that high male status in contemporary society correlates with a man's number of sexual encounters but not reproductive success (Vining, 1986).

Developmental research on the ontogeny of decisions regarding consumption, fertility, sexual fidelity, and investment in children would also be useful. Do experiences taking care of infants and children during childhood and adolescence, investment of time and resources by parents, marital status of parents, exposure to media, and school composition affect desired levels of consumption and desire to have and/or rear children? To what extent are differences in selectivity of partner choice, relationship fidelity, willingness to invest in children after marital separation, and willingness to invest in stepchildren associated with developmental experience?

In a similar vein, it would be useful to investigate how information is evaluated and how those processes of evaluation affect the diffusion of information and behavioral changes through networks and communities (see Bock, 1999, for a discussion). How do people evaluate messages about breast-feeding or the risks associated with teen pregnancy? For example, do they simply weight messages by their frequency of occurrence, according to the prestige of the source, or according to some perceived relevance to their own individual situation? Do people actively choose to participate in networks or expose themselves to media that increase or decrease the likelihood of receiving different messages?

In terms of the interaction of those decision-making processes with socioecological/socioeconomic conditions, the major research implication is that micro-level studies of budgetary allocations and fertility should be designed in terms of their contribution to an integrated and general theory. An integrated theory in this sense does not imply a unicausal model of transitions (such as mortality change, economic development, or access to birth control), but rather an understanding of how constellations of factors jointly determine outcomes through their impacts on an organized response system.

The framework introduced here is designed to provide guidance for such research. It will be critical to analyze and measure how resources are acquired, the impacts of investments on resource acquisition, mortality rates and the impacts of investments on mortality, complementarity of male and female inputs, and variation among and within individuals over time in access to resources.

There is still much to be learned from the study of traditional societies. While the impacts of breast-feeding frequency and intensity on reproductive physiology have received considerable attention, the factors determining their patterning have not been systematically investigated but rather relegated to unexplained cultural differences. What determines the timing of solid food introduction, the duration of breast-feeding, and its diurnal rhythm, both across and within cultures? To what extent do features of the ecology in terms of work, child care, and food resources explain the cross-cultural variation? To what extent does its patterning respond to the individual condition of mother or baby within communities? Is it the baby's or the mother's behavior that exerts the most influence over the process? Similar questions can be asked of the regulation of work and food sharing with children and adolescents. Such microecological studies should provide insights into the evolved psychology underlying parent-offspring interactions and how ecology translates into varying demographic outcomes.

Another important research area in traditional societies is the study of social status and social capital. Since it is possible that concerns about relative social standing exert strong influence on modern consumption behavior and fertility decisions, an understanding of its role in contexts without material wealth should provide new insights. For example, anthropologists who have witnessed groups during the early phases of exposure to material goods, such as wrist watches, jewelry, and radios, are often impressed by how quickly those items are adopted in apparent displays of social status. What are the determinants of social standing when there is no stored wealth? Why are people motivated to pursue it? What are the costs and benefits of its pursuit? It is possible that behavior relevant to social standing had little direct impact on the regulation of fertility decisions in the past but now plays a greater role because the two trade off against one another with modern budgets.

There is still considerable debate about the relationships between men and women in traditional societies. According to one view (Hawkes and Bliege Bird, 2002), the provisioning of meat by men is actually generalized mating effort, not parental effort. Meat is acquired and shared with the whole band, and men gain access to women through the social prestige it confers. The view presented here is that men do provision their families, either directly or through return shares of food (Gurven et al., 2000), and complementarity in parental investment has led to pair bonding and specialized capital investment trajectories by men and women. Further research to resolve this debate should provide general insights into the factors affecting parental investment and mating systems.

The framework may also be applied to critical contrasts in historical and modern contexts. For example, it could be used to investigate why in the early 19th century couples in France had reduced marital fertility, whereas delays to marriage had larger impacts on fertility in England (Szreter and Garrett, 2000). One hypothesis is that differences in the labor markets between the two countries, with women in France juggling work and reproduction simultaneously and women in England working until marriage. The framework could also be applied to below-replacement fertility. Is very low fertility in Eastern and Southern Europe due to the same costs and benefits, or are there different factors leading to similar outcomes? For the most part, world population projections are based on statistical trends from the past and guesses about convergence on stable total fertility rates (Lutz et al., 2001). A deeper understanding of the relationship between conditions and fertility behavior would be useful for making population projections, especially in light of changing conditions.

The global growth of the matrifocal family is perhaps the most critical area for comparative research. Following the World Population Conference in Cairo (1994), the major policy emphasis has been on improving women's education and autonomy in work, family, and reproductive decision making. Such policies fail to consider the relationships between men's economic opportunities, mating systems, and the investment that children receive. We need a better understanding of men's and women's criteria for choice of mates and how those criteria vary with socioeconomic conditions and how the dynamics of mating systems affect exchanges between men and women and between men and their genetic children and stepchildren. To what extent are men's motivations and behavior regarding investments in children determined by their relationships with the child's mother versus parental concerns, and how does that mix vary with socioeconomic conditions (see Anderson et al., 1999a, 1999b, for a discussion)?

The framework also has implications for research into the emergence of institutions and the interplay between institutions and individual behavior. Rather than viewing institutions (such as despotic systems of political control) as exogenous social determinants of individual behavior, the framework treats them as the emergent outcomes of interactions between individuals. In modern contexts, this suggests that increased research attention should be directed toward understanding the reciprocal influences of public and private investments and policies. For example, to what extent were increased public investments in health and education in the 20th century due to increased individual interest in such investments? Similarly, to what extent do government policies with regard to family planning reflect the individual behavior and interests of policy makers? How representative are policy makers of individuals in the general population? Since those institutional developments affect the costs and benefits of individual actions, there is clearly a route for reciprocal influence. We need better understanding of those reciprocal influences and of the relationship between micro- and macrolevel outcomes.

Evolutionary demography is best viewed not as an alternative to traditional approaches but as a general theoretical framework that can inform and enhance existing research endeavors. Economic modeling is fundamental to evolutionary analysis. Economists are primarily concerned with conscious, rational decision-making processes, but such processes are only a subset of the regulatory mechanisms of controlling fertility. In addition, there is no generally accepted causal theory of human utility in economics; natural selection is a causal process that constrains the types of utility functions that may evolve. Feminist demography details the conflicts of interest between men and women and how they vary with social context. A more basic evolutionary understanding of why men and women differ in their life histories and reproductive careers and how socioecology affects the extent to which the behavior and goals of the two sexes converge and diverge will enrich such insights. Most of human behavior is not instinctual, nor even the result of simple trial-and-error learning. Since information about the costs and benefits of alternative behavioral options is often socially acquired, understanding cultural diffusion is critical. Evolutionary logic provides a framework for analysis of the active role that people play in determining which ideas they choose to adopt.

ACKNOWLEDGMENTS

This paper was written with support from the National Institute on Aging. The authors also wish to acknowledge the contributions of Kim Hill to the datasets and their analyses on the comparative diets and demography of chimpanzees and foragers published in a previous paper (Kaplan et al., 2000). We also thank Kim Hill and Magdalena Hurtado for their data on resource acquisition by age and sex among Hiwi and Ache. These datasets and analyses formed a critical base for part of this paper. We also wish to thank Monique Borgerhoff Mulder for her careful and extensive suggestions for revision of a draft of this paper.

REFERENCES

Anderson, K., H. Kaplan, D. Lam, and J. Lancaster
1999a Paternal care by genetic fathers and stepfathers II: Reports by Xhosa High School students. *Evolution and Human Behavior* 20:433-452.

Anderson K.G., H. Kaplan, and D. Lam
2001 Grade repetition, schooling attainment and family background in South Africa. Unpublished manuscript. Population Studies Center, University of Michigan, Ann Arbor.

Anderson, K.G., H. Kaplan, and J. Lancaster
1999b Paternal care by genetic fathers and stepfathers I: Reports from Albuquerque men. *Evolution and Human Behavior* 20:405-432.

Bailey, R.C., M.R. Jenike, P.T. Ellison, G.R. Bentley, A.M. Harrigan, and N.R. Peacock
1992 The ecology of birth seasonality among agriculturalists in Central Africa. *Journal of Biosocial Science* 24:393-412.

Becker, G.S.
1975 *Human Capital.* New York: Columbia University Press.

Becker, G.S., and R.J. Barro
1988 A reformulation of the economic theory of fertility. *Quarterly Journal of Economics* 103:1-25.

Bentley, G.R., R.R. Paine, and J.L. Boldsen
2001 Fertility changes with the prehistoric transition to agriculture. Pp. 203-232 in *Reproductive Ecology and Human Evolution.* P.T. Ellison, ed. Hawthorne, NY: Aldine de Gruyter.

Betzig, L.
1986 *Despotism and Differential Reproduction: A Darwinian View of History.* Hawthorne, NY: Aldine de Gruyter.
1992a Roman monogamy. *Ethology and Sociobiology* 13:351-383.
1992b Roman polygyny. *Ethology and Sociobiology* 13:309-349.

1993 Sex, succession and stratification in the first six civilizations: How powerful men reproduced, passed power on to their sons, and used their power to defend their wealth, women and children. Pp. 37-74 in *Social Stratification and Socioeconomic Inequality*. L. Ellis, ed. New York: Praeger.

Binford, L.R.
2001 *Constructing Frames of Reference*. Berkeley: University of California Press.

Bird, D.W., and R. Bliege Bird
2002 Children on the reef: Slow learning or strategic foraging. *Human Nature* 13:269-297.

Bliege Bird, R., and D.W. Bird
2002 Constraints of knowing or constraints of growing? Fishing and collecting among the children of Mer. *Human Nature* 13:00-00.

Blake, J.
1989 *Family Size and Achievement*. Los Angeles: University of California Press.

Blurton Jones, N.G., K. Hawkes, and J. O'Connell
1989 Modeling and measuring the costs of children in two foraging societies. Pp. 367-390 in *Comparative Socioecology of Humans and Other Mammals*. V. Standen and R.A. Foley, eds. London: Basil Blackwell.

Blurton Jones, N.G., K. Hawkes, and P. Draper
1994a Differences between Hadza and !Kung children's work: Original affluence or practical reason. Pp. 189-215 in *Key Issues in Hunter-Gatherer Research*. E.S. Burch, ed. Oxford: Berg.
1994b Foraging returns of !Kung adults and children: Why didn't !Kung children forage? *Journal of Anthropological Research* 50:217-248.

Bock, J.
1995 The Determinants of Variation in Children's Activities in a Southern African Community. Ph.D. dissertation, University of New Mexico, Albuquerque.
1999 Evolutionary approaches to population: Implications for research and policy. *Population and Environment* 21:193-222.
2002 Learning, life history, and productivity: Children's lives in the Okavango Delta, Botswana. *Human Nature* 13:161-198.

Bongaarts, J., and R.G. Porter
1983 *Fertility, Biology and Behavior: An Analysis of Proximate Determinants*. New York: Academic Press.

Boone, J.
1986 Parental investment and elite family structure in preindustrial states: A case study of late medieval-early modern Portuguese genealogies. *American Anthropologist* 88:259-278.
1988 Parental investment, social subordination and population processes among the 15th and 16th century Portuguese nobility. Pp. 201-220 in *Human Reproductive Behavior: A Darwinian Perspective*. L. Betzig, P. Turke, and M. Borgerhoff Mulder, eds. Cambridge: Cambridge University Press.

Boone, J.L., and K.L. Kessler
1999 More status or more children? Social status, fertility reduction, and long-term fitness. *Evolution and Human Behavior* 20:257-277.

Borgerhoff Mulder, M.
1988 Kipsigis bride wealth payments. In *Human Reproductive Behavior*. L. Betzig, M. Borgerhoff Mulder, and P. Turke, eds. Cambridge: Cambridge University Press.
1989 Early maturing Kipsigis women have higher reproductive success than late maturing women and cost more to marry. *Behavioral Ecology and Sociobiology* 24:145-153.

1991 Behavioural ecology of humans: Studies of foraging and reproduction. Pp. 69-98 in *Behavioural Ecology*. J.R. Krebs and N.B. Davies, eds. Oxford: Blackwell Scientific Publications.

1992 Demography of pastoralists: Preliminary data on the Datoga of Tanzania. *Human Ecology* 20:383-405.

1995 Bride wealth and its correlates: Quantifying changes over time. *Current Anthropology* 36:573-603.

1998 Brothers and sisters: How sibling interactions affect optimal parental investment. *Human Nature* 9:119-162.

2000 Optimizing offspring: The quantity-quality tradeoff in agropastoral Kipsigis. *Evolution and Human Behavior* 21:391-410.

Boserup, E.

1970 *Women's Role in Economic Development*. London: Allen and Unwin.

Boswell, J.

1990 *The Kindness of Strangers: The Abandonment of Children in Western Europe from Late Antiquity to the Renaissance*. New York: Vintage Books.

Brown, J.K.

1970 A note on the division of labor by sex. *American Anthropologist* 72:1073-1078.

Burck, C.G.

1976 A group profile of the Fortune 500 child executives. Fortune (May Issue):173-177.

Burman, S., and E. Preston-Whyte, eds.

1992 *Questionable Issue: Illegitimacy in South Africa*. Cape Town: Oxford University Press.

Burman, S., and P. Reynolds, eds.

1986 *Growing Up in a Divided Society: The Contexts of Childhood in South Africa*. Johannesburg: Ravan Press.

Burton, L.

1990 Teenage childbearing as an alternative life-course strategy in multigenerational black families. *Human Nature* 1:123-144.

Chagnon, N.A.

1979 Is reproductive success equal in egalitarian societies? Pp. 374-401 in *Evolutionary Biology and Human Social Behavior: An Anthropological Perspective*. N.A. Chagnon and W. Irons, eds. North Scituate, MA: Duxbury Press.

1988 Life histories, blood revenge, and warfare in a tribal population. *Science* 239:985-992.

2000 Manipulating kinship rules: A form of male Yanomamo reproductive competition. Pp. 115-132 in *Adaptation and Human Behavior: An Anthropological Perspective*. L. Cronk, N. Chagnon, and W. Irons, eds. Hawthorne, NY: Aldine de Gruyter.

Charnov, E.L.

1993 *Life History Invariants: Some Explanations of Symmetry in Evolutionary Ecology*. Oxford: Oxford University Press.

Child Trends, Inc.

1995 *Teen Births and Births to Unmarried Women: Facts at a Glance*. Washington, DC: Author.

1996 *New Data from Child Trends, Inc: Facts at a Glance*. Washington, DC: Author.

Clarke, A.L. and B.S. Low

1992 Ecological correlates of human dispersal in 19th century Sweden. *Animal Behavior* 44:677-693.

2001 Testing evolutionary hypotheses with demographic data. *Population and Development Review* 27:633-660.

Clutton-Brock, T.H.
1991 *The Evolution of Parental Care*. Princeton, NJ: Princeton University Press.

Clutton-Brock, T.H., and G.A. Parker
1992 Potential reproductive rates and the operation of sexual selection. *Quarterly Review of Biology* 67:437-456.

Coale, A.J., and R. Treadway
1986 A summary of the changing distribution of overall fertility, marital fertility and the proportion married in the provinces of Europe. Pp. 31-181 in *The Decline of Fertility in Europe*. A.J. Coale and S.C. Watkins, eds. Princeton, NJ: Princeton University Press.

Colson, E.
1960 *Social Organization of the Gwembe Tonga*. Manchester: Rhodes-Livingstone Institute.

Cromer, A.
1993 *Uncommon Sense: The Heretical Nature of Science*. New York: Oxford University Press.

Crook, J.H., and S.J. Crook
1988 Tibetan polyandry: Problems of adaptation and fitness. Pp. 97-114 in *Human Reproductive Behavior: A Darwinian Perspective*. L. Betzig, M. Borgerhoff Mulder, and P. Turke, eds. Cambridge: Cambridge University Press.

Curtin, P.D.
1989 *Death by Migration: Europe's Encounter with the Tropical World in the Nineteenth Century*. Cambridge: Cambridge University Press.

Dickemann, M.
1979a The ecology of mating systems in hypergynous dowry societies. *Social Science Information* 18:163-195.
1979b Female infanticide and the reproductive consequences of stratified human societies. In *Evolutionary Societies and Human Social Behavior*. N.A. Chagnon, and W. Irons, eds. North Scituate, MA: Duxbury Press.
1981 Paternal confidence and dowry competition: A biocultural analysis of purdah. In *Natural Selection and Social Behavior*. R.D. Alexander and D.W. Tinkle, eds. New York: Chiron Press.

DiVale, W., and M. Harris
1976 Population, warfare, and the male supremacist complex. *American Anthropologist* 80:21-41.

Downey, D.B.
1995 When bigger is not better: Family size, parental resources, and children's education performance. *American Sociological Review* 60:746-761.

Draper, P.
1992 Room to maneuver: !Kung women cope with men. Pp. 43-63 in *Sanctions and Sanctuary: Cultural Perspectives on the Beating of Wives*. D. Counts, J.K. Brown, and J. Campbell, eds. Boulder, CO: Westview Press.

Dunbar, R.I.M.
1991 Sociobiological theory and the Cheyenne case. *Current Anthropology* 32:169-173.

Ellison, P.T.
2001a *On Fertile Ground: A Natural History of Human Reproduction*. Cambridge, MA: Harvard University Press.

Ellison, P.T., ed.
2001b *Reproductive Ecology and Human Evolution.* Hawthorne, NY: Aldine de Gruyter.

Ember, C.R.
1983 The relative decline in women's contributions to agriculture with intensification. *American Anthropologist* 85:285-304.

Gaulin, S., and J. Boster
1990 Dowry as female competition. *American Antrhopologist* 92:994-1005.

Geronimus, A.T.
1996 What teen mothers know. *Human Nature* 7:323-352.

Geronimus, A.T., J. Bound, and T.A. Waidmann
1999 Health inequality and population variation in fertility timing. *Social Science and Medicine* 49:1623-1636.

Geronimus, A.T., and S. Korenman
1992 The socioeconomic consequences of teen childbearing reconsidered. *The Quarterly Review of Economics* 107:1187-1214.

Godfray, H.C.J., L. Partridge, and P.H. Harvey
1991 Clutch size. *Annual Review of Ecology and Systematics* 22:409-429.

Goodale, J.C.
1971 *Tiwi Wives.* Seattle: University of Washington Press.

Goody, J.
1973 Bride wealth and dowry in Africa and Eurasia. In *Bride Wealth and Dowry.* J.R. Goody and S.J. Tambiah, eds. Cambridge: Cambridge University Press.
1976 *Production and Reproduction: A Comparative Study of the Domestic Domain.* Cambridge: Cambridge University Press.
1983 *The Development of the Family and Marriage in Europe.* Cambridge: Cambridge University Press.

Grafen, A.
1991 Modeling a behavioural ecology. Pp. 5-31 in *Behavioural Ecology: An Evolutionary Approach.* J.R. Krebs and N.B. Davies, eds. Oxford: Blackwell Scientific.

Gurven, M., K. Hill, H. Kaplan, M. Hurtado, and R. Lyles
2000 Food transfers among Hiwi foragers of Venezuela: Tests of reciprocity. *Human Ecology* 28:171-218.

Gwyne, D.T.
1991 Sexual competition among females: What causes courtship role reversal. *Trends in Evolution and Ecology* 6:118-1222.

Gwyne, D.T., and L.W. Simmons
1990 Experimental reversal of courtship roles in an insect. *Nature* 346:172-174.

Haaga, J.G.
2001 Comment: The pace of fertility decline and the utility of evolutionary approaches. In *Global Fertility Transition*, R.A. Bulatao, and J.B. casterline, eds. *Population and Development Review* (suppl) 27:53-59.

Haddix, K.
2001 When polyandry falls apart: Leaving your wife and your brothers. *Evolution and Human Behavior* 22:47-60.

Harpending, H.
1994 Infertility and hunter-gatherer demography. *American Journal of Physical Anthropology* 93:385-390.

Hart, B., and T. Risley
1995 *Meaningful Differences in the Everyday Experience of Young American Children.* Baltimore, MD: Brookes.

Hart, C.W.M., and A.R. Pilling
1960 *The Tiwi of North Australia*. New York: Holt, Rinehart and Winston.

Hartung, J.
1982 Polygyny and the inheritance of wealth. *Current Anthropology* 23:1-12.

Hawkes, K., and R.Bliege Bird
2002 Showing off, handicap signaling, and the evolution of men's work. *Evolutionary Anthropology* 11:58-67.

Hawkes, K., J.F. O'Connell, and H.G. Blurton Jones
1995 Hadza children's foraging: Juvenile dependency, social arrangements and mobility among hunter-gatherers. *Current Anthropology* 36:688-700.

Herrnstein, R.J., and C. Murray
1994 *The Bell Curve: Intelligence and Class Structure in American Life*. New York: Free Press.

Hill, K., and A.M. Hurtado
1991 The evolution of reproductive senescence and menopause in human females. *Human Nature* 2:315-350.
1996 *Ache Life History: The Ecology and Demography of a Foraging People*. Hawthorne, NY: Aldine.

Hoff-Ginsberg, E., and T. Tardiff
1995 Socioeconomic status and parenting. In *The Handbook of Parenting*. M. Bornstein, ed. Hillsdate, NJ: Erlbaum.

Hrdy, S.B.
1994 Fitness tradeoffs in the history and evolution of delegated mothering with special reference to wet-nursing, abandonment, and infanticide. In *Infanticide and Parental Care*. S. Parmigiani and F.S. vom Saal, eds. Chur, Switzerland: Harwood Academic Publishers.
1999 *Mother Nature: A History of Mothers, Infants, and Natural Selection*. New York: Pantheon.

Hrdy, S.B., and D. Judge
1993 Darwin and the puzzle of primogeniture: An essay on biases in parental investment after death. *Human Nature* 4:1-45.

Hughes, A.L.
1986 Reproductive success and occupational class in eighteenth-century Lancashire, England. *Social Biology* 33:109-115.

Hurtado, A.M., K. Hawkes, K. Hill, and H. Kaplan
1985 Female subsistence strategies among Ache hunter-gatherers of Eastern Paraguay. *Human Ecology* 13:29-47.

Hurtado, A.M., and K. Hill
1990 Seasonality in a foraging society: Variation in diet, work effort, fertility, and the sexual division of labor among the Hiwi of Venezuela. *Journal of Anthropological Research* 46:293-345.

Irons, W.
1979a Cultural and biological success. Pp. 257-272 in *Natural Selection and Social Behavior*. N.A. Chagnon and W. Irons, eds. North Scituate, MA: Duxbury Press.
1979b Investment and primary social dyads. Pp. 181-213 in *Evolutionary Biology and Human Social Behavior*. N.A. Chagnon and W. Irons, eds. North Scituate, MA: Duxbury Press.

Isbell, L.A.
1991 Contest and scramble competition: Patterns of female aggression and ranging behavior among primates. *Behavioral Ecology* 2:143-155.

Jasienska, G.
2000 Why energy expenditure causes reproductive suppression in women. Pp. 59-84 in *Reproductive Ecology and Human Evolution.* P. Ellison, ed. Hawthorne, NY: Aldine de Gruyter.

Jerison, H.
1973 *Evolution of the Brain and Intelligence.* New York: Academic Press.
1976 Paleoneurology and the evolution of mind. *Scientific American* 234:90-101.

Kaplan, H.S.
1996 A theory of fertility and parental investment in traditional and modern human societies. *Yearbook of Physical Anthropology* 39:91-135.

Kaplan, H.S., and K. Hill
1985 Hunting ability and reproductive success among male Ache foragers. *Current Anthropology* 26:131-133.

Kaplan, H.S., and J.B. Lancaster
2000 The evolutionary economics and psychology of the demographic transition to low fertility. Pp. 238-322 in *Human Behavior and Adaptation: An Anthropological Perspective.* L. Cronk, W. Irons, and N. Chagnon, eds. Hawthorne, NY: Aldine de Gruyter.

Kaplan, H., K. Hill, A.M. Hurtado, J. Lancaster, and R. Robson
2001a *Embodied Capital and the Evolutionary Economics of the Human Lifespan.* Albuquerque: University of New Mexico.

Kaplan, H.S., K. Hill, A.M. Hurtado, and J.B. Lancaster
2001b The embodied capital theory of human evolution. Pp. 293-318 in *Reproductive Ecology and Human Evolution.* P.T. Ellison, ed. Hawthorne, NY: Aldine de Gruyter.

Kaplan, H., K. Hill, J.B. Lancaster, and A.M. Hurtado
2000 A theory of human life history evolution: Diet, intelligence, and longevity. *Evolutionary Anthropology* 9:156-185.

Kaplan, H.S., J. Lancaster, J. Bock, and S. Johnson
1995 Does observed fertility maximize fitness among New Mexican men? A test of an optimality model and a new theory of parental investment in the embodied capital of offspring. *Human Nature* 6:325-360.

Kaplan, H.S., J.B. Lancaster, W.T. Tucker, and K.G. Anderson
2002 An evolutionary approach to below replacement fertility. *American Journal of Human Biology* 14:1-24.

Kaplan, H.S., and A. Robson
2002 The emergence of humans: the coevolution of intelligence and longevity with intergenerational transfers. *Proceedings of the National Academy of Sciences* 99(15):10221-10226.

Keeley, L.H.
1996 *War Before Civilization: The Myth of the Peaceful Savage.* Oxford: Oxford University Press.

Kirwin, M.
1979 *African Widows.* Maryknoll: Orbis.

Kozlowski, J., and R.G. Weigert
1987 Optimal age and size at maturity in the annuals and perennials with determinant growth. *Evolutionary Ecology* 1:231-244.

Kramer, K.
2002 Variability in the duration of juvenile dependence: The benefits of Maya children's work to parents. *Human Nature* 13:299-325.

Kuzawa, C.W.
1998 Adipose tissue in human infancy and childhood: An evolutionary perspective. *Yearbook of Physical Anthropology* 41:177-209.

Lack, D.
1968 *Ecological Adaptations for Breeding in Birds*. London: Methuen.

Lancaster, C.S.
1981 *The Goba of the Zambezi: Sex Roles, Economics, and Change*. Norman, OK: University of Oklahoma Press.

Lancaster, J.B.
1989 Evolutionary and cross-cultural perspectives on single parenthood. Pp. 63-72 in *Sociobiology and the Social Sciences*. R.W. Bell and N.J. Bell, eds. Lubbock: Texas Tech University Press.
1997 The evolutionary history of human parental investment in relation to population growth and social stratification. Pp. 466-489 in *Feminism and Evolutionary Biology*. P.A. Gowaty, ed. New York: Chapman and Hall.

Lancaster, J.B., and H. Kaplan
1992 Human mating and family formation strategies: The effects of variability among males in quality and the allocation of mating effort and parental investment. In *Topics in Primatology: Human Origins*. T. Nishida, W.C. McGrew, P. Marler, M. Pickford, and F. de Waal, eds. Tokyo: University of Tokyo Press.

Lancaster, J.B., H. Kaplan, K. Hill, and A.M. Hurtado
2000 The evolution of life history, intelligence and diet among chimpanzees and human foragers. Pp. 47-72 in *Perspectives in Ethology: Evolution, Culture and Behavior*. F. Tonneau and N.S. Thompson, eds. New York: Plenum.

Lawrence, M., and R.G. Whitehead
1988 Physical activity and total energy expenditure of child-bearing Gambian village women. *European Journal of Clinical Nutrition* 42:145-160.

Low, B.S.
1990 Occupational status, landownership, and reproductive behavior in 19th-century Sweden: Tuna parish. *American Anthropologist* 92:457-468.
1991 Reproductive life in nineteenth century Sweden: An evolutionary perspective on demographic phenomena. *Ethology and Sociobiology* 12:411-448.
1994 Men in the demographic transition. *Human Nature* 5:223-253.
2000 *Why Sex Matters: A Darwinian Look at Human Behavior*. Princeton, NJ: Princeton University Press.

Lummaa, V., and T. Clutton-Brock
2002 Early development, survival and reproduction in humans. *Trends in Ecology and Evolution* 17:141-147.

Luttbeg, B., M. Borgerhoff Mulder, and M.S. Mangel
2000 To marry again or not: A dynamic model for demographic transition. Pp. 345-368 in *Adaptation and Human Behavior: An Anthropological Perspective*. L. Cronk, N.A. Chagnon, and W. Irons, eds. Hawthorne, NY: Aldine de Gruyter.

Lutz, W., W. Sanderson, and S. Scherbov
2001 The end of world population growth. *Nature* 412:543-545.

Mace, R.
2000 An adaptive model of human reproductive rate where wealth is inherited: Why people have small families. Pp. 261-282 in *Adaptation and Human Behavior: An Anthropological Perspective*. L. Cronk, N.A. Chagnon, and W. Irons, eds. Hawthorne, NY: Aldine de Gruyter.

Manson, J., and R. Wrangham
1991 Intergroup aggression in chimpanzees and humans. *Current Anthropology* 32:369-390.

McDade, T.W.
2001 Parent-offspring conflict and the cultural ecology of breast feeding. *Human Nature* 12:9-25.

Mueller, U.
2001 Is there a stabilizing selection around average fertility in modern human populations? *Population and Development Review* 27:469-498.

Murdock, G.P.
1967 Ethnographic atlas: A summary. *Ethnology* 6:109-236.

Newcomer, M.
1955 *The Big Business Executive: The Factors that Made Him, 1890-1950.* New York: Columbia University Press.

Orians, G.H.
1969 On the evolution of mating systems in birds and mammals. *American Naturalist* 103:589-603.

Partridge, L., and P. Harvey
1985 Costs of reproduction. *Nature* 316:20-21.

Pennington, R.
2001 Hunter-gatherer demography. Pp. 170-204 in *Hunter-Gatherers: An Interdisciplinary Perspective.* C. Panter-Brick, R.H. Layton, and P. Rowley-Conwy, eds. Cambridge: Cambridge University Press.

Pike, I.L.
1999 Age, reproductive history, seasonality, and maternal body composition during pregnancy for nomadic Turkana of Kenya. *American Journal of Human Biology* 11:658-672.

Poppitt, S.D., A.M. Prentice, E. Jequier, Y. Schutz, and R.G. Whitehead
1993 Evidence of energy sparing in Gambian women during pregnancy: A longitudinal study using whole-body calorimetry. *American Journal of Clinical Nutrition* 57:353-364.

Potts, M.
1997 Sex and the birth rate. *Population and Development Review* 23:1-19.

Prentice, A.M., and R.G. Whitehead
1987 The energetics of human reproduction. *Symposium of the Zoological Society of London* 57:275-304.

Preston, S., and M. Haines
1991 *Fatal Years: Child Mortality in Late Nineteenth Century America.* Princeton, NJ: Princeton University Press.

Promislow, D.E.L., and P.H. Harvey
1990 Living fast and dying young: A comparative analysis of life history variation among mammals. *Journal of Zoology* 220:417-437.

Retherford, R.D.
1993 *Demographic Transition and the Evolution of Intelligence: Theory and Evidence.* Honolulu: East-West Center.

Robson, A., and H.S. Kaplan
2003 The coevolution of intelligence and life expectancy in hunter-gatherer economies. *American Economics Review* (in press).

Rogers, A.
1993 Why menopause? *Evolutionary Ecology* 7:406-420.

Scott, S., and C.J. Duncan
1999 Reproductive strategies and sex-biased investment. *Human Nature* 10:85-108.

Sear, R., R. Mace, and I.A. McGregor
2001 Determinants of fertility in rural Gambia: An evolutionary ecological approach. Paper presented at the General Population Conference, International Union for the Scientific Study of Population.
Sellen, D.W., and R. Mace
1997 Fertility and mode of subsistence: A phylogenetic analysis. *Current Anthropology* 38:878-889.
Sellen, D.W., and D.B. Smay
2001 Relationship between subsistence and age at weaning in "pre-industrial" societies. *Human Nature* 12:47-87.
Shanley, D.P., and T.B.L. Kirkwood
2000 Calorie restriction and aging: A life-history analysis. *Evolution* 54:740-750.
Smith, C.C., and S.D. Fretwell
1974 The optimal balance between size and number of offspring. *American Naturalist* 108:499-506.
Stack, C.
1974 *All Our Kin: Strategies for Survival in a Black Community*. New York: Harper & Row.
Sterck, E.H.M., D.P. Watts, and C.P. van Schaik
1997 The evolution of female social relationships in nonhuman primates. *Behavioral Ecology and Sociobiology* 41:291-309.
Svedberg, P.
1990 Undernutrition in Sub-Saharan Africa: Is there a gender bias? *Journal for Development Studies* 26:469-486.
Szreter, S., and E. Garrett
2000 Reproduction, compositional demography, and economic growth in early modern England. *Population and Development Review* 26:45-80.
Tatar, M., D.W. Grey, and J.R. Carey
1997 Altitudinal variation in senescence in a Melanoplus grasshopper species complex. *Oecologia* 111:357-364.
Towner, M.
1999 A dynamic model of human dispersal in a land-based economy. *Behavioral Ecology and Sociobiology* 46:82-94.
2001 Linking dispersal and resources in humans: Life history data from Oakham, Massachusetts (1750-1850). *Human Nature* 12:321-350.
Trivers, R.L.
1972 Parental investment and sexual selection. In *Sexual Selection and the Descent of Man, 1871-1971*. B. Campbell, ed. Chicago: Aldine.
Tucker, M.B., and C. Mitchell-Kernan
1995 *The Decline in Marriage Among African Americans: Causes, Consequences, and Policy Implications*. New York: Russell Sage Foundation.
Vining, D.R.
1986 Social versus reproductive success: The central theoretical problem of human sociobiology. *Behavioral and Brain Sciences* 9:167-216.
Vinovskis, M.A.
1994 Education and the economic transformation of nineteenth century America. Pp. 171-196 in *Age and Structural Lag: Society's Failure to Provide Meaningful Opportunities in Work, Family, and Leisure*. M.W. Riley, R.L. Kahn, and A. Foner, eds. New York: John Wiley & Sons.
Voland, E.
1990 Differential reproductive success with the Krummhorn population (Germany, 18th and 19th centuries). *Behavioral Ecology and Sociobiology* 26:65-72.

2000 Contributions of family reconstitution studies to evolutionary reproductive ecology. *Evolutionary Anthropology* 9:134-146.

Voland, E., and A. Chasiotis

1998 How female reproductive decisions cause social inequality in male reproductive fitness: Evidence from eighteenth- and nineteenth-century Germany. Pp. 220-238 in *Human Biology and Social Inequality*. S.S. Strickland and P.S. Shetty, eds. Cambridge: Cambridge University Press.

Voland, E., and R.I.M. Dunbar

1995 Resource competition and reproduction: The relationship between economic and parental strategies in the Krummhorn Population (1720-1874). *Human Nature* 6:33-49.

1997 The impact of social status and migration of female age at marriage in an historical population in north-west Germany. *Journal of Biosocial Science* 29:355-360.

Voland, E., R.I.M. Dunbar, C. Engel, and P. Stephan

1997 Population increase and sex-biased parental investment: Evidence from 18th and 19th Century Germany. *Current Anthropology* 38:129-135.

Voland, E., and C. Engel

1990 Female choice in humans: A conditional mate selection strategy of the Krummhorn women (Germany, 1720-1874). *Ethology* 84:144-154.

Voland, E., E. Suegrekjiwm, and C. Engel

1991 Cost/benefit oriented parental investment by high status families: The Krummhorn case. *Ethology and Evolutionary Biology* 12:105-118.

Weiss, Y., and R.J. Willis

1985 Children as collective goods and divorce settlements. *Journal of Labor Economics* 3:268-292.

Werner, E.E.

1986 Amphibian metamorphosis: Growth rate, predation risk and the optimal time to transform. *American Naturalist* 128:319-341.

White, D.R., and M.L. Burton

1988 Causes of polygyny: Ecology, economy, kinship, and warfare. *American Anthropologist* 90:871-887.

Williams, G.C.

1957 Pleitropy, natural selection and the evolution of senescence. *Evolution* 11:398-411.

Willis, R.J.

1987 Public and private intergenerational transfers, economic growth and demographic transition. Pp. 717-740 in *Conference on Economic Development and Social Welfare in Taiwan*. Taipei, Taiwan: Institute of Economics, Academica Sinica.

1994 Economic analysis of fertility: Micro foundations and aggregate implications. Pp. 139-171 in *Population, Economic Development, and the Environment*. K.L. Kiessling and H. Landberg, eds. New York: Oxford University Press.

Willis, R.J., and J.G. Haaga

1996 Economic approaches to understanding nonmarital fertility. In *Fertility in the United States: New Patterns, New Theories*. J.D. Casterline, R.D. Lee, and K.A. Foote, eds. New York: The Population Council.

Wood, J.W.

1994 *Dynamics of Human Reproduction: Biology, Biometry and Demography*. New York: Aldine de Gruyter.

8

Sexually Antagonistic Coevolution: Theory, Evidence, and Implications for Patterns of Human Mating and Fertility

Steven W. Gangestad

Reproduction in humans, as in most species, involves sex. For an individual in a sexually reproducing animal species to reproduce, he or she typically must attract a mate, find a mate sufficiently attractive to have sex with him or her, and be adequately compatible genetically with the mate to produce a viable offspring. In many species, including humans, successful propagation of one's genes through sexual reproduction also requires an investment by one or both parents of time and energy into the well-being of the offspring for at least part of the period from conception to the offspring's own reproduction. Each of these components of reproduction is a product of evolution and is under selective pressures. Although much about human fertility patterns can be learned in the absence of an evolutionary framework, many details cannot be appreciated except in the light of an understanding of how selection has shaped mating and parenting.

In any specific instance, sexual reproduction is a task that can clearly benefit both the male and the female involved. After all, both individuals' genes are passed on to an offspring they jointly conceive, and hence the offspring is a vehicle through which each individual's genes can be propagated. Nonetheless, reproduction should by no means be thought of as a purely cooperative enterprise between mates. Selection will favor individuals' treating their mates' outcomes just as important as one's own when each individual can possibly reproduce only with that particular mate. In such a case, the death of the mate ends the individual's reproductive career just as surely as does the individual's own death. By creating living groups of just two individuals—one member of each sex—experimental biologists have created these circumstances in laboratory populations. In nearly all natural populations, however, this circumstance rarely if ever exists. Instead, although an ordering of events in terms of the extent to which they would promote or diminish the lifetime reproductive success of an individual may substantially covary with an ordering of events in terms of the extent to which they would promote or diminish the lifetime reproductive success of an individual's mate, there is rarely perfect covariation. Mismatches in these orderings represent genetic conflicts of interest between the sexes within mateships. These genetic conflicts of interest can produce selection for characteristics of members of one sex that promote the fitness of that sex at the expense of the fitness of the other. The outcome of such selection is referred to as *sexually antagonistic adaptation* (Rice, 1996). Although sexual conflicts of interest have long been recognized in evolutionary biology, only in the past several years have evolutionary biologists come to appreciate the dramatic ways by which the selection they fuel can influence the dynamics of mating, affect patterns of fertility, and explain outcomes that otherwise appear inexplicable.

This chapter paper has several aims. First, I discuss experimental work on the effects of sexual conflicts of interest in laboratory and field populations. Second, I summarize, at a conceptual level, the main consequences of selection fueled by sexual conflicts of interest. Third, I provide an overview of work suggesting that sexual conflicts of interest may have been common in ancestral human populations and hence had opportunity to affect selection on human mating and reproduction. Fourth, I describe three examples of how sexual conflicts of interest have affected specific phenotypic characteristics and mechanisms that, in turn, affect patterns of fertility. Finally, I will discuss the important ways by which sexual conflicts may have varied ancestrally in systematic ways, such that the outcomes of selection fueled by them may be expressed contingently, depending on particular circumstances.

EXPERIMENTAL DEMONSTRATIONS OF SEXUAL CONFLICTS OF INTEREST

Evolving Male Lines, with No Selection Mediated by Female Success

In 1996, William Rice published a spectacular demonstration of sexually antagonistic adaptation fueled by sexual conflicts of interest. Though an ingenious procedure, he allowed *Drosophila melanogaster* males to evolve while preventing females from evolving counteradaptations. Females in the line were always taken from a nonresponding target stock, whereas males were taken from the adapting-male line. Furthermore, artificial selection procedures ensured that males in the line always passed on the genes they inherited from their fathers rather than their mothers.). After 30 generations, a series of tests of the relative fitness of males in the experimental line and control males was performed. There was substantial evidence for male adaptation in the experimental line to the target females. Males in the experimental line had increased capacity for remating with females who had previously mated with competitor males taken from the control line. At the same time, competitor males had decreased ability to remate with females previously mated with experimental males and to displace sperm inseminated by experimental males, even when experimental males were not present at the time females were presented with competitor males. In mixed groups the reproductive success of experimental males was 24 percent greater than that of control competitor males.

Additional evidence showed that male adaptation evolved at the expense of female fitness. Females that mated with experimental males experienced a death rate greater than that experienced by females mated to control males. No compensating increase in fecundity of females mated to experimental males was observed. Previous research had shown that the protein in male *Drosophila melanogaster* seminal fluid are a low-level toxin to females (e.g., Fowler and Partridge, 1989; Chapman et al., 1995). Evidence in Rice's experiment suggested that the mortality cost to females was mediated by both an increase in the remating rate (and hence greater exposure to seminal proteins) and enhanced toxicity of male seminal proteins.

The toxicity of male seminal fluids to females is unlikely to be an effect that is itself selected. Rather, evidence suggests that the harmful effect is an incidental by-product of beneficial effects on male reproductive success. The proteins can harm other males' sperm and hence facilitate sperm competition (Clark et al., 1995; Harshman and Prout, 1994). Furthermore, some seminal proteins appear to enter the female's circulatory system and thereby influence her neuroendocrine system in ways that benefit the male (e.g., by reducing her remating rate; Aigaki et al., 1991). The costly effects on females are thus to be understood as sexually antagonistic outcomes of male adaptation.

Effects of Enforced Monogamy on Sexually Antagonistic Adaptation

Wild *Drosophila melanogaster* typically mate promiscuously, and males make frequent attempts to induce remating on the part of females. Following the dramatic direct demonstration of sexually antagonistic adaptation, Holland and Rice (1999) asked whether enforced monogamy, which relaxes intersexual conflict and increases the benefits of male benevolence toward females, might yield reduced male traits antagonistic to females, thereby reducing a cost of mating to females. They established two replicate populations. In the control population, a single female was housed with three males (which parallels the sex ratio that takes place during mating episodes in natural populations). In the other population, a single female was housed with a single male. In the latter situation, male reproductive success did not depend on males' ability to outcompete other males for access to or insemination of a single female. In fact, it depended as much as his mate's well-being as on his own. Holland and Rice therefore predicted that in the monogamously mated population the seminal fluid proteins would evolve to be less toxic to females, male remating efforts would become less intense, and the net reproductive rate (the number of adult progeny produced per female) would increase.[1]

All predictions were supported. After 45 generations, test females that had mated once to a male sampled from the monogamous population had greater survival compared to those that mated once to a male sampled from the control population. At the same time, females in the monogamous line died faster than control females when housed with control males. Males in the monogamous line courted females less than those in the control line when housed with females with whom they had evolved. Finally, females in the monogamous line produced a greater number of offspring surviving to adulthood than did control females when females were mated to males with whom they had evolved. Subsequent work has furthermore demonstrated that females mated to males evolved in a monogamous line produce offspring at a higher rate after a single mating than do females mated to control males, purportedly due to the evolution of male benevolence toward females in monogamous lines (Pitnick et al., 2001).

Evolution of Female Sexually Antagonistic Adaptations

Sexual conflict should be expected to produce female traits that are sexually antagonistic as well as male traits. Hosken et al. (2001) evolved two lines of dung flies: one in which strict genetic monogamy was enforced, the other allowing female polyandry. As expected, males in the polyandrous line had testes of greater size, reflecting the fact that they had evolved to invest greater effort in the production of sperm or other seminal products, which may be involved in sperm competition (see also Pitnick et al., 2001). At the same time, females in this line evolved larger sex accessory glands. These glands produce a spermicidal secretion and thereby influence female ability to affect the paternity of her offspring. Perhaps as a result,

[1]As Holland and Rice (1999) note, polyandry could have benefits due to mate choice that outweigh the costs of sexually antagonistic adaptation, and in some species that appears to be the case. Holland and Rice did not observe that outcome in their own experiment, however.

males who mated second with a female from this line had reduced success compared to males mated second with a female from the monogamous line.

Sexually Antagonistic Coevolution and Parental Investment

Sexual conflicts of interest arise not only in the area of sperm competition and its effects on female well-being but also arise over levels of parental investment. Recently, Royle et al. (2002) demonstrated their effects on parental investment in zebra finches. Male and female pairs of zebra finches typically share parental investment responsibilities of feeding and protecting young. Because rates of adult mortality are appreciable, however, young not uncommonly have a single parent investing in them. Royle et al. were interested in whether the parenting effort of single parents is greater or lesser than that of individuals biparentally investing in offspring. Female birds raised young in two experimental conditions: First, they raised two young to the age of 35 days by themselves; second, the same females raised four young with the father of the offspring to the age of 35 days. The order of these conditions was counterbalanced and controlled.

If parents work equally and dedicate as much effort to care in biparental conditions as in uniparental conditions, offspring in the two situations should have fared equally well. If there are nonadditive returns to investment by two parents (e.g., because of greater optimization of own or offspring feeding times owing to sharing of parental duties), offspring in biparental conditions could fare better even if parents exert equal amounts of time and energy to parental duties in the two situations. In fact, however, the opposite pattern was observed: The amount of food consumed per chick when offspring were fed by only the mother was greater than the amount consumed when they were fed by two parents. This difference apparently yielded meaningful fitness effects; as adults, sons raised by single mothers were more attractive to females than were sons raised by two parents. This pattern could occur if fathers typically feed chicks less than mothers do. But comparison of maternal and paternal rates of feeding offspring revealed that fathers provide similar or greater amounts of food to chicks.

The likely explanation of these results is that sexual conflicts of interest over rates of feeding result in a net reduction of feeding per chick when two parents share feeding duties. In such circumstances, parents presumably negotiate the extent to which each will feed offspring. Because each parent's genetic interests are not identical (as neither parent's future reproductive success is fully dependent on the well-being of the other parent), each parent gains if the other parent takes on a greater proportion of the parental investment in the brood. Modeling of the negotiation game that determines levels of parental investment in situations in which conflicts exist indicates that it can often result in less investment per parent than the optimal level of parenting by a single parent (McNamara et al., 1999, in press). In effect, each parent may gain by sharply responding to deficits in investment ("free-riding") by the other parent by their own reductions in effort. (See also Parker et al., 2002.)

A CONCEPTUALIZATION OF SEXUALLY ANTAGONISTIC ADAPTATION AND ITS IMPLICATIONS

It has long been recognized that species may coevolve with other species in their environments in either a mutualistic or antagonistic fashion. Cases that involve interspecific antagonism are perhaps the more widely recognized and dominate: for example, the coevolution of predator-prey, host-pathogen, or competitors for the same food source. When antagonistic coevolution prevails, new adaptations in one species (e.g., a trait in predators that increases their ability to capture prey) evoke selection on the other species (e.g., on prey) to evolve counteradaptations (e.g., defenses), which may then produce selective pressures on the first species to counter those counteradaptations, and so on. Potentially, antagonistic coevolution of adaptation and counteradaptation can continue through a long period of evolutionary time, resulting in persistent evolutionary change in both species. Antagonistic coevolution is now widely known as the Red Queen process (Van Valen, 1962). This character in *Alice in Wonderland* claimed that she had to keep running simply to stay in the same place, and so too species must continually evolve to stay competitive against their enemies.

Just as genes within two species' genomes can coevolve in response to their interaction, so too can genes in a single species can coevolve. The more widely recognized and probably dominant case here is mutualistic coevolution. Alleles that "work well" with alleles at other loci are very often selected over alternatives, as illustrated by many commonsense examples. Sonar was more likely to evolve in a flying noctural animal, such as a bat, than in a terrestrial diurnal animal. Penguin wings were more likely to evolve into structures that function much like fins (ineffective for flying) once penguins entered water to feed.

Intraspecific genomic coevolution may be antagonistic as well, however. Rice and Holland (1997) refer to such coevolution as interlocus contest evolution, of which sexually antagonistic coevolution is a prime example. Consider, for simplicity's sake, genes that are sex limited and therefore expressed in only one sex. Genes expressed only in males will be selected for benefits that they provide males. Genes expressed only in females will be selected for benefits that they provide females. Alleles at male sex-limited genes that have negative effects on their male carriers' mates may nonetheless spread in the population if they benefit males. The evolution of the adaptations they beget (e.g., seminal proteins that affect female remating), however, set the stage for the evolution of adaptations due to female sex-limited genes that counter those adaptations and their negative effects (e.g., resistance to the effects of the seminal proteins). Such counteradaptation may then evoke selection for male counters to those counteradaptations (e.g., production of a more intense form or dose of seminal proteins). Ultimately, persistent antagonistic coevolution of male and female sex-limited genes (and the adaptations they beget) in a single species' genome—that is, an *intraspecific* Red Queen process—may be the outcome (Rice and Holland, 1997).[2]

Red Queen processes—including intraspecific ones and hence ones fueled by sexual conflicts of interest—give rise to some predictable evolutionary outcomes. Below, I describe several evolutionary outcomes of sexually antagonistic adaptation that are of note.

Relatively Rapid Evolution

If, as might be expected, evolution of a new allele at one locus involved in sexually antagonistic selection leads to selection for new alleles at loci that counteract its effects (i.e., are expressed in the other sex), loci involved in sexually antagonistic selection should be characterized by relatively rapid evolution. (Put otherwise, sexually antagonistic adaptations should be less likely to be evolutionarily stable, as they are subject to counteradaptation in the other sex.) As reproductive traits may often be sexually antagonistic adaptations, these traits should and apparently do evolve at rapid rates. For instance, gamete proteins in a variety of species, including mammals, evolve at extremely rapid rates (e.g., Palumbi and Metz, 1991; Vanquier and Lee, 1993; Metz and Palumbi, 1996; Tsaur et al., 2001; Swanson et al., 2001a, 2000b). Furthermore, characteristics of reproductive tracts tend to evolve faster than other traits (and hence, for instance, are more likely to discriminate closely related species than other traits; e.g., Eberhard, 1996). Recent findings show that rapid divergence of reproductive genes has occurred in primates and is marked in the

[2]Sex limitation is not required nor necessarily expected of genes evolved through sexually antagonistic coevolution. Perhaps not atypically, genes that benefit one sex in intersexual conflicts actually impose costs when expressed in the other sex (e.g., genes that adaptively increase hormone action in one sex may maladaptively do so in the other sex). These *sexually antagonistic genes* may be selected if the net benefits to one sex outweigh the costs to the other. Selection should favor modifier genes that limit expression of the gene to the sex benefited by it. Because genes involved in sexually antagonistic adaptations rapidly evolve, however, periods of stable selection on the sex necessary for the evolution of complete sex limitation may not be common. Sexually antagonistic genes compromise the design of each sex away from its optimum. See Chippendale et al. (2001).

divergence of chimpanzees and humans (Wyckoff et al., 2000). This divergence appears to be largely due to positive selection for new alleles (as is expected if antagonistic coevolution is involved) rather than simply relaxation of negative selection against alleles coupled with drift (Wyckoff et al., 2000; see also Swanson et al., 2001a, 2001b). (For theoretical treatments, see also Gavrilets, 2000, and Van Doorn et al., 2001.)

Interindividual Variation

A corollary of rapid evolution is interindividual variation. In cases of adaptations that represent evolutionarily stable solutions, selection may drive the alleles that map onto the adaptations to near fixation (at least with respect to functionally significant, i.e., nonneutral, variation, the exception being a small proportion of deleterious alleles due to mutation). In the case of sexually antagonistic adaptations, however, rapid evolution may lead to variation being maintained. If selection changes so rapidly that an allele B at locus Z that becomes favored by selection over a predominant alternative allele A at time t_1 has not gone to fixation by the time t_2, at which a new allele C becomes favored over allele B, then throughout the period during which B was favored (t_1 to t_2; and, in all likelihood, some period of time thereafter) the population will have always been characterized by variation at locus Z. Even if rapid evolution leads to this situation, only a small-to-moderate proportion of the time, traits affected by multiple loci, each with a nonnegligible probability of being polymorphic at each point in time, may possess significant genetic variation.

Fitness traits, including fecundity, typically possess much more genetic variation than ordinary morphological traits and traits known to be understabilizing selection (e.g., Houle, 1992). For instance, whereas human height possesses a coefficient of additive genetic variation (CV_A; square root of genetic variation times 100 over trait mean) of about 5, human fecundity appears to possess a CV_A greater than 20 (e.g., Burt, 1995; Rodgers et al., 2001). (The same pattern can be observed for traits of *Drosophila*; Houle, 1992.) Some of the genetic variation in fitness traits can be accounted for by mutation-selection balance (e.g., Charlesworth and Hughes, 1998, who estimate that a CV_A of about 8 in *Drosophila* fitness could be due to mutation-selection balance). Nonetheless, best estimates suggest that not all genetic variation in fitness is owing to mutation. For reproductive traits, coevolution of sexually antagonistic adaptation is a prime candidate to account for a meaningful amount of variation.[3]

---

[3]Aside from the fact that rapid evolution maintains allelic variation, it may select for a higher rate of mutation and a lack of canalizing processes that modify and narrow the range of gene expression (e.g., Williams and Hurst, 2000). See also note 2.

A Nonnegligible Level of Maladaptation Within Populations

It is no wonder that humans have not evolved surefire immunity to pathogen-mediated disease. The pathogens against which we should be selected to defend ourselves are consistently evolving new ways to defeat our defense. Any solution to their attacks is thus likely to be only temporary. Rapid coevolution thus tends not only to produce interindividual variation in adaptation, but the mean level of adaptation to coevolving antagonists in the population will tend to be less than the mean level of adaptation to stable aspects of the environment. Just as this statement should hold true of interspecific coevolution (e.g., host-pathogen coevolution), it should hold true of intraspecific coevolution, such as sexually antagonistic coevolution. Naturally, if individuals vary in the extent to which they possess newly evolving offensive or defensive traits involved in antagonistic coevolution, the load of maladaptation in the population is carried disproportionately by some subset of individuals. Nonetheless, considering the fact that many antagonistic adaptations may be involved, all individuals may be likely to carry some of this load.

In the past decade, appreciation of antagonistic coevolution between mothers and the fetuses they carry has led to explanations for why pregnancy appears to be a process that ends in a perhaps surprisingly large proportion of reproductively poor outcomes, in light of the strength of the selection pressures one might expect on reproductive traits. The optimal flow of nutrients from the mother to the fetus from the viewpoint of fetal genes exceeds the optimal flow of nutrients from the viewpoint of maternal genes (Trivers, 1974). Maternal traits and fetal traits may hence antagonistically coevolve as suites of counter-adapted characteristics. Evidence strongly argues for such a coevolutionary process (see Haig, 1993). For instance, human placental lactogen produced under fetal control increases maternal resistance to insulin and thereby acts to maintain longer periods of high blood glucose levels. This effect is countered, however, by increased maternal production of insulin. Haig (1993) has argued that many of the common maladies associated with pregnancy (e.g., hypertension, preeclampsia, gestational diabetes) should be understood as maladaptive byproducts of antagonistic coevolution.

Reproductive traits involved in mating and conception may also be antagonistic and hence responsible for high levels of maladaptation. The fact that *Drosophila melanogaster* experience increased reproductive success, even based on single matings, when evolved in monogamous pairs provides indirect evidence for this proposition. Below I discuss one possible area of sexually antagonistic coevolution that may contribute to infertility in humans.

Favorable Outcomes That Depend on the Compatibility of Male and Female Traits

There is at least one way in which some intraspecific antagonistic coevolution differs from interspecific antagonistic coevolution. All else equal, an individual of one species (e.g., a predator) experiences reproductive success to the extent that the individual succeeds in the conflict with individuals of antagonistic species (e.g., prey). By contrast, individuals can suffer reproductive costs by dominating too severely a contest with an intraspecific rival. Mothers who are well adapted to restrict transfer of nutrients to a fetus may suffer fitness costs if her fetus is not particularly well suited to obtain nutrients from a resistant mother. A fetus that is well adapted to restrict maternal peripheral blood flow may cause the mother's death and, ultimately, its own demise if the mother is not well adapted to counter the fetal adaptations. Similarly, male *Drosophila* with seminal proteins too toxic to his female partner may cause her death prior to her laying fertilized eggs. Females who produce spermicidal secretions that kill sperm of all her mates do not reproduce. Because, on average in the population, genes for antagonistic adaptations may be favored and evolve despite some poor outcomes due to severe overdominance. Compatibilities between male and female features, however, may also affect outcomes. These comparibilities are to be understood as interactions between male and female features on reproductive success.

As argued by Zeh and Zeh (2001), compatibility effects caused by sexually antagonistic coevolution may invoke subsequent selection on mate choice to seek mates who possess features compatible with one's own. Selection for compatible mates appears to be responsible for preferences for mates who possess dissimilar (and thereby compatible) major histocompatibility complex (MHC) genes in mice and rats (for a review, see Penn and Potts, 1999) and perhaps humans (Wedekind et al., 1995; Wedekind and Furi, 1997; but see Jacob et al., 2002; Thornhill et al., in press). This form of compatibility is not obviously one that is the outcome of sexually antagonistic coevolution, however. A recent review by Tregenza and Wedell (2000) noted that several studies show indirect evidence for choice of genetically compatible mates; female choice in some species leads to greater offspring fitness with no clear evidence that their mates provide material benefits or intrinsically good genes. The authors note that there is little evidence for specific sources of genetic compatibility that might drive mate choice for genetic compatibility (the MHC effects being an exception), although they emphasize this area has yet to be well investigated.

THE POTENTIAL FOR SEXUALLY ANTAGONISTIC COEVOLUTION IN HUMANS

Thus far I have discussed the general notion of sexually antagonistic coevolution, experimental demonstrations of its effects in populations of laboratory animals, and evolutionary implications of sexually antagonistic selection. The remainder of this chapter examines potential causes and effects of sexually antagonistic coevolution in humans.

Human Females: Monogamous or Polyandrous?

As noted above, the dramatic reproductive costs of sexually antagonistic coevolution have become widely appreciated in biology only in the past decade. Multiple matings on the part of females (polyandry) increase sexual conflicts of interest and ensuing antagonistic adaptation in the processes that determine conception; female monogamy decreases these conflicts.[4] It is ironic, then, that also during the past decade, biologists have come to appreciate the prevalence and level of polyandry, even in species formerly thought to be relatively monogamous. The case of socially monogamous birds is now well documented. On average in these species, the extra-pair paternity rate (percentage of offspring sired by a father other than a female's social mate, as estimated through DNA fingerprinting) is 10 to 15 percent, with rates of 25 percent or greater not uncommon (Birkhead and Møller, 1995). Zeh and Zeh (2001:1051) have gone so far as to declare an ongoing "paradigm shift" in behavioral ecology, "with the traditional concepts of the choosy, monogamous female and the coadapted gene complex increasingly giving way to the realization that sexual reproduction . . . promotes polyandry . . . ." Whether a true paradigm shift is underway might be debated. Without doubt, however, is the fact that, as the costly outcomes of multiple mating have become appreciated, behavioral ecologists have become all the more aware of the high probability that, at least in many circumstances (including ones in which males provide substantial parental care), polyandry must have substantial benefits to offset these costs and hence is an option that females often pursue strategically.

Research on the benefits of polyandry (most notably when it is in the form of extra-pair mating and hence where females have social mates investing in offspring) has identified several possible benefits that fall into two broad categories: material benefits (benefits that directly increase the reproductive success of females) and genetic benefits (benefits that indirectly increase female reproductive success by increasing the viability or

[4]As discussed later, multiple matings by both males and females can increase sexual conflicts of interest regarding parental investment.

mating success of offspring). Traditionally, material benefits have been more widely accepted: for instance, direct nutritional benefits, physical protection, confusion of paternity (see Zeh and Zeh, 2001). In recent years, however, genetic benefits have garnered considerable support (for a review, see Jennions and Petrie, 2000). These benefits fall into three main categories: (1) intrinsic good genes: choice of an extra-pair mate who has genes that additively enhance offspring fitness independently of maternal genes (e.g., lack of mutations, favorable disease resistance genes involved in antagonistic interaction with pathogens, favorable genes involved in sexually antagonistic interaction, as discussed in this paper); (2) compatible genes: choice of an extra-pair mate who has genes that are compatible with female genes (with compatibility possibly the outcome of sexually antagonistic coevolution) and thereby enhance offspring fitness; (3) diverse genes: choice of an extra-pair mate whose genes will diversify the genetic makeup of the female's offspring, which may have any number of benefits (e.g., a hedge against environmental uncertainty, reduced chances of an intrafamilial disease epidemic). (For more fine-grained discriminations, see Jennions and Petrie, 2000; Zeh and Zeh, 2001.) It is beyond this chapter to review the relative strength of evidence for these benefits. It should be noted, however, that the benefits of polyandry need not be mutually exclusive; within single species, multiple benefits may account for extra-pair mating.

Published studies that have estimated the extra-pair paternity rate in human populations based on DNA or serological data are scant. Only two full reports exist. One estimated a rate of less than 1 percent in a Swiss population (Sasse et al., 1994). The other estimated a rate of 11 percent in a population from Monterrey, Mexico (Cerda-Flores et al., 1999). In the latter study, the extra-pair paternity rate varied as a function of socioeconomic status. Whereas it was about 5 percent in the high socioeconomic status population, it was estimated to be 20 percent in the low socioeconomic status population. Obviously, generalizations from data on only two populations are risky. They do suggest, nonetheless, that (1) the extra-pair paternity rate can be very substantial in human populations and (2) its range across populations is very considerable. One possibility is that ecological and socioecological circumstances that moderate the benefits of polyandry account for the variability through expression of environmentally contingent mating and parenting strategies of humans, a possibility explored in greater detail in a later section.

Another Source of Evidence for Polyandrous Tendencies: Design for Polyandry

Sexually antagonistic coevolution of adaptations in modern humans would have occurred in ancestral populations. A tack for addressing whether ancestral females engaged in polyandry as a strategic option is to look for evidence that women possess features apparently designed for obtaining benefits through polyandry. Several years ago, Randy Thornhill and I proposed to look for a set of features in women that may have design for obtaining genetic benefits from extra-pair men (Gangestad and Thornhill, 1998). Specifically, we proposed that, if ancestral women could have obtained genetic benefits through extra-pair sex but at some risk of cost (perhaps largely due to loss of a mate's parental investment in her offspring), selection may have forged preferences for phenotypic indicators of those genetic benefits to be conditional and depend on women's phase of the menstrual cycle: be most pronounced during the fertile phase of the cycle, when such benefits could be garnered, and subdued outside the fertile phase. As Penton-Voak et al. (1999) added, this shift should be most notable in women's preferences for a sex partner (or "short-term" partner) and perhaps absent in women's preferences for a long-term mate. The straightforward evolutionary economic reasoning is that, if there are no benefits to be gained, there is no sense in paying costs. Benefits can only possibly exceed costs when the possibility that they can be garnered is nonzero.

We and others have largely applied this reasoning to look for a design for obtaining intrinsically good genes, though more recently we have looked for a design for obtaining MHC-compatible genes. Several preference shifts across the cycle have now been demonstrated and in some instances replicated multiple times:

1. *Preference for the scent of symmetry.* Fluctuating asymmetry (FA) is lack of symmetry on bilateral traits that are symmetrical at the population level and is thought to be the outcome of developmental instability, errors in development due to perturbations such as mutations, pathogens, and toxins (for a review, see Møller and Swaddle, 1997). It appears to be partly heritable (Gangestad and Thornhill, 1999, in press-b; but see also Fuller and Houle, in press). We measure 10 such traits in humans and sum the standardized asymmetries to form a single index of FA as a measure of developmental instability. Our studies show that men who possess low FA tend to have greater numbers of sex partners (Gangestad et al., 2001, 2002b; Gangestad and Thornhill, 1997a; Thornhill and Gangestad, 1994), an effect that appears to be partly mediated by phenotypic traits such as social status and intrasexual competitiveness (e.g., Gangestad and Thornhill, 1997b; Simpson et al., 1999). In three studies we have found that normally ovulating women (those not using hormone-based contraception) prefer the scent of symmetrical men, though only when in the fertile phase of the cycle (Gangestad and Thornhill, 1998; Thornhill et al., 2002; Thornhill and Gangestad, 1999). The correlation between preference for the scent of symmetrical men and fertility risk estimated from the day of the cycle and actuarial data when all samples are aggregated is .40. The regression-based

estimated preference when fertility is zero is close to nil. This effect has been replicated in a fourth study performed in Vienna (Rikowski and Grammer, 1999).

2. *Preference for male facial masculinity*. By manipulating digital images, Penton-Voak et al. (1999) created male faces varying with respect to masculinity and femininity. Three studies (two in the United Kingdom, one in Japan) have shown that the face women find most attractive just prior to ovulation is more masculine than the one they most prefer outside the fertile phase (Penton-Voak et al., 1999; Penton-Voak and Perrett, 2000). Using a somewhat different methodology, Johnston et al. (2001) replicated this effect in the United States and, importantly, found that women's ratings of female facial attractiveness was not affected by menstrual phase. Penton-Voak et al. explicitly asked women to rate men's attractiveness as a short-term mate (i.e., a sex partner) and a long-term mate. Fertility risk interacted with relationship context to affect preferences. Greater preference for masculinity just prior to ovulation was observed only when women were rating attractiveness as a short-term mate. Men's facial masculinity covaries with their body symmetry (Gangestad and Thornhill, in press-a), and hence shifts in preference for facial masculinity and the scent in symmetry are shifts in preference for correlated indicators.

3. *Preference for men's behavioral displays*. Gangestad et al. (2002a) had women view brief videotaped segments of men interviewed for a potential lunch date by an attractive female and rate the attractiveness of each man as a sex partner and long-term mate. A large number of nonverbal and verbal features of the interviews were coded, and, through principal components analysis, two major dimensions discriminating men's performance were identified: social presence (e.g., direct eye contact, lack of downward gaze, confidence) and direct intrasexual competitiveness (e.g., derogation of a competitor male, direct comparisons of self with the competitor). A fertility risk by relationship context interaction effect on preferences for these two sorts of displays was found, one paralleling that reported by Penton-Voak et al. When at high fertility risk, women particularly preferred men who evidenced social presence and direct intrasexual competitiveness as short-term mates. Fertility risk did not influence preference for the displays in long-term mates. Based on these same interviews, Simpson et al. (1999) reported that men's direct intrasexual competitiveness covaries with their symmetry, and, thus once again, these preference shifts concern features that at least partly overlap with other features for which preferences shift.[5]

---

[5]In an effort to test whether women might also seek compatible genes at midcycle, Thornhill et al. (2002) examined menstrual cycle effects on women's scent preference for MHC dissimilarity. They found no evidence for shifts across the cycle and, in fact, did not replicate previous findings that women prefer the scent of individuals dissimilar at MHC (Wedekind et al. 1995; Wedekind and Furi, 1997). See also Jacob et al. (2002).

Gangestad et al. (2002b) asked women how often in the past 2 days they had experienced sexual attraction to or fantasized about men other than a primary partner as well as their primary partners twice during the cycle: once within 4 days before or a day after a lutenizing hormone surge (i.e., at high fertility risk) and once in the mid-to-late luteal phase. As might be expected, if women found a suite of features particularly sexy (attractive in a short-term partner) just prior to ovulation, they reported greater sexual interest in men other than primary partners just prior to ovulation. No comparable shift in women's interest in their own partners was detected. Naturally, these shifts in sexual interest may only occasionally lead women to have extra-pair sex. Nonetheless, when they do, they might well be more likely to do so midcycle. Bellis and Baker (1990) surveyed British women and found precisely that pattern. By contrast, women's sex with their primary partners was more evenly distributed across the cycle.[6]

These studies suggest that, like females of many other species, polyandry may have been part of the tactical repertoire in the reproductive strategy of ancestral females (albeit one whose expression evolved to be conditional on environmental circumstances). Although to evolve as a reproductive tactic, female polyandry must have had benefits, it also had costs. Many of those costs should be understood as the outcomes of sexually antagonistic coevolution.

A premise of the expectation that female interest in markers of genetic benefits in sex partners should be contingent on female fertility risk was that females could pay costs by engaging in extra-pair sex, largely because their male partners will be less willing to invest in their partners' offspring if they know or suspect that their partners have engaged in extra-pair sex. The decision process that underlies male willingness to invest in offspring can itself be thought of as a coevolved counteradaptation to female polyandry. In fact, the same study that found that female interest in extra-pair men is contingent on female cycle phase found evidence that male counteradaptation to female polyandry is similarly honed by selection to be sensitive to the female cycle phase. Women were asked the extent to which their primary partners had, in the past 2 days, engaged in a number of "mate retention tactics," such as vigilance (frequent checking up on them) and monopolization of their time. Women reported that their partners had been both more proprietary (e.g., vigilant) and attentive (e.g., monopolizing of time) during the high-fertility days prior to ovulation than during the luteal phase (Gangestad et al., 2002b). Although men could be interested in spend-

[6]The sample in this study was highly self-selected, as female readers of *Parade* magazine were asked to respond to a survey. It is unclear how the nonrepresentative nature of the sample would generate the observed interaction between relationship type (extra-pair vs. in-pair) and menstrual phase. Nonetheless, the findings bear replication.

ing time with their partners for any number of reasons, interestingly the men most likely to have increased interest in doing so midcycle tended to be those with partners who expressed increased sexual interest in extra-pair men—not their primary partners—during this same period. The pattern of findings suggests that either (a) men have evolved to respond to whatever residual cues of fertility status (e.g., scent; Singh and Bronstad, 2001) exist by engaging in greater mate guarding when the costs of their partners' extra-pair sex are greatest, particularly when cues suggest risk that their partners may have extra-pair sex at that time, or (b) men have evolved to the cues that their partners have increased interest in extra-pair men themselves. In either case, the outcome should be understood as a counteradaptation to polyandry.

The Effects of Polygyny on Sexual Conflicts of Interest

Female multiple matings create sexual conflicts of interest in the area of fertilization processes. Whereas an individual male benefits from having his own sperm father a female's offspring, the female's interests may be best served by having another sire for her offspring. Polygyny (male multiple matings) in the absence of polyandry can also create conflicts of interest. For instance, males may benefit from rates or lengths of mating bouts different from those that would optimize female fertility. These effects on sexually antagonistic coevolution, however, are probably small in comparison to the effects of female multiple matings. Female multiple matings create conflicts over paternity, in which case whether a male reproduces at all is at stake. It is unlikely that male multiple matings can impact female reproductive success as dramatically.

When males invest in offspring, however, male multiple matings can foster conflicts of interest over parental care. From the male's point of view, there is some optimal mixture of effort dedicated to parenting and effort to seek additional mates. This mixture deviates from the optimal allocation of male effort from the female's point of view, which includes no effort dedicated to seeking additional mates. Conflict hence arises over the allocation of effort that males exert on parenting and, conversely, efforts to seek other mates. As noted above, when conflicts of interest over parenting effort exist, the negotiation process can lead to lower allocations of parenting effort than single parents would expend.

Human males have probably evolved to invest considerable amounts of time and effort toward enhancing the well-being and productive development of offspring (e.g., Kaplan et al., 2000), albeit contingently based on a variety of factors (e.g., Geary, 2000). Naturally, male parental effort would not have evolved had it not had a considerable impact on offspring quality or the rate at which female mates could reproduce. At the same time, however, men probably also evolved to seek additional mating opportunities, albeit also conditionally (e.g., dependent on his success in attracting additional mates; Buss and Schmitt, 1993; Gangestad and Simpson, 2000; Trivers, 1972). Indeed, if, as argued above, ancestral women sometimes benefited from extra-pair matings with men who did not invest in resulting offspring, it stands to reason that men would have evolved to seek and compete for those mating opportunities. Studies of human sexual interest reliably find that men's interest in sexual variety and multiple matings exceeds that of women. One study, for instance, found that, on average, college men reported that they would optimally have 10 sexual partners in the next 3 years (Buss and Schmitt, 1993; see also Schmitt et al., 2001). By contrast, women reported that they would optimally have, on average, two partners over the same time period. As men's efforts to seek additional mates would not have increased their primary mates' reproductive success, male-female conflicts of interest over men's efforts to seek multiple mates should have existed. These conflicts should have resulted in the evolution of sexually antagonistic adaptations used in the negotiation of parenting effort.[7]

As discussed earlier, outcomes of sexually antagonistic adaptation in one sex may have clear fitness costs for the other sex, either in the form of reduced viability or reduced fecundity. The next section discusses three examples of antagonistic adaptation with such costs that may have evolved in humans.

ILLUSTRATIONS OF ADAPTATION AND COUNTER-ADAPTATION IN HUMAN SEXUALLY ANTAGONISTIC COEVOLUTION

Potentially, many human features have evolved through sexually antagonistic coevolution. Every tactic of persuasion that, if successful, increases the persuader's reproductive success at the expense of the reproductive success of the target of persuasion should eventually be met by evolved resistance to the persuasion. Across the animal world, courtship rituals may be packed with such counter-adapted complexes. Undoubtedly, some advertisements in the biological world (such as the peacock's tail; Petrie, 1994) are honest indicators of underlying quality that members of the other

[7]Because female multiple matings could potentially take away from parenting effort, it stands to reason that multiple matings may also have fueled some conflict over parenting. Because females should not be expected to have to pay the same heavy costs in mating effort that men do (because men should be motivated to seek opportunistic matings with women), however, the effect of female multiple mating on the negotiation of allocation of effort to parenting (independent of its effects on paternity) should be small relative to the effect of male multiple matings. When females do engage in mating effort at the expense of parenting, however, it should naturally be a source of conflict between mates.

sex benefit from valuing. Nonetheless, each sex may have sensory biases that favor certain displays that offer no quality of true value to the chooser. Selection should lead choosers to resist being influenced by these advertisements. Ironically, however, one possible outcome of one sex's resistance to the other sex's displays is evolved exaggeration of the display (see Holland and Rice, 1998, on "chase-away sexual selection"; but see also Getty, 1999, and Rice and Holland, 1999). It seems likely that the human courtship repertoire possesses coevolved elements of false advertisement and resistance, but this issue has hardly been explored. Another potential area of conflict in the domain of fertility-related behavior is the frequency and timing of intercourse. When the probability of female multiple matings is nonzero, the optimal rate and timing of intercourse for male and female members of a pair may differ (with males preferring a higher rate).

Three particular potential sets of adaptations that evolved through sexually antagonistic coevolution are discussed below. The first two concern processes directly involved in the mechanics of reproduction: pregnancy and conception. I have chosen them as illustrations because (1) they involve physiological mechanisms that have been observed or are, in principle, directly observable; (2) they are directly involved in reproduction; (3) at least potentially they have fertility (and possibly other) costs that, by all reasonable inference, are part of the reproductive load imposed by sexual conflicts of interest; and (4) although a variety of predictions can be derived from well-reasoned theory, most of these predictions have not yet been assessed, and hence these examples illustrate how theory about sexually antagonistic coevolution can guide future research. The last illustration concerns parenting efforts, a realm that may importantly affect fertility outcomes in humans.

Genomic Imprinting

Genomic imprinting refers to differential expression of genes depending on the parent of origin. In the instance of nonimprinted genes, both the paternally derived and maternally derived alleles are active. In the case of imprinted genes (of which there appear to be approximately 100 in mammals; Mochizuki et al., 1996), either the paternal or the maternal copy of the gene is more active than the other. In many cases the less active allele is completely silent. The evolutionary theory of imprinting that is most accepted to date, both because of its logical coherence and empirical support for it, is Haig's kinship theory (for a recent review, see Haig, 2000). This theory states that imprinting evolved because of conflicts of interest of offspring genes with maternal genes that differ depending on whether they are derived from the mother or the father. Although this conflict may arise in a number of different contexts (see Trivers and Burt, 1999), the most clearly supported is in the fetal-maternal conflict over parental investment in the offspring. Maternally derived genes will occur in the mother's future offspring 50 percent of the time. In the absence of strict genetic monogamy, paternally derived alleles will occur in the mother's future offspring less than 50 percent of the time. (In the extreme case in which mothers and fathers produce at most one offspring together, this value is 0 percent. As noted by Parker et al., 2002, however, even when mothers are sexually monogamous, sexual conflicts can exist because males can potentially mate with other females, and hence their future reproduction need not depend on the well-being of a single female.) It follows that genes that affect the growth of a fetus and hence its nutritional demands on the mother are strong candidates to be imprinted, with growth promoters expected to be active when paternally derived and growth suppressors expected to be active when maternally derived. In fact, a host of imprinted genes in both humans and mice follow this pattern.[8]

Imprinting (the silencing of gene expression) requires special machinery, which begins in the production of male and female gametes. At least in many cases it involves methylation of DNA (e.g., REF). DNA methylation of alleles in the production of gametes requires the action of a gene that applies this imprint (or genes that do so), which may be *cis*-acting or *trans*-acting (on the same chromosome or a different chromosome, respectively). For genes to differentially apply imprints to maternally or paternally derived copies, they must be differentially expressed in the male and female, that is sex limited in their expression. Hence, the evolution of imprinting involves sexually antagonistic coevolution of male and female imprinter genes (see Zeh and Zeh, 2001). Paternal imprinters can be construed as adaptations that increase the viability of the fetus at the cost of the mother's viability. Evolution of these adaptations sets the stage for counteradaptation involving maternal imprinting.[9]

We should expect that, like other antagonistic coevolutionary processes, the coevolution of imprinting should yield the evolutionary outcomes discussed earlier.

---

[8]Genes on the Y chromosome, like paternally imprinted genes, are expressed only as paternal copies. As expected, the genes that favor fetal growth tend to accumulate on Y. The Y thus is expected to accumulate genes that enhance fetal demands on maternal resources. Moreover, in instances in which a mother's offspring do often have the same father, Y genes will be selected to favor subsequent brothers at the expense of sisters because brothers share Y, whereas sisters do not. Maternally active genes on X may evolve to counteract selfish growth factors on Y, and paternally active X genes (passed on only to daughters) may evolve to favor sisters. For details and other complications with sex chromosomes, see Trivers and Burt (1999), Haig (2000), and Hurst (1994).

[9]One interesting complication not dealt with here is that imprinter genes can be in conflict with the genes they imprint. See Burt and Trivers (2000).

1. *Imprinter and/or imprinted genes should evolve rapidly.* Although some analyses suggest that imprinted genes are characterized by frequent positive selection for functional DNA substitutions, the evidence to date is not compelling (Trivers and Burt, 1999). Little is known about the rate of evolution of imprinter genes.

2. *Imprinter and/or imprinted genes should be characterized as substantial allelic variation.* Little appears to be known about the polymorphism of imprinter genes. A recent study examined expressed polymorphisms in blood for three imprinted human genes, IGF2 (insulin-like growth factor II), SNRPN (nuclear ribonucleoprotein N), and IMPT1 (multimembrane-spanning polyspecific transporter-like gene 1) in a normal Japanese sample (Sakitani et al., 2001). The first two genes are paternally active, while the latter is maternally active. Consistently, only the paternal copy of SNRPN was expressed. By contrast, notable variation in the expression of the maternal copy of IGF2 was observed, and there was very substantial variation in the degree to which the paternal copy of IMPT1 was expressed. It is not known at this time whether the individual variation in expression of these imprinter genes is due to allelic variation in imprinter genes, though that is one possibility.

Of the many genes whose allelic variation has been examined in relation to IQ, the only one whose association has been multiply replicated is IGF2R (insulin-like growth factor 2 receptor), a maternally active imprinted gene (Chorney et al., 1998). One possibility is that the current variation we observe is but a snapshot in an evolutionary scenario in which one allele is replacing another through positive Darwinian selection driven by sexually antagonistic genetic interests. This possibility has not been evaluated.

3. *The antagonistic coevolution of interests of maternally and paternally derived fetal genes (and the sex-limited imprinter genes that account for imprinting) should be a source of maladaptation.* As discussed earlier, antagonistic adaptations that evolved in response to the maternal-fetal conflict appear to be responsible for a variety of poor reproductive outcomes of pregnancy. One should expect that some of the fetal adaptations antagonistic to maternal well-being are paternally active imprinted genes. The genetic bases of many of these adaptations (e.g., manipulation of hormone levels in the maternal bloodstream, partly responsible for gestational diabetes and hypertension) is unknown.

4. *Favorable outcomes should partly be a function of compatibility between maternal and paternal imprints.* Imprinted genes evolve in a context in which only one copy of the gene is (typically) expressed. Paternally active alleles should be selected to be strongly expressed when maternal copies are silenced. But the optimal situation from the standpoint of the paternally derived genes is not unfettered expression. In principle, the fetus

may grow at a rate far greater than optimal even from the perspective of paternally derived genes, for the result may be spontaneous abortion or death of the mother (see Haig, 1993). Similarly, the fetus may demand resources at a level far less than is optimal from the standpoint of growth-suppressing maternally imprinted genes, for the fetus may be deprived. Fetuses differing in their relative expression of paternally active imprinted genes may optimally thrive when paired with different maternally active imprinted genes. On average, for instance, the success of strongly expressed paternally active genes may be maximized when paired with maternally active imprinted genes that are expressed more strongly than those that would maximize the success of more weakly expressed paternally active genes (Zeh and Zeh, 2001). Mismatches in expression of imprinted genes are expected to account for a meaningful proportion of poor pregnancy outcomes.

Conflict Over Immunosuppression in the Female Reproductive Tract

As discussed earlier, proteins in male *Drosophila* seminal fluid are low-level toxins to females, effects that are at least partly by-products of selection for ability to effectively engage in competition against other males' sperm. In addition, some seminal fluid proteins in *Drosophila* are absorbed into the female bloodstream, mimic her hormones, and thereby manipulate her responses. Human seminal fluid also carries a host of products (e.g., proteins, fatty acids) with sperm into the female reproductive tract. As far as is known, these products do not have directly toxic effects on females. Moreover, there is no compelling evidence that components of human seminal fluid play a major role in sperm competition (cf. Baker and Bellis, 1995). Seminal products presumably have evolved functions, however, and it should not be surprising if some of these functions have been selected through sexually antagonistic coevolution, with deleterious effects on female viability and/or fecundity.[10]

Vaginal, cervical, and uterine mucosa are rich in immunological factors, including leucocytes, cytokines, immunoglobulins, and antimicrobial peptides (e.g., Quayle et al., 1998; Yeaman et al., 1998). A primary function of their presence is likely as a defense against sexually transmitted diseases (STDs). Indeed, a recent comparative analysis of primates found that, controlling for group size and exposure to soilborne pathogens, white

[10]Mimicry of female hormones and manipulation of responses should not be discounted as a possibility; after all, prostaglandins are primarily female hormones in humans and importantly function during pregnancy, with large concentrations in men found only in the prostate, where they are manufactured for release into seminal fluid.

blood cell counts are greater in species in which females have more mating partners and hence species in which STDs are a greater risk, suggesting that STDs have been a significant selective pressure on the evolution of primate immune systems (Nunn et al., 2000). Cell-mediated and humoral immune responses in the reproductive tract, however, may attack not only pathogens but also sperm subject to attack or trapping (e.g., Hirano et al., 1999). Female immune responses can, in principle, eliminate the possibility of successful fertilization and indeed appear to play a role in some instances of infertility (e.g., Harrison et al., 1998; Mazumdar and Levine, 1998; Hirano et al., 1999). Immunological defense in the reproductive tract, then, has both benefits and costs, and presumably there is some optimal trade-off maximizing net benefit.

From the male perspective, these same costs and benefits may also operate, particularly when there is some probability of having subsequent offspring with his female mate. Nonetheless, because (1) in the absence of strict monogamy, his future reproductive success need not be tied to hers, (2) immunological factors in the female reproductive tract probably function to prevent male-to-female transmission of STDs more so than female-to-male transmission; (3) there may be greater reproductive costs of STDs to females than males (due to greater association with sterility [Westrom, 1994], possibly an effect that evolved to benefit sexually transmitted pathogens), it seems likely that the level of immunological capacity in the female reproductive tract maximizing male reproductive success is less than what is optimal from the female point of view. In all likelihood, there is a sexual conflict of interest in this area.

In recent years, medical research has shown that a variety of products in human male seminal plasma have immunosuppressive effects. For instance, prostaglandins, which are major constituents of seminal plasma, stimulate the production of the antiinflammatory cytokine interleukin-10 (IL-10; Kelly et al., 1997; Denison et al., 1999) and inhibit the production of the proinflammatory cytokine IL-12 (Kelly et al., 1997). IL-10 inhibits the killing activity of T-cells and natural killer cells and thereby suppresses cell-mediated immune responses, whereas IL-12 promotes cell-mediated immunity. Jeremias et al. (1998) similarly reported that human semen produces messenger RNA for IL-10 in female blood cells and, furthermore, can inhibit production of IFN-g, a proinflammatory cytokine. Some effects appear contrary to the general trend (e.g., prostaglandins may also enhance production of IL-8, a proinflammatory cytokine; Denison et al., 1999); possibly, the overall effect is more complexly patterned than simply a general immunosuppressive effect. (For instance, it may be that the capacity to attack viruses and foreign antigens in particular is suppressed, with attacks triggered by bacterial chemical trails unchanged or enhanced.) At present, however, it does seem clear that at least some components of seminal plasma function to suppress both cell-mediated and humoral immune responses (Kelly, 1997).

Immunosuppressive functions make perfect sense when viewed through the lens of sexually antagonistic coevolution. Indeed, if there exists a sexual conflict of interest over the capacity for immunological responses in the female reproductive tract, one should expect males to have evolved to suppress these immune functions, females to have countered by increasing allocation of effort to them, males to have responded by increasing immunosuppressive efforts, and so on, in an escalating coevolutionary tug-of-war. Evidence for such a tug-of-war could be that females counteract male immunosuppressive activity by, for instance, disabling those functions. Alternatively, females may have undermined attempts to suppress immune function by evolving immunostimulators that are enhanced by the same male products evolved to suppress activity. (Indeed, one possible explanation for certain immunostimulatory effects of male seminal plasma is precisely this counteradaptation; future research may address this possibility.) At the present time, there is neither evidence strongly in favor or against antagonistic coevolution, as it appears that research in this area has proceeded blind of these ideas. Rice's (1996) seminal article has been cited approximately 150 times in the scientific literature but not once in a journal concerning human reproduction or fertility. Where evident, the prevailing functional framework in this literature starkly contrasts with sexually antagonistic coevolution: that reproduction is characterized by a cooperative division of labor in which the sexes have similar if not identical interests in the endeavor (e.g., Denison et al., 1999).

One piece of evidence is mildly suggestive of antagonistic coevolution. Female immunological responsivity appears to vary across the menstrual cycle. Cervical production of immunoglobulin A, the major immunoglobulin responsible for humoral immune reactions in the reproductive tract, is greatest 2 to 3 days prior to ovulation (Kutteh et al., 1996), days associated with peak fertility (Wilcox et al., 1995). Furthermore, antigen presentation by mucousal tissues in the reproductive tract is highest in the days just prior to ovulation, a time at which copulation can lead to conception (though it falls at ovulation itself; Prabhala and Wira, 1995). If female interests were driven solely by trade-offs between immune defense and fertilization, one would expect that immunocompetence would be reduced as fertility risk increased. The fact that certain forms of immunocompetence increase at high fertility risk suggests that other factors operate. As discussed above, ancestral females were more likely to have sex with extra-pair males near midcycle, mates who (1) probably were more likely to present novel STDs to females than their in-pair mates and (2) because of their lower likelihood of having multiple offspring with the female would be in greater conflict with her over level of immunosuppression. Possibly, then, women accordingly evolved to increase their allocation of effort toward reproductive tract immune function during this time. An interesting and testable empirical question is whether men counter by increasing seminal levels of immunosuppressive factors when their mate is near mid-cycle. Such a pattern would constitute strong evidence for a coevolutionary tug-of-war between the sexes, quite possibly over female immune function.[11]

If male and female efforts to control immune function have antagonistically coevolved, we should expect rapid evolution and notable genetic variation of male seminal products and female immunological factors in the reproductive tract. We should furthermore expect that the struggle for control not infrequently leads to poor outcomes, either in the form of infertility or compromised female defense against STDs. Finally, the success of outcomes should partly be a function of the match between male ability to suppress female immune function and female ability to maintain it. These predictions may be explored in future research.

Conflict Over Parenting Effort

A large literature on the transition to parenthood has accumulated over the past two decades—the transition that individuals and couples experience during pregnancy, birth, and rearing of a first child (for a review, see, e.g., Gottman and Notarius, 2000). A robust finding across a large number of studies and multiple cultures is that, on average, men's and women's satisfaction with their marriages and their partners declines during the year following the birth of a first child (e.g., Terry et al., 1991; Crohan, 1996; El Giamal, 1997; Bottcher and Nickel, 1998; Gloger-Tippelt and Huerkamp, 1998; Morse et al., 2000; Wadsby and Sydsjo, 2001). As should be expected if explicit or implicit negotiation over responsibilities for child care and other household tasks entails conflicts, declines in marital satisfaction appear to substantially if not largely stem from perceptions that the partner does not meet expectations of responsible sharing in child care or that household tasks are allocated unfairly (Belsky and Hsieh, 1998; El Giamal, 1997; Grote and Clark, 2001).

If sexual conflicts of interest affected the evolution of negotiation strategies involved in these conflicts, we should perhaps expect that these conflicts revolve around the father's allocation of time and effort to parenting

[11]The possibility that female immune responses against sperm are not merely a by-product of selection for defense against pathogens but rather are partly due to selection for their own benefits should also be considered. Lu and Zha (2000) found that seminal plasma from men with normal sperm inhibited antisperm antibodies more effectively than seminal plasma from men with abnormal sperm. Possibly, then, production of antisperm antibodies is a means whereby females increase the probability of conceiving with men with normal sperm.

more so than the mother's. As noted above, in most mammalian species (probably including humans), males pay a heavier cost of mating (searching for and attracting mates) than do females. Hence, even if both sexes may be motivated to engage in extra-pair mating, males in all likelihood pay a larger cost to seek it. As a result, the conflict over allocation of time and effort to parenting a new child is more likely to be around a father's allocation of time to it (as opposed to effort to seek or attract new mates) than a mother's (though it should be emphasized that mothers may provide or withhold care as tactics in the negotiation process). A number of findings are consistent with this expectation. Terry et al. (1991) found that an increase in females' marital satisfaction across the transition to parenthood was predicted by a perception that her partner fairly participated in household tasks. Furthermore, a decline in women's affection for their partners was evident only for those dissatisfied with their partner's postpartum performance as a father and cooperative caretaker. By contrast, there was no evidence that men's marital dissatisfaction was predicted by how well they perceived their partner's performance as a mother. Similar findings were reported by Shapiro et al. (2000). In a study of couples from diverse socioeconomic backgrounds, Levy-Shiff (1994) found that fathers' caregiving, play, and affiliative behaviors predicted stable or positive (as opposed to declining) marital satisfaction of both sexes. Maternal behaviors did not similarly predict satisfaction. (In fact, mothers' caregiving actually predicted men's marital satisfaction negatively, perhaps because it reflected greater caregiving by fathers themselves.) Rholes et al. (2001) reported that women preoccupied with concerns over their partners' love and commitment to them who also entered parenthood concerned about the level of support they would receive from their husbands experienced particularly large declines in marital satisfaction. Again, no such effects were found for men. Finally, a study of Turkish couples with young first-born children revealed that a pattern of resolving conflicts (presumably often over child care and other household responsibilities) favoring the wife was associated with greater satisfaction of both spouses with their marriages; a pattern of conflict resolution in which the husband's view prevailed predicted negative feelings toward the spouse (Hortacsu, 1999). These findings need not suggest that paternal involvement in child care and household responsibilities directly and unconditionally *affects* both parents' satisfaction. They are consistent with the possibility that circumstances that favor paternal interest in participating in child care and household responsibilities lead to reduced conflict and increased marital satisfaction *in these circumstances*. (Factors that may influence paternal interest in participating in child care and household responsibilities are discussed below.)

Conflicts ultimately arising from diverging interests of the sexes pertaining to parenting may influence fertility-related behaviors in a variety of ways. First, they may directly affect child outcomes. Marital conflict is associated with parental parenting strategies, and Margolin et al. (2001) reported evidence consistent with coparenting processes (cooperation and conflict between parents over parental tasks) mediating this association. Marital conflict and conflictual coparenting in turn predict child problem behaviors (e.g., acting out, lack of impulse control; Schoppe et al., 2001), which may be adaptive or maladaptive responses to (from the child's standpoint) low levels of parental care and guidance. (It should be emphasized that these familial associations may be due to shared genetic influences on behavior rather than direct effects of parenting strategies; unfortunately, no genetically informative study capable of separating these sources of influence has been conducted.) In economically disadvantaged populations in which nutritional stress is common, compromises to parental care owing to sexual conflicts of interest may affect the growth and developmental health of children. Second, these conflicts may influence processes that affect the interbirth interval (as well as, in certain circumstances completed family size). One might expect that heightened conflict between spouses over child care duties may delay willingness on the part of one or both partners to have another child or, in natural fertility populations, increase the interbirth interval by, for instance, increasing the age at weaning. Third, anticipation of conflicts of interest may influence desires to have children with a current partner and hence motivation to start a family.

Although research has extensively documented heightened conflict between new parents, we know very little about the nature of the tactics that partners use in attempts to enhance participation in parenting by the other parent or countertactics to subvert these attempts. Similarly, we know very little about the costs of these tactics to parenting and thereby children. We should expect that these tactics revolve more around controlling how the male partner allocates his time and effort than around how the female partner does so. Because women may withdraw parental investment to enhance male participation, however, conflicts over female parenting may also arise. Furthermore, although the initial arena of conflict may concern parental efforts, influence tactics may spread to other aspects of the relationship, as partners reinforce parenting efforts (or punish lack of such efforts) by introducing contingencies on other valued behaviors (e.g., if the male partner prefers a higher rate of sexual behavior, females may initiate or respond to male attempts to initiate sex contingent on male parenting efforts).

As noted earlier, the optimal allocation of male effort to parenting should (or ancestrally should have) depended on payoffs to parenting as well as payoffs to other activities (e.g., those related to seeking additional mating opportunities). Because work on the transition to parenthood has not been informed by an evolutionary perspective on sexual conflicts of interest (but rather has tended to view this transition as a normal period of "adjustment" that parents undergo), research has not systematically examined the impact of factors that moderate these payoffs on conflicts. Males who possess characteristics that make them more attractive to females in general may be more reluctant to engage in parenting efforts (for an avian example, see Smith, 1995). If so, do they experience more conflict with their partners over parenting? Or, just as females in a number of bird species increase parenting efforts with more attractive males (for a review, see Sheldon, 2000), might the negotiation process lead to greater allocation of effort on the part of their partners (see Boussière, 2002, on cost-benefit modeling)? Because men with partners who would be difficult to replace may perceive greater costs to efforts to seek other mating opportunities, female features (e.g., attractiveness) should also affect the degree of and resolution of conflict over parenting. Finally, conflict may also depend on characteristics of the child. The perceived marginal gain as a function of parenting may differ for children of different developmental qualities or health. For these offspring, then, fewer benefits from other activities are necessary for those activities to compete with parenting effort, and conflict over their care may be greater. These possibilities may be explored in future research.

Just as coevolutionary processes may be responsible for variation in men's and women's control over immunologic activity in the female reproductive tract, they may have created differences in men's and women's influence over the negotiation process regarding parenting. And just as matching of men's and women's abilities to control immunologic activity may affect fertility outcomes, matching of men's and women's influence over the negotiation process may importantly affect parenting and thereby child outcomes.

FACULTATIVE EXPRESSION OF SEXUALLY ANTAGONISTIC ADAPTATIONS IN HUMANS?

Sexually antagonistic coevolution is fueled by differences in the genetic interests of male and female mates in the absence of strict genetic monogamy. When strict or relative monogamy reigns, whether in natural or laboratory populations, males and females should evolve relative benevolence toward mates. As mating departs from monogamy, conflicts increase, selection for sexually antagonistic traits is strengthened, and a reproductive load on mortality or fecundity should result (Holland and Rice, 1999).

Women show evidence of design for strategic polyandry. Furthermore, at least one modern human population is characterized by a rate of extra-pair paternity that would fuel considerable sexual conflicts of interest. Not unlikely, many ancestral human groups were exposed to similar levels of sexual conflict. At the same time, at least one modern population is characterized by a very low rate of extra-pair paternity, and, not unlikely, some ancestral human groups were similarly exposed to low levels of sexual conflict. Quite possibly, humans have evolved patterns of mating and parental investment that are variable in nature and contingently expressed as a function of ecological and/or socioecological factors. (See Gross, 1996, for a discussion of conditional mating strategies.) In part, the contingent expression of reproductive tactics should be a function of factors that affect the benefits and costs of polyandry, which may include, but not be limited to, (a) the degree to which men vary with regard to intrinsic genetic benefits (e.g., the prevalence of parasites or environmental stress, both of which may potentiate expression of fitness-relevant genetic variation; Gangestad and Simpson, 2000) and (b) the degree to which paternal investment adds to offspring fitness, possibly as a function of the extent to which maternal and paternal investment multiplicatively influence offspring fitness (e.g., through division of labor; Kaplan et al., 2000).

Just as mating and parenting tactics in general may have evolved to be facultatively expressed, so too sexually antagonistic tactics may have evolved to be contingent responses in men's and women's reproductive strategies. Hence, just as male *Drosophila* evolve to be more benevolent toward their mates when strict monogamy is enforced, men and women may be more benevolent when conditions favor relative monogamy. By contrast, just as male *Drosophila* impose a reproductive load on females when mating is promiscuous, men and women may express adaptations that impose reproductive costs on the other sex when conditions favor multiple matings. With regard to the three illustrations sketched above, one might expect that (a) the expression of imprinter genes may be adaptively contingent on environmental factors, such that imprinting, maternal-fetal conflict, and the reproductive load (e.g., fetal insufficiency, maternal stress) that results increase as a function of factors favoring polyandry and ease as a function of factors favoring relative monogamy (see Haig, 1993, and Trivers and Burt, 1999, for related remarks); (b) the struggle over control of immune function in the reproductive tract and its reproductive load (e.g., infertility, spread of STDs) are enhanced by factors favoring polyandry and eased as a function of factors favoring relative monogamy; (c) conflicts between parents will be reduced, care and provisioning will be more efficiently and effectively provided to offspring, and offspring health and features of adaptive functioning affected by parental care will be enhanced under circumstances in which men are motivated to engage in parental care rather than seek multiple mating opportunities.

SUMMARY

Sexual mates have correlated interests in favorable reproductive outcomes. Because their interests do not perfectly correspond, however, sexual conflicts of interest also exist. These conflicts can lead to sexually antagonistic coevolution, in which each sex evolves adaptations that benefit mates of that sex at the expense of the interests of mates of the other sex. This coevolution process typically results in a reproductive load on the species, reducing the efficiency by which sexual pairs produce and care for offspring. An understanding of fertility-related behavior and processes can be informed by an appreciation of how sexual conflicts of interest have manifested in sexually antagonistic features.

Only under conditions of true genetic monogamy (in which each sex can potentially reproduce with one mate only) do sexual conflicts of interest fail to exist. Multiple matings by members of both sexes (whether serially or simultaneously) create sexual conflicts of interest. In species in which females are inseminated, polyandry fuels sexual conflicts of interest over control of paternity. In these species in which both sexes invest in offspring, polygyny fuels sexual conflicts of interest over coparenting efforts. Polyandry and polygyny both contribute to sexual conflicts of interest over the flow of resources from mothers to offspring. Evidence for adaptations that result from each of these conflicts of interest in a variety of nonhuman species are well documented. Adaptations underlying human fertility-related behavior and processes that may have been shaped by sexually antagonistic coevolution are an area ripe for exploration.

REFERENCES

Aigaki, T., I. Fleischmann, P.S. Chen, and E. Kubli
1991 Ectopic expression of sex peptide alters reproductive behavior of female *Drosophila melanogaster*. *Neuron* 7:557-563.

Baker, R.R., and M.A. Bellis
1995 *Human Sperm Competition: Copulation, Masturbation, and Infidelity*. London: Chapman and Hall.

Bellis, M.A., and R.R. Baker
1990 Do females promote sperm competition? Data for humans. *Animal Behavior* 40:997-999.

Belsky, J., and K.H. Hsieh
1998 Patterns of marital change during the early childhood years: Parent personality, coparenting, and division-of-labor correlates. *Journal of Family Psychology* 12:511-528.

Birkhead, T.R., and A.P. Møller
1995 Extra-pair copulation and extra-pair paternity in birds. *Animal Behavior* 49:843-848.

Bottcher, A., and H. Nickel
1998 Maternal attitudes and family changes across the transition to parenthood in a cross-cultural perspective: Studies on first-time and second-time mothers in West Germany, Georgia US, and Korea. *Psychologie in Erziehung und Unterricht* 45:92-112.

Boussière, L.F.
2002 A model of the interaction between "good genes" and direct benefits in the provisioning of offspring: When do males of high genetic quality invest less? *Philosophical Transactions of the Royal Society of London* B357:309-317.

Burt, A.
1995 Perspective: The evolution of fitness. *Evolution* 49:1-8.

Burt, A., and R. Trivers
2000 Genetic conflicts in genomic imprinting. *Proceedings of the Royal Society of London* B265:2393-2397.

Buss, D.M., and D.P. Schmitt
1993 Sexual strategies theory: A contextual evolutionary analysis of human mating. *Psychological Review* 100:204-232.

Cerda-Flores, R.M., S.A. Barton, L.F. Marty-Gonzalez, F. Rivas, and R. Chakraborty
1999 Estimation of nonpaternity in the Mexican population of Nueveo Leon: A validation study with blood group markers. *American Journal of Physical Anthropology* 109:281-293.

Chapman, T., F. Lindsay, F. Liddle, J. Kalb, M.F. Wolfner, and L. Partridge
1995 Cost of mating in *Drosophila melanogaster* females is mediated by male accessory gland products. *Nature* 373:241-244.

Charlesworth, B., and K.A. Hughes
1998 The maintenance of genetic variation in life history traits. In *Evolutionary Genetics from Molecules to Morphology*. R.S. Singh and C.B. Krimbas, eds. Cambridge: Cambridge University Press.

Chippendale, A.K., J.R. Gibson, and W.R. Rice
2001 Negative genetic correlation between adult fitness for the sexes reveals ontogenetic conflict in *Drosophila*. *Proceedings of the National Academy of Sciences* 98:1671-1675.

Chorney, M.J., K. Chorney, N. Seese, M.J. Owen, J. Daniels, P. McGuffin, L.A. Thompson, D.K. Detterman, C. Benbow, D. Lubinski, T. Eley, and R. Plomin
1998 A quantitative trait locus associated with cognitive ability in children. *Psychological Science* 9:159-166.

Clark, A., G.M. Agoude, T. Prout, L. Harshman, and C.H. Langley
1995 Variation in sperm displacement and its association with accessory gland protein loci in *Drosophila melanogaster*. *Genetics* 139:189-201.

Crohan, S.E.
1996 Marital quality and conflict across the transition to parenthood in African American and white couples. *Journal of Marriage and the Family* 58:933-944.

Denison, F.C., V.E. Grant, A.A. Calder, and R.W. Kelly
1999 Seminal plasma components stimulate interleukin-8 and interleukin-10 release. *Molecular Human Reproduction* 5:220-226.

Eberhard, W.G.
1996 *Female Control: Sexual Selection by Cryptic Female Choice*. Princeton, NJ: Princeton University Press.

El Giamal, M.
1997 Changes in marital satisfaction and coping during the transition to parenthood: A review of current studies. *Psychologie in Erziehung und Unterricht* 44:256-275.

Fowler, K., and L. Partridge

1989 A cost of mating in female fruitflies. *Nature* 338:760-761.

Fuller, R.C., and D. Houle

In press Inheritance of developmental instability. Pp. 157-184 in *Developmental Instability: Causes and Consequences*. M. Polak, ed. Cambridge: Cambridge University Press.

Gangestad, S.W., K. Bennett, and R. Thornhill

2001 A latent variable model of the developmental instability in relation to men's sexual behavior. *Proceedings of the Royal Society of London* B268:1677-1684.

Gangestad, S.W., and J.A. Simpson

2000 The evolution of human mating: The role of trade-offs and strategic pluralism. *Behavioral and Brain Sciences* 23:675-687.

Gangestad, S.W., J.A. Simpson, A.J. Cousins, C.E. Garver, and P.N. Christensen

2002a Menstrual cycle variation in female preferences for male behavioral displays. Manuscript submitted for publication.

Gangestad, S.W., and R. Thornhill

1997a The evolutionary psychology of extrapair sex: The role of fluctuating asymmetry. *Evolution and Human Behavior* 18:69-88.

1997b Human sexual selection and developmental stability. Pp. 169-195 in *Evolutionary Personality and Social Psychology*. J.A. Simpson and D.T. Kenrick, eds. Hillsdale, NJ: Erlbaum.

1998 Menstrual cycle variation in women's preference for the scent of symmetrical men. *Proceedings of the Royal Society of London* B265:927-933.

1999 Individual differences in developmental precision and fluctuating asymmetry: A model and its implications. *Journal of Evolutionary Biology* 12:402-416.

In press-a Facial masculinity and fluctuating asymmetry. *Evolution and Human Behavior*.

In press-b Fluctuating asymmetry, developmental instability, and fitness: Toward model-based interpretation. Pp. 165-216 in *Developmental Instability: Causes and Consequences*. M. Polak, ed. Cambridge: Cambridge University Press.

Gangestad, S.W., R. Thornhill, and C. Garver

2002b Changes in women's sexual interests and their partners' mate retention tactics across the menstrual cycle: Evidence for shifting conflicts of interest. *Proceedings of the Royal Society of London* B 269:975-982.

Gavrilets, S.

2000 Rapid evolution of reproductive barriers driven by sexual conflict. Nature *403:886-889.*

Geary, D.C.

2000 Evolution and proximate expression of human paternal investment. *Psychological Bulletin* 126:55-77.

Getty, T.

1999 Chase-away selection as noisy reliable signaling. *Evolution* 53:299-302.

Gloger-Tippelt, G.S., and M. Huerkamp

1998 Relationship change at the transition to parenthood and security of infant-mother attachment. *International Journal of Behavioral Development* 22:633-655.

Gottman, J.M., and C.L. Notarius

2000 Decade review: Observing marital interaction. *Journal of Marriage and Family* 62:927-947.

Gross, M.R.

1996 Alternative reproductive strategies and tactics: Diversity within sexes. *Trends in Ecology and Evolution* 11:92-98.

Grote, N.K., and M.S. Clark
2001 Perceiving unfairness in the family: Cause or consequence of marital distress? *Journal on Perspectives in Social Psychology* 80:281-293.

Haig, D.
1993 Genetic conflicts in human pregnancy. *Quarterly Review of Biology* 68:495-532.
2000 The kinship theory of genomic imprinting. *Annual Review of Ecological Systems* 31:9-32.

Harrison, S., G. Hull, and S. Pillai
1998 Sperm acrosome status and sperm antibodies in infertility. *Journal of Urology* 159:1554:1558.

Harshman, L.G., and T. Prout
1994 Sperm displacement without sperm transfer in *Drosophila melanogaster. Evolution* 48:758-756.

Hirano, M., M. Kamada, M. Maegawa, H. Gima, and T. Aono
1999 Binding of human secretory leukocyte protease inhibitor in uterine cervical mucus to immunoglobulins: Pathophysiology in immunologic infertility and local immune defense. *Fertility and Sterility* 71:1108-1114.

Holland, B., and W.R. Rice
1998 Chase-away sexual selection: Antagonistic seduction versus resistance. *Evolution* 52:1-7.
1999 Experimental removal of sexual selection reverses intrasexual antagonistic coevolution and removes a reproductive load. *Proceedings of the National Academy of Sciences USA* 96:5083-5088.

Hortacsu, N.
1999 Transition to parenthood: The Turkish case. *Journal of Social Behavioral Perspectives* 14:325-343.

Hosken, D.J., T.W.J. Garner, and P.L. Ward
2001 Sexual conflict selects for male and female reproductive characters. *Current Biology* 11:489-493.

Houle, D.
1992 Comparing evolvability and variability of traits. *Genetics* 130:195-204.

Hurst, L.D.
1994 Embryonic growth and the evolution of the mammalian Y chromosome: 1. The Y as an attractor for selfish growth factors. *Heredity* 73:223-232.

Jacob, S., M.K. McClintick, B. Zelano, and C. Ober
2002 Paternally inherited HLA alleles are associated with women's choice of male odor. *Nature Genetics* 30:175-179.

Jennions, M.D., and M. Petrie
2000 Why do females mate multiply? A review of the genetic benefits. *Biology Reviews* 75:21-64.

Jeremias, J., S. Mockel, and S.S. Witkin
1998 Human semen induces interleukin 10 and 70 kDa heat shock protein gene transcription and inhibits interferon-gamma messenger RNA production in peripheral blood mononuclear cells. *Molecular Human Reproduction* 4:1084-1088.

Johnston, V.S., R. Hagel, M. Franklin, B. Fink, and K. Grammer
2001 Male facial attractiveness: Evidence for hormone medicated adaptive design. *Evolution and Human Behavior* 22:251-267.

Kaplan, H.S., K. Hill, J.B. Lancaster, and A.M. Hurtado
2000 A theory of human life history evolution: Diet, intelligence, and longevity. *Evolutionary Anthropology* 9:156-185.

Kelly, R.W.
1997 Prostaglandins in primate semen: Biasing the immune system to benefit spermatozoa and virus? *Prostaglandins, Leukotrienes & Essential Fatty Acids* 57:113-118.

Kelly, R.W., and H.O.D. Critchley
1997 Immunomodulation by human seminal plasmas: A benefit for spermatozoon and pathogen? *Human Reproduction* 12:2200-2207.

Kutteh, W.H., S.J. Prince, K.R. Hammond, C.C. Kutteh, and J. Mestecky
1996 Variations in immunoglobulins and IgA subclasses of human uterine cervical secretions around the time of ovulation. *Clinical and Experimental Immunology* 104:538-542.

Lu, N.Q., and S.W. Zha
2000 Inhibitory effects of human seminal plasma on an ELISA used to detect antisperm antibodies: Implications for the determination of sperm quality. *Journal of Reproductive Immunology* 47:33-40.

Levy-Shiff, R.
1994 Individual and contextual correlates of marital change across the transition to parenthood. *Developmental Psychology* 30:591-601.

Margolin, G., E.B. Gordis, and R.S. John
2001 Coparenting: A link between marital conflict and parenting in two-parent families. *Journal of Family Psychology* 15:3-21.

Mazumdar, S., and A.S. Levine
1998 Antisperm antibodies: Etiology, pathogenesis, diagnosis, and treatment. *Fertility and Sterility* 70:799-810.

McNamara, J. M., C. E. Gasson, and A. I. Houston
1999 Incorporating rules for responding into evolutionary games. *Nature* 401:368-371.

McNamara, J. M., A. I Houston, Z. Barta, J.-L. Osorno
In press Should young ever be better off with one parent than two? *Behavioral Ecology*.

Metz, E.C., and S.R. Palumbi
1996 Positive selection for sequence rearrangements generates extensive polymorphism in the gamete recognition protein binding. *Molecular Biology and Evolution* 13:391-406.

Mochizuki, A., Y. Takeda, and Y. Iwasa
1996 The evolution of genomic imprinting. *Genetics* 144:1283-1295.

Møller, A.P., and J.P. Swaddle
1997 *Asymmetry, Developmental Stability and Evolution*. Oxford: Oxford University Press.

Morse, C.A., A. Buist, and S. Durst
2000 First-time parenthood: Influences on pre- and postnatal adjustment in fathers and mothers. *Journal of Psychosomatic Obstetrics and Gynecology* 21:109-120.

Nunn, C.L., J.L. Gittleman, and J. Antonovics
2000 Promiscuity and the primate immune system. *Science* 290:1168-1170.

Palumbi, S.R., and E.C. Metz
1991 Strong reproductive isolation between closely related tropical sea urchins (genus *Echinometra*). *Molecular Biology and Evolution* 8:227-239.

Parker, G.A., N.J. Royle, and I.R. Hartley
2002 Intrafamilial conflict and parental investment: A synthesis. *Philosophical Transactions of the Royal Society of London* B357:295-307.

Penn, D., and W.K. Potts
1999 The evolution of mating preferences and major histocompatibility genes. *American Naturalist* 153:145-164.

Penton-Voak, I.S., and D.I. Perrett
2000 Female preference for male faces changes cyclicallyæfurther evidence. *Evolution and Human Behavior* 21:39-48.

Penton-Voak, I.S., D.I. Perrett, D. Castles, M. Burt, T. Koyabashi, and L.K. Murray
1999 Female preference for male faces changes cyclically. *Nature* 399:741-742.

Petrie, M.
1994 Improved growth and survival of offspring of peacocks with more elaborate trains. *Nature* 371:598-599.

Pitnick, S., W.D. Brown, and G.T. Miller
2001 Evolution of female remating behaviour following experimental removal of sexual selection. *Proceedings of the Royal Society of London* B268:557-563.

Prabhala, R.H., and C.R. Wira
1995 Sex-hormone and IL-6 regulation of antigen-presentation in the female reproductive tract mucosal tissues. *Journal of Immunology* 155:5566-5573.

Quayle, A.J., E.M. Porter, A.A. Nussbaum, Y.M. Wang, C. Brabec, K.P. Yip, and S.C. Mok
1998 Gene expression, immunolocalization, and secretion of human defensin-5 in human female reproductive tract. *American Journal of Pathology* 152:1247-1258.

Rholes, W.S., J.A. Simpson, L. Campbell, and J. Grich
2001 Adult attachment and the transition to parenthood. *Journal on Perspectives in Social Psychology* 81:421-435.

Rice, W.R.
1996 Sexually antagonistic male adaptation triggered by experimental arrest of female evolution. *Nature* 381:232-234.

Rice, W.R., and B. Holland
1997 The enemies within: Intragenomic conflict, interlocus contest evolution (ICE), and the intraspecific Red Queen. *Behavioral Ecology and Sociobiology* 41:1-10.
1999 Reply to comments on the chase-away model of sexual selection. *Evolution* 53:302-306.

Rikowski, A., and K. Grammer
1999 Human body odour, symmetry, and attractiveness. *Proceedings of the Royal Society of London B* 266:869-874.

Rodgers, J.L., K. Hughes, H.P. Kohler, K. Christensen, D. Doughty, D.C. Rowe, and W.B. Miller
2001 Genetic influence helps explain variation in human fertility: Evidence from recent behavioral and molecular genetic studies. *Current Directions in Pyschosocial Sciences* 10:184-188.

Royle, N.J., I.R. Hartley, and G.A. Parker
2002 Sexual conflict reduces offspring fitness in zebra finches. *Nature* 416:733-736.

Sakitani, T., M. Wei, K. Motonobu, C. Okita, D. Wada, K. Mitsuya, M. Meguro, M. Ikeguchi, H. Ito, B. Tycko, and M. Oshimura
2001 Epigenetic heterogeneity at imprinted loci in normal populations. *Biochemical and Biophysical Research Communications* 283:1124-1130.

Sasse, G., H. Muller, R. Chakraborty, and J. Ott
1994 Estimating the frequency of nonpaternity in Switzerland. *Human Heredity* 44:337-343.

Schmitt, D.P., T.K. Shackleford, J. Duntley, W. Tooke, and D.M. Buss
2001 The desire for sexual variety as a key to understanding basic human mating strategies. *Personal Relationships* 8:425-455.

Schoppe, S.J., S.C. Mangelsdorf, and C.A. Frosch

2001 Coparenting, family process, and family structure: Implications for preschoolers' externalizing behavior problems. *Journal of Family Psychology* 15:526-545.

Shapiro, A.F., J.M. Gottman, and S. Carrere

2000 The baby and the marriage: Identifying factors that buffer against decline in marital satisfaction after the first baby arrives. *Journal of Family Psychology* 14:59-70.

Sheldon, B.C.

2000 Differential allocation: Tests, mechanisms and implications. *Trends In Ecology and Evolution* 15:397-402.

Simpson, J.A., S.W. Gangestad, P.N. Christensen, and K. Leck

1999 Fluctuating asymmetry, sociosexuality, and intrasexual competitive tactics. *Journal on Perspectives in Social Psychology* 76:159-172.

Singh, D., and P.M. Bronstad

2001 Female body odour is a potential cue to ovulation. *Proceedings of the Royal Society of London* B268:797-801.

Smith, H.G.

1995 Experimental demonstration of a trade-off between mate attraction and paternal care. *Proceedings of the Royal Society of London B* 260:45-51.

Swanson, W.J., A.G. Clark, H.M. Waldrip-Dail, M.F. Wolfner, and C.F. Aquadro

2001a Evolutionary EST analysis identifies rapidly evolving male reproductive proteins in Drosophila. *Proceedings of the National Academy of Sciences* 98:7375-7379.

Swanson, W.J., Z.H. Zhang, M.F. Wolfner, and C.F. Aquadro

2001b Positive Darwinian selection drives the evolution of several female reproductive proteins in mammals. *Proceedings of the National Academy of Sciences* 98:2509-2514.

Terry, D.J., T.A. McHugh, and P. Noller

1991 Role dissatisfaction and the decline in marital quality across the transition to parenthood. *Australian Journal of Psychology* 43:129-132.

Thornhill, R., and S.W. Gangestad

1994 Fluctuating asymmetry and human sexual behavior. *Psycholgical Science.* 5:297-302.

1999 The scent of symmetry: A human sex pheromone that signals fitness? *Evolution and Human Behavior* 20:175-201.

Thornhill, R., S.W. Gangestad, R. Miller, G. Scheyd, J. K. McCollough, and M. Franklin

In press MHC, symmetry, and body scent attractiveness in men and women. *Behavioral Ecology.*

Tregenza, T., and N. Wedell

2000 Genetic compatibility, mate choice and patterns of parentage: Invited review. *Molecular Biology* 9:1013-1027.

Trivers, R.L.

1972 Sexual selection and parental investment. In *Sexual Selection and the Descent of Man, 1871-1971.* B. Campbell, ed. Chicago: Aldine.

1974 Parent-offspring conflict. *American Zoologist* 14:249-264.

Trivers, R., and A. Burt

1999 Kinship and genomic imprinting. Pp. 1-21 in *Genomic Imprinting: An Interdisciplinary Approach.* R. Ohlsson, ed. Heidelberg: Springer.

Tsaur, S.C., C.T. Ting, and C.I. Wu
2001 Sex in *Drosophila mauritiana*: A very high level of amino acid polymorphism in a male reproductive protein gene, Acp26Aa. *Molecular Biology and Evolution* 18:22-26.

Van Doorn, G.S., P.C. Luttikhuizen, and F.J. Weissing
2001 Sexual selection at the protein level drives the extraordinary divergence of sex-related genes during sympatric speciation. *Proceedings of the Royal Society of London* B268:2155-2161.

Van Valen, L.
1962 A study of fluctuating asymmetry. *Evolution* 10:139-146.

Vanquier, V.D., and Y.-H. Lee
1993 Abalone sperm lysine: An unusual mode of evolution of a gamete recognition protein. *Zygote* 1:181-196.

Wadsby, M., and G. Sydsjo
2001 From pregnancy to parenthood: A study of couples' relationship. *Nordisk Psykologi* 53:275-288.

Wedekind, C., and S. Furi
1997 Body odor preference in men and women: Do they aim for specific MHC combinations or simply heterozygosity? *Proceedings of the Royal Society of London* B264:1471-1479.

Wedekind, C., T. Seebeck, F. Bettens, and A.J. Paepke
1995 MHC-dependent mate preferences in humans. *Proceedings of the Royal Society of London* B260:245-249.

Westrom, L.V.
1994 Sexually-transmitted diseases and infertility. *Sexually Transmitted Diseases* 21: S32-S37.

Wilcox, A.J., C.R. Weinberg, and B.D. Baird
1995 Timing of sexual intercourse in relation to ovulation. *New England Journal of Medicine* 333:1517-1521.

Williams, E.J.B., and L.D. Hurst
2000 The proteins of linked genes evolve at similar rates. *Nature* 407:900-903.

Wyckoff, G.J., W. Wang, and C.L. Wu
2000 Rapid evolution of male reproductive genes in the descent of man. *Nature* 403: 304-309.

Yeaman, G.R., H.D. White, A. Howell, R. Prabhala, and C.R. Wira
1998 The mucosal immune system in the human female reproductive tract: Potential insights into the heterosexual transmission of HIV. *AIDS Research and Human Retroviruses* 14:S57-S62.

Zeh, J.A., and D.W. Zeh
2001 Reproductive mode and genetic benefits of polyandry. *Animal Behavior* 612: 1051-1063.

9

Pubertal Maturation, Adrenarche, and the Onset of Reproduction in Human Males

Benjamin Campbell

Despite their essential participation in the reproductive process, the role of males in fertility variation has tended to be downplayed by demographers, who are primarily interested in fertility differentials between groups, though there is increasing interest in the role of men (see, for instance, Bledsoe et al., 2000). A focus on females makes sense for all of the standard reasons in terms of reproductive accounting because of maternal certainty and the fact that females have more constrained reproductive spans and fertility. However, the benefits of this accounting approach begin to decline as we move further afield to consider factors less directly related to pregnancy, such as behavior. Here there is more room for other perspectives with which to orient our thinking.

From an evolutionary point of view, male humans, as the sex with greater variation in reproductive success, can be expected to be subject to more intense selection (Bateman, 1948). Recently, genetic evidence supports the idea that male reproductive genes undergo more rapid evolution than females (Wyckoff et al., 2000), though it is unclear if this represents greater mutation rates in the male germ line because of more replication events (Vogel and Ratherberg, 1975) or the impact of other processes such as methylation of genes (Huttley et al., 2000) or incorporation of transposable elements (Erlandsson et al., 2000).

The impact of selection on male reproductive biology is evident in morphological differences in male genitalia across species (see Eberhard, 1985, for graphic examples), as well as functional differences in sperm production. Across primate species the ratio of testes size to body size (Harcourt et al., 1981) and even the morphology of sperm themselves

(Anderson and Dixson, 2002) vary between monogamous and polygynous mating systems as a result of selection for sperm competition. For instance, seasonally breeding rhesus macaques have 60 percent larger testes than do the closely related and similarly sized nonseasonally breeding pigtailed macaques, a result of the greater mating competition during seasonal breeding. In addition, rhesus males have 60 percent larger abdominal fatfolds than pigtail males (Muhlenbein et al., 2002), suggesting that substantial energy reserves are needed to offset the energetic costs of male-male competition, among male rhesus.

Such findings are powerful evidence for the impact of selection on sperm production and delivery across species. However, the relatively small testicular to body size ratio exhibited by humans suggests that sperm competition in human males has played only a small role in human evolution (Dixson, 1998; Smith, 1984). Furthermore, the low percentage of normal sperm in human ejaculates is comparable to that of gorillas and very different from that of chimpanzees (Small, 1988), suggesting that the human male reproductive strategy has more in common with preinsemination mate guarding among gorillas than the postinsemination sperm competition of the chimpanzee. Thus, the fact that the size of male ejaculates has been shown to vary with time since exposure to their partners is less evidence for sperm competition in humans (Baker and Bellis, 1989) per se than it is for the importance of mate guarding.

However, in the case of humans, the role of paternal investment in offspring means that selection on males includes not only behavior leading to sex, and aspects of the male reproductive tract associated with insemination, but also behaviors related to pair bonding and the provisioning of offspring. Anecdotal evidence that testosterone increases in males exposed to mates after a prolonged absence (Bribiescas, 2001) suggests a role for testosterone in sexual behavior and pair bonding (see Young, this volume). Recent reports of lower testosterone levels in fathers of young children than in nonfathers (Berg and Wynne-Edwards, 2001; Storey et al., 2000) suggest that changes in testosterone may play a role in shifting behavior from mating to parenting.

With that brief orientation toward the critical elements of male reproductive strategies among humans, I turn to the central focus of this paper, the role of reproductive maturation in the development of male sexual behavior, pair bonding, and parenting.

Here I argue that this process can be considered to have two major dimensions: 1) sexual behavior that is related to reproductive maturation and somatic growth and that is organized by testosterone as part of the reproductive axis, and 2) social behavior that is related to early childhood experience and to the adrenal axis, which produces cortisol and dehydroepiandrosterone and its sulfate DHEA/S. Briefly put, maturation of the reproductive axis is crucial to sexual behavior, whereas development of the adrenal axis is crucial to social behavior and attachment and hence the expression of sexual behavior, as fertility and family formation. It is only by understanding the separate roles of these two important domains of human behavior and their interaction during maturation that we can get a differentiated account of the development of male reproductive behavior.

Of course, any such model represents a vast simplification of all that goes into male reproductive maturation. At the same time, it is intended to be a human model in the essential sense of the word, a model that integrates factors we encounter as part of our everyday existence, without necessarily experiencing them fully or in isolation. As such it should be applicable to variation across societies, including variation in social structures, and biological differences in the timing of adolescent maturation, as well as cultural practices that may have independent effects on behavior.

Finally, much of what will be discussed here is necessarily speculative. Thus, I conclude with recommendations for research that might elaborate and test how these hormones mediate the interaction of biological, psychological, and social levels of fertility behavior in human males.

THE SCOPE OF MALE REPRODUCTIVE MATURATION

Most biological analyses of male reproductive maturation focus exclusively on adolescence because of the obvious connection between pubertal maturation and the onset of sexual behavior. However, the onset of reproductive capacity and sexual behavior may be considered a necessary, but not sufficient, condition for reproduction among human males for whom pair bonding and paternal investment play an additional role (Lancaster and Lancaster, 1987). Thus, changes in familial relationships (Bee, 1997), cognition (Nelson, 1996), and the subjective sense of self (Herdt and McClintock, 2000) that begin prepubertally may be considered as part of the reproductive transition.

In addition, reproduction among males is generally associated with young adulthood and family formation, which do not take place until the early 20s. For instance, in the United States only 3 percent of births are fathered by men under the age of 20, while traditional Kikuyu men marry and become fathers around the age of 25 (Bogin, 2001). Thus, the establishment of productive skills and the development of social position can also be considered part of the process of male reproductive maturation (see Kaplan and Lancaster, this volume).

Furthermore, juvenile, adolescent, and young adult stages appear to be linked as a coherent biological process by increases in the production of DHEA/S by the adrenal gland (because of the close relationship of the two hormones, I will refer to them here collectively as DHEA/S unless discussing

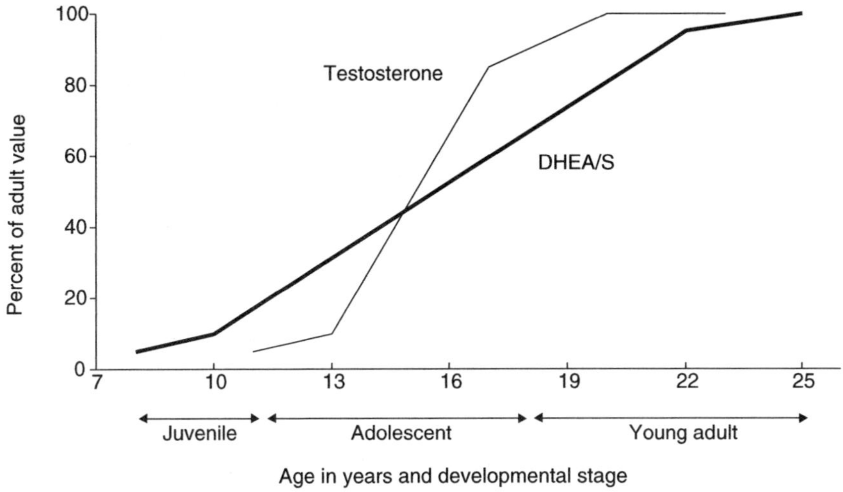

FIGURE 9-1 Temporal relationship of adrenarche and puberty in human males. NOTE: This graph indicates the relative role of changes in DHEA/S and testosterone at different stages of the development of males from age 8 to 25. Both the young adult and juvenile stages are marked by changes in DHEA/S without changes in testosterone, whereas during adolescent both hormones are increasing.

results that are specifically based on one of the two hormones). Based on Western populations, increases in the production of DHEA/S by the adrenal gland, a process referred to as adrenarche, begin around age 8 and continue until the mid-20s (Worthman, 1999), thus bracketing the progression of pubertal development from roughly ages 10 to 18 (see Figure 9-1). Furthermore, the increase of DHEA/S in males appears to extend some 5 years beyond that for females (Worthman, 1999) suggesting important sex differences in the onset of reproduction.

DHEA/S is the most common hormone in the human body. Yet despite its well-known importance as a precursor for estrogen production during fetal development (Parker 1999) and its rise during maturation (Orentreich et al., 1992), a functional understanding of DHEA/S's role in postnatal development remains hazy. DHEA/S is a neurosteroid, meaning that it is produced in the brain as well as the adrenal gland (Baulieu, 1998), though a specific DHEA/S receptor is lacking (Robel and Baulieu et al., 1995). However, DHEA/S is known to occupy receptors for the neurotransmitter gamma aminobutyric acid type (GABA-A) acting as an antagonist (Majewska, 1995) and presumably influencing neural mechanisms in this way.

In addition, DHEA/S is converted to estrogen and testosterone in peripheral tissues (Labrie et al., 1995), meaning that it may also have effects through testosterone and estrogen receptors, not only within the brain but also on immune function and bone and muscle growth. For instance, males with 21-hydroxylase deficiency, a condition that leads to the overproduction of DHEA/S, have reduced fertility, as a result of increased estrogen concentrations suppressing gonadotropin stimulation of the testes (Cabrera et al., 2001; Stikkelbroeck et al., 2001). However, such individuals are also likely to have testicular tumors, clouding the implication of these findings for normal maturation.

DHEA/S is known to have a variety of physiological effects during maturation, including promoting muscle and bone growth (Argquitt et al., 1991; Zemel and Katz, 1986) and disease resistance (Kurtis et al., 2001), as well as playing a role in mood (Goodyer et al., 1996). In addition premature adrenarche has been shown to have effects on both cognition and psychosocial development (Dorn et al. 1999; Nass et al. 1990). Though it is unclear how far findings on cognition can be generalized, Goodyer et al. found that DHEA/S hyposecretion was related to major depression in a sample of 8- to 16-year olds, suggesting that DHEA/S does have important effects on mood during development in normal children.

BIOLOGY OF REPRODUCTIVE MATURATION IN HUMAN MALES

To understand the role of reproductive maturation in the development of reproductive behavior in human males, its important to separate various strands, including reproductive maturation, pubertal development, and somatic growth. Reproductive maturation involves maturation of the hypothalamic-pituitary testicular axis. This starts with gonadarche or the beginning of testicular growth and the onset of spermatogenesis and testosterone production by the testes, which plays some role in libido. Pubertal maturation, or the development of secondary sexual characteristics as a consequence of increasing testosterone levels, represents the outward appearance of reproductive maturation and plays a role in changing social status.

Both reproductive maturation and pubertal maturation are necessary conditions for adult maturation common to mammalian species. Somatic growth, on the other hand, is not essential to the beginning of reproduction; in fact, in many species reproductive maturation begins when somatic growth has reached its nadir. In contrast, for humans somatic growth during adolescence includes a reacceleration of growth in both weight and height that has been slowing down ever since infancy, suggesting that the pubertal growth spurt may be a specifically human adaptive feature (Bogin, 1999).

However, more recent work suggests that other primate species exhibit a similar growth spurt (Leigh, 1998) in weight, especially among sexually dimorphic species. Chimp males, for instance, show important gains in weight during reproductive maturation (Leigh and Shea, 1996). Thus, the distinctive element of the adolescent growth spurt in humans is not increased growth per se but, more specifically, the dramatic increases in stature. This is easily attributable to our bipedality, which makes height a more salient dimension of size.

Unfortunately, definitive fossil evidence for the origins of the adolescent growth spurt in height during human evolution is not available. Current speculations focus on *Homo ergaster* when increases in size and loss of sexual dimorphism suggest important changes in the timing of maturation (Hawkes, 2002). However, interpretation of the almost complete skeleton of the Nariokotome boy at 1.8MYA does not provide conclusive evidence for the existence of a growth spurt during this time period. Smith (1993) argues that the relationship between dental and postcranial developmental timing demonstrated by the specimen is at variance with that seen in modern humans, while Clegg and Aiello (1999) argue that it is, in fact, within the range of variation found in modern humans. Thus, the temporal origin of the human growth spurt remains an open issue.

In addition to the pubertal growth spurt, the existence of adrenarche as part of human maturation deserves attention as a distinctive clue to the human life course. Again, adrenarche is not uniquely a human attribute but rather one we share with other great apes (Collins et al., 1981; Smail et al., 1982) that may take on a distinctively human pattern. Importantly, adrenarche follows the completion of brain growth around the age of 7 and precedes the onset of puberty (Bogin, 1999), suggesting that it plays some role between the energetic demands of brain growth and those of puberty.

While adrenarche was once thought to be directly related to the onset of puberty, there is no evidence for an obligate role of adrenarche in the onset of pubertal maturation, and adrenarche and gonadarche are considered functionally separate processes. Instead it appears that adrenarche may be more directly related to processes of brain maturation. DHEA/S has an impact on Gamma-aminobutyric acid (GABA(a)) neurons (Majewska, 1995) that act to inhibit dopaminergic neurons in the prefrontal cortex that regulate judgment and the control of behavioral impulses (Niehoff, 1999). In addition, the impact of DHEA/S on GABA(a) neurons in the hypothalamus may act to inhibit GnRH production and retard the onset of puberty (Genazzani et al., 2000). Thus, while adrenarche and gonadarche are fundamentally separate processes, they are not unrelated, a point that comes home when we consider the role of energetics in reproductive maturation.

ENERGETICS AND MALE REPRODUCTIVE MATURATION

For males, increases in stature and muscle mass come well after the onset of testicular growth and the onset of spermatogenesis (Tanner, 1978).

This is in clear contrast to human females for whom menarche, the first clear sign of reproductive function, occurs after peak height velocity. At the broadest level, this difference in the relative timing of reproductive maturation and somatic growth between the sexes can be explained in terms of energetics. Reproduction is energetically costly in females and so reproductive function matures only after the energetic demands of growth are nearly finished. In contrast, the low relatively energetic cost of sperm production in males means that its early onset does not detract from further growth in stature and muscle mass (Ellison, 2001).

This energetic perspective can be applied to understanding the process of reproductive maturation in males as well. As mentioned earlier, previous attempts to link adrenarche and pubertal onset have focused on the potential role of adrenarche in the onset of pubertal maturation. Increases in adrenal androgens were thought to desensitize the hypothamalus to negative feedback from gonadal steroids thus allowing gonadal production to rise and initiating puberty (Grumbach et al., 1974; see Figure 9-2A). However, it is now clear that adrenarche is not necessary for pubertal maturation (Counts et al., 1987), and the idea of adrenarche as a specific event that causes the onset of pubertal maturation has been largely discarded (Parker, 1999).

Nonetheless, adrenarche and gonadarche may be related by a third factor on which both depend—energetic status, as suggested by the model presented in Figure 9-2B. In this model the timing of adrenarche and gonadarche is the product of two separate processes: maturation of the hypothalamus and pituitary and maturation of the adrenal gland and the testes. Hypothalamic and pituitary maturation appears to be a largely internal process reflecting more general developmental processes extending back to the womb. More importantly, maturation of the hypothalamus and pituitary appears to precede maturation of the adrenal gland and testes, suggesting that variation in the timing of adrenarche and gonadarche is largely dependent on development of adrenal gland and gonadals.

In fact, the onset of adrenal and gonadal androgen production has been tied to variations in energetic availability, specifically fat stores. Recent evidence indicates that the timing of adrenarche is associated with maximum increases in body mass index (Remer, 2000; Remer and Manz, 1999), while the timing of pubertal onset—that is, testicular growth—is directly related to fat stores (Vizmanos and Marti-Henneberg, 2000). Thus, greater food availability would lead to earlier onset of adrenarche as well as an earlier onset of puberty and a correlation of testosterone and DHEA/S levels without any direct relationship between the two processes.

Once testosterone production has begun, pubertal development and somatic growth are related to both increasing testicular production of testosterone and energetic availability through the effects of blood glucose, insulin, and activity, as shown in Figure 9-2B. Continued increases in

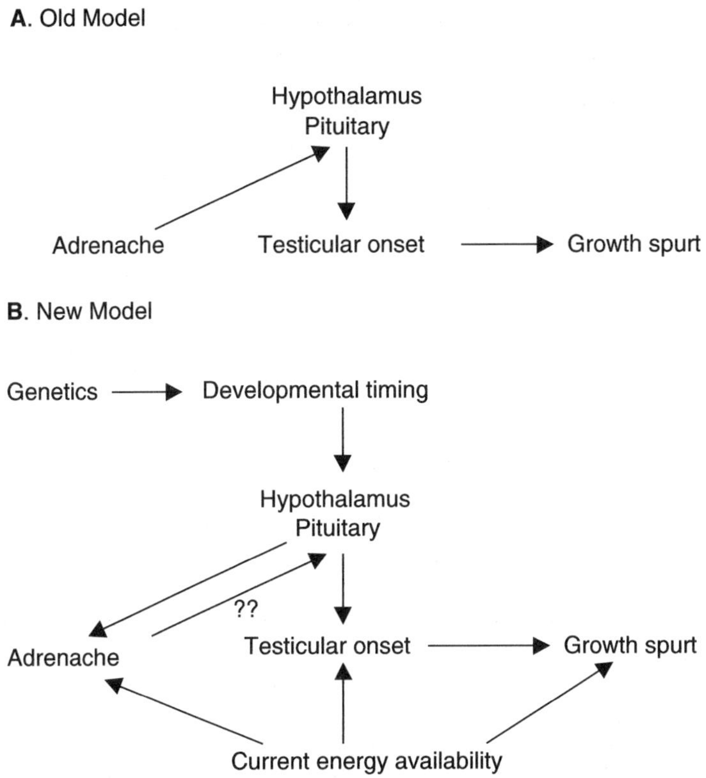

FIGURE 9-2 Causal relationship of adrenarche and pubertal maturation.
NOTE: The old model suggests that adrenal androgens produced by adrenarche are necessary for desensitizing the hypothalamus to the feedback effects of gonadal androgens thus allowing testicular production of testosterone to begin to rise. The new model incorporates both genetic and environmental factors in the onset of adrenarche and gonadarche. In addition to variation in the timing of hypothalamic and pituitary maturation, the onset of adrenal production of DHEA/S and gonadal production of testosterone are also related to energy availability, most likely in the form of fat storage. Adrenal production of DHEA/S may also alter hypothalamic-pituitary control of gonadotropins. The pubertal growth spurt is a product of both the onset of testicular production of testosterone and energy available for bone and muscle growth.

DHEA/S contribute to the development of somatic growth as well, though their role appears to be negligible compared to that of testosterone. However, in populations where energetic constraints lead to lowered testosterone levels, the contribution of DHEA/S to the progression of pubertal maturation may increase.

EVOLUTIONARY EXPLANATIONS OF HUMAN REPRODUCTIVE MATURATION

The model of energetics and pubertal timing outlined above suggests that, in the case of humans, energetic constraints on the simultaneous development of the brain and reproductive maturation acted as the primary selective force in the development of the maturation process beginning with adrenarche and marked by continuing increases in DHEA/S. It is difficult to be sure when changes in human life history evolved. In the scenario suggested here, changes in life history patterns associated increased size, slowed childhood growth, and changes in the relative metabolic costs of the gut versus the brain would have started with the origins of *Homo ergaster* (Aiello and Wells, 2002). Initially, the increased metabolic demands of the brain may have been met by an increase in caloric intake, involving dietary shift, changes in relative size of the gut, and slower childhood growth.

With further increases in brain size subsequent to *Homo ergaster* full development of a larger brain would have required additional energy and time. In order to allow for continued brain development without engendering the energetic costs of reproductive maturation, increases in DHEA/S production would have promoted development of the prefrontal cortex, while suppressing GnRH production and the onset of pubertal maturation. At younger ages, reproductive suppression may have been complete, creating a juvenile phase in which the brain could develop without the competing demands of reproductive maturation. However, continued increases in DHEA/S would allow for further brain maturation even as reproductive maturation and sexual behavior commenced, thus allowing the integration of sexual impulses and their behavioral expression.

BEHAVIORAL IMPLICATIONS

Bogin (1994) has argued that the adolescent growth spurt in human males reflects the results of male-male competition. He suggests that, once males exhibit the somatic cues of maturity, they enter into a competitive world of adult males that inevitably carries costs, including the risk of injury. Thus it would be beneficial to delay development of full secondary sexual characteristics, including growth, until one is as competitive as possible so that the benefits of engaging in male-male competition are more likely to outweigh the costs. Bercovitch and Ziegler (2002) make a similar argument for primates.

Among orangutans the presence of adult males does directly suppress the development of secondary sexual characteristics in developing males without suppressing reproductive function (Maggioncalda et al., 2002), suggesting that the presence of older males is a critical social signal of reproductive opportunities. There is no evidence for such reproductive suppression in humans and the role of male-male competition during adolescence seems secondary to the role of energetic factors. However, the fact that the presence/absence of the father during early childhood has been linked to hormonal profiles (Flinn et al., 1996) suggests that male parental care may play a role as a social cue about later reproductive opportunities (see section on Cultural Variation).

Nonetheless, male-male competition would make adolescence a stressful time. In addition to a potential role in suppressing the onset of reproductive maturation, increased DHEA/S production during reproductive maturation may have been selected for because of its protective role in the stress response. Under conditions of stress such as those associated with major life transitions (Dorn and Chrousos, 1997), elevated cortisol is associated with anxiety (Frankenhaeuser, 1980), which may in turn interfere with social interaction and learning. As Fredrickson (2000) has put it, activation of the hypothalamic-pituitary-adrenol (HPA) axis may be associated with execution of narrow behavioral programs mediated by the limbic system. In contrast, DHEA/S has been associated with improved mood among HIV-positive men (Cruess et al., 1999) and improved mood and cognition in aging men (van Niekerk et al., 2001). Furthermore Boudarene and Legos (2002) report that low anxiety levels are associated with increased levels of DHEA/S during cognitive stress tests.

Importantly, DHEA/S is a cortisol antagonist, meaning that it acts to block the effects of cortisol on neurons in the brain (Kimonides et al., 1999; Yoo et al., 1996). Given these actions of cortisol and DHEA on the hippocampus for learning and memory (McEwen, 1999), increased levels of DHEA would alleviate the effects of cortisol in narrowing concentration (Stansbury and Gunnar, 1994) and lead to increased inputs to the hippocampus from the cortex allowing for greater possibility of flexible behavior and increased learning.

In the case of adolescent males for whom increased testosterone levels are associated with increases in sexual behavior (Halpern et al., 1998), learning may be very much focused on interactions with the opposite sex as well as competitive interactions with other males (Weisfield, 1999). Increasing levels of testosterone can be thought of as making such interactions increasingly salient and promoting impulses toward sex and aggression. Cortisol and DHEA/S may be thought of as having contrasting effects on the execution of these impulses. Increased levels of DHEA/S would promote their expression and relate them to a wider arrange of social inputs through its effects on the prefrontal cortex. Cortisol, on the other hand, would interfere with the broader associations of such behavior by blocking the formation of new memories by the hippocampus (see Figure 9-3 for a diagrammatic representation).

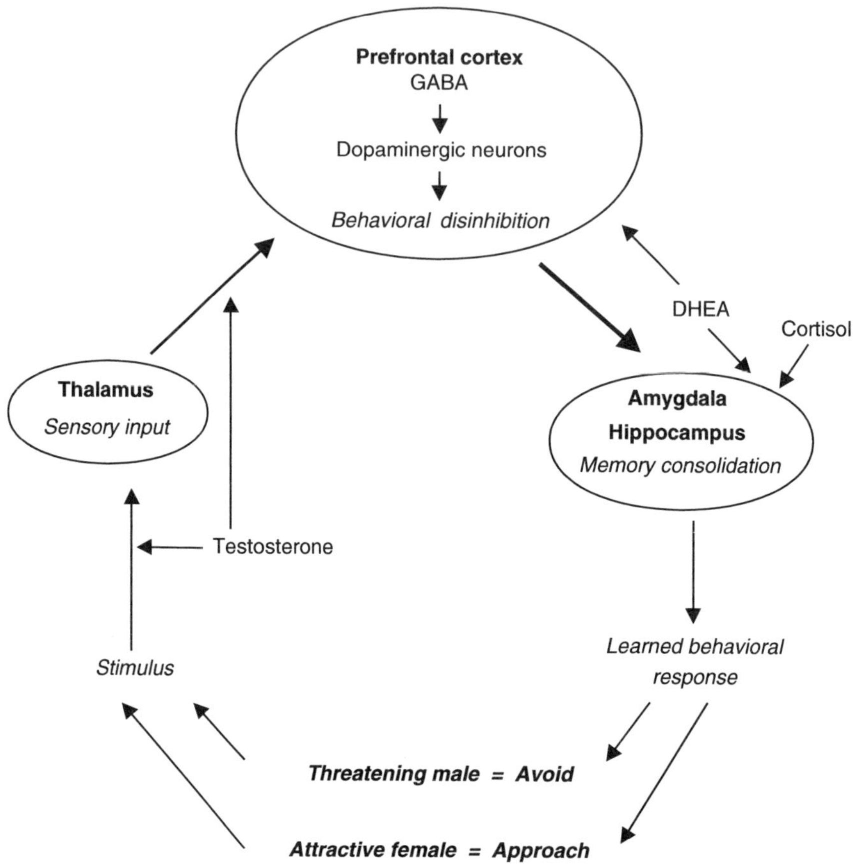

FIGURE 9-3 Schematic representation of the impact of gonadal and adrenal hormones on reproductive strategies.
NOTE: This diagram, loosely based on Ledoux (1998) and Zuckerman (1995) suggests that testosterone, DHEA/S, and cortisol all play different roles in brain mechanisms that underlie the expression of sexual behavior. Testosterone is related to the perception of sexual stimuli and associated sexual impulses. DHEA/S, on the other hand, is related to disinhibition of behavior in the precortex, whereas cortisol acts on the formulation of memories in the amygdala and hippocampus and the development of learned behavioral responses to sexual interaction.

In more human terms, Weisfield (1999) has argued that adolescence represents a time in which social emotions become associated with sexual behavior and the social relationships that go with them. In particular he argues that pride and shame have important roles as males start to judge achievement in terms of their ability to attract mates. If, as Damassio

(1999) argues, emotions involve the cognitive appraisal by the cortex of emotional impulses generated by the limbic system, testosterone would potentiate the original impulses involved in attracting and competing for mates. DHEA/S would act to expand these impulses by promoting neural pathways that incorporate the positive judgment of social factors that lead to pride while cortisol would tend to lead to the negative awareness of social factors contained in shame. Such a process might also underlie the creativity that Miller (2000) argues is the basis of courtship in human males.

So far, I have argued, on largely theoretical grounds, that the existence of adrenarche in humans gives us special reason to expand our understanding of the processes involved in human reproductive maturation beyond simply the development of sexual behavior. The next section follows through on this argument by considering empirical evidence for gonadal and adrenal hormones in the sexual behavior of adolescent boys. We start with findings on the role of pubertal maturation and testosterone in the onset of sexual behavior and then move to evidence that both cortisol and DHEA/S may have a role in aspects of social behavior important for the full expression of sexual behavior.

HORMONES AND ADOLESCENT SEXUAL BEHAVIOR

Udry has developed a biosocial model of the determinants of sexual behavior among adolescent boys (Udry et al., 1985; Udry and Billy, 1987). In its original formulation the model argued that increasing levels of testosterone during puberty will result in increasing levels of endogenous sexual motivation in boys. To the extent that sexual motivation is not socially controlled, it will result in the onset of sexual behavior in boys. And compared to girls, it appears that there are relatively few social controls on boys.

PUBERTAL MATURATION

The role of testosterone in pubertal maturation remains hard to pin down. Halpern (1997) was able to demonstrate a direct relationship between salivary testosterone and sexual behavior in adolescent boys, though an earlier analysis found that secondary sexual characteristics, not serum testosterone, was the more important predictor (Halpern et al., 1993). Differentiating behavior and physical effects of testosterone is difficult because testosterone levels rise quite quickly in individual boys (Nielsen et al., 1986). Thus, changes in motivation associated with testosterone stimulation of the brain may happen in the absence of social opportunities for sexual behavior.

Fortunately, the distinction between direct and indirect effects of testosterone may not be crucial to understanding the role of pubertal maturation in the onset of sexual behavior. To the extent that increases in testosterone are important to development of the nervous system and secondary sexual characteristics, their effects will be synchronized, and a general measure of pubertal timing may be sufficient to represent the effects of testosterone.

RISK TAKING

A model of adolescent sexual behavior based entirely on the biological effects of pubertal maturation and the role of testosterone is, however, clearly insufficient to capture the process of sexual initiation. Sexual behavior includes an important element of social behavior, including risk taking. This is most apparent in early adolescence when sexual behavior is not a normative behavior and is associated with socially proscribed risk-taking behaviors such as smoking, drinking, and stealing (Mott and Haurin, 1988; Rosenthal et al., 1999; Tapert et al., 2001; Tubman et al., 1996; Wagner, 2001). Even later in adolescence sexual behavior generally involves initiation on the part of the male, which may be considered a form of risk taking.

Though testosterone may play a role in sensation-seeking and impulsivity (Virkkunen et al., 1994), risk taking is more closely related to adrenal hormones, particularly cortisol. Cortisol has been shown to be inversely related to novelty seeking in Vietnam veterans with posttraumatic stress disorder (Wang et al., 1997) and sensation seeking in college-age men (Rosenblitt et al., 2001). In addition, increased cortisol reactivity has been associated with social inhibition and anxiety among adolescents (Granger et al., 1994) and internalizing symptoms (Klimes-Dougan et al., 2001). In contrast, boys with conduct disorder exhibit low cortisol on average (McBurnett et al., 2000).

There is less evidence demonstrating how the role of cortisol in behavioral inhibition (or lack of it) may be related to sexual behavior. However, Halpern et al. (2002) have shown that cortisol reactivity is inversely related to the number of sex partners and frequency of condom use in a sample of 18- to 25-year old males. In addition, cortisol reactivity was also related to substance use, suggesting that individual differences in the HPA axis may underlie the relationship between various aspects of risk taking in adolescent boys.

BIOLOGICAL MODEL: INTEGRATING PUBERTAL MATURATION AND RISK TAKING

Given the evidence outlined above, pubertal maturation and risk taking can be conceived of as two separate dimensions of adolescent sexual behavior, associated with gonadal and adrenal steroids, respectively. Pubertal

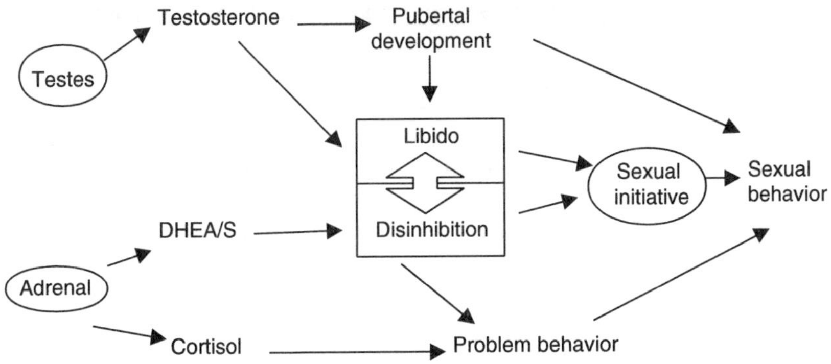

FIGURE 9-4 Conceptual model of biological dimension of adolescent sexual behavior.
NOTE: This figure proposes a two-dimensional model of biological influences on the onset of sexual behavior among adolescent males. Increasing levels of testosterone are known to promote sexual behavior in adolescent males through two separate pathways: by increasing secondary sexual characteristics, which are a sign of social maturity, and through libido, which plays a role in sexual initiation. On the other hand, individual variation in cortisol has been related to problem behavior that is known to be related to adolescent sexual behavior. Initiative in sexual behavior is seen here as a form of risk taking. Together sexual opportunity and sexual initiation result in sexual behavior. The role of DHEA/S in sexual behavior is largely unknown. However, it may have direct effects on the disinhibition of social behavior. In addition, DHEA/S antiglucocorticoid actions may reduce the inhibiting effects of cortisol on behavior.

maturation is associated with increases in testosterone that are related to the development of secondary sexual characteristics and the onset of sexual motivation. As such it is related to sexual opportunities.

Risk taking, on the other hand, is associated with socially problematic behavior. As such it may be related to taking advantage of sexual opportunities when such behavior is not normative. Risk taking is related to cortisol, and low cortisol is related to acting on impulse. However, in contrast to testosterone, cortisol levels do not change dramatically at puberty (Walker et al., 2001) and represent a stable individual characteristic preceding puberty.

In the model proposed here, the two dimensions of pubertal maturation and risk taking come together to produce sexual behavior with cortisol modifying the expression of developing sexual impulses produced by increasing testosterone levels, as shown in Figure 9-4.

IMPLICATIONS FOR ADULT FERTILITY BEHAVIOR

Timing of reproductive maturation by itself seems unlikely to play a major role in fertility behavior in males. In many societies reproduction does not start until the mid-20s long after reproductive maturation is complete and late maturers have had a chance to catch up with early maturers in terms of the impact of testosterone and its behavioral and somatic effects. For instance, early maturers start the pubertal growth spurt earlier and go through it with greater intensity; they are not taller than late maturers at the end of puberty (Bourguignon, 1988; Vizmanos et al., 2001). Thus, although height has been related to male fertility (Pawlowski et al., 2000) as well as sperm count (Manning et al., 1998), variation in height is not established at puberty.

Instead, pubertal timing in males is likely a proxy for individual variation in the activity of the hypothalamic-pituitary-testicular axis established early in development and persisting into adulthood (Bribiescas, 2001). Variations in testosterone levels as well as production rates in Western populations are quite heritable (Handelsman, 1997; Meikle et al., 1997), suggesting that individual differences in testosterone and its effects on behavior go back at least to prenatal development. For instance, testosterone has been related to aggression in both preschool boys (Sanchez-Martin et al., 2000) and prepubertal adolescent males (Gerra et al., 1998). Scerbo and Kolko (1994) report that testosterone was related to aggression in a sample of disruptive prepubertal children, although Constantino et al. (1993) did not find elevated testosterone and aggression in 18 highly aggressive prepubertal boys compared to normal controls.

Such a developmental model may help explain recent findings of genetic influences on the timing of first intercourse among adolescent boys (Miller et al., 1999; Rodgers et al., 1999). Rodgers et al.'s findings fail to account for the effects of pubertal timing, which presumably has genetic elements in boys, as it does in girls (Campbell and Udry, 1995). On the other hand, Miller et al.'s findings that variation in genes for dopamine receptor type helps account for variation in age at first sexual intercourse in a sample of non-Hispanic European American men and women, even controlling for a variety of psychosocial factors, is compatible with individual variation in risk taking, given evidence for dopamine in impulsivity among adolescents with attention-deficit disorder with hyperactivity (Rosa Neto et al., 2002).

However, Rodger et al.'s genetic findings hold for European American males, but not females and not African American males, suggesting an important interaction of genetic factors with the social context in which behavior is expressed. We will come back to this point in our discussion of cultural variation in the development of male fertility behavior.

The fact that both testosterone (Handelsman, 1997; Meikle et al., 1997) and cortisol (Meikle et al., 1988) levels are heritable suggests that individual variation in these two hormones may play a role in the sexual behavior of adult males, just as they do in adolescents. In the case of testosterone, levels decline gradually with age, suggesting that they may underlie age-related declines in sexual behavior. At the same time, cortisol levels change little with age, suggesting a relatively fixed effect of individual variation. However, sexual behavior in adults depends much more heavily on the development of long-term relationships, in which the role of libido and risk taking in sexual behavior may be very different and may lead to changes in the observable effects of testosterone and cortisol.

In fact, individual variation in testosterone does appear to be related to the maintenance of sexual relationships and marriage. For instance, Bogaert and Fischer (1995) reported a small positive effect of testosterone on the number of sex partners among young adult men, even controlling for psychological variables such as disinhibition. Furthermore, several studies have documented lower testosterone levels in married men compared to unmarried men (Booth and Dabbs, 1993; Booth and Osgood, 1993; Gray et al., 2002). Finally, testosterone increases around the time of divorce and then declines, suggesting that it may respond to increased competition associated with marital dissolution (Mazur and Michalek, 1998).

At a more mechanistic level, testosterone has demonstrable effects on sexual awareness and arousal in adult males (Alexander and Sherwin, 1991; Anderson et al., 1992). At the same time, recent experimental work using exogenous testosterone provides little evidence to sustain an important effect of testosterone levels on the frequency of sexual behavior among adult men (Bhasin et al., 2001; Buena et al., 1993). Anderson et al. reconcile this difference by pointing to the possibly constraining influence of sex partners. Unfortunately, similar evidence for the role of cortisol in male sexual or social behavior is lacking.

CULTURAL VARIATION

Draper and Harpending (1982) have suggested that variation in social structure has an important impact on the sexual and parenting behaviors of human males. They argue that so-called father-absent societies would produce males who would tend to put their energy into mating effort over paternal investment in offspring, while males in father-present societies put their energy into parental investment over mating effort.

Given that males in father-absent societies grow up to be absent fathers, Draper and Harpending's argument might seem almost tautological. However, the important question is whether there is a biological mechanism translating variation in early childhood experience into predictable behavioral predispositions underlying mating in adulthood. Belsky et al. (1991) offered one such mechanism in the case of girls; internalizing behavior associated with early stress would lead to increased eating, hasten age at reproductive maturation, and lead to a greater number of sexual partners. The data do not bear out this mechanism (Belsky et al., 1991; Campbell and Udry, 1995).

However, another potential mechanism relating early experience to adult behavior in boys is the impact of father absence on the development of the adrenal axis (Flinn et al., 1996). In humans, several studies have shown that cortisol reactivity in infancy is related to attachment (Gunnar et al., 1996; Hertsgaard et al., 1995). Furthermore, there are sex differences in cortisol reactivity from infancy (Davis and Emory, 1995), and the effects of childhood trauma appear to increase cortisol responsiveness in women (Heim et al., 2002) while leading to decreased cortisol levels among males (Dawes et al., 1999; Moss et al., 1999).

The lack of a father in the household may result in disruption of maternal care and hence poorer attachment and subsequent changes in adrenal reactivity. In the case of boys, early childhood stress associated with poor maternal care and physical abuse is more likely to lead to low cortisol levels in some samples of boys (Dawes et al., 1999; Moss et al., 1999), which in turn is related to the acting out of problem behavior.

Flinn et al. (1996) also found that boys from father-absent homes exhibited lower cortisol levels in a sample from Bwa Mawego, a village on the Island of Dominica, suggesting the cross-cultural generalizability of such effects. In fact, because fetal undernutrition results in elevated cortisol levels (Clark et al., 1996; Levitt et al., 2000; Phillips et al., 1998, 2000; Reynolds et al., 2001), the effects of father absence in food-limited populations may act through both prenatal development and early childhood attachment, thus multiplying its impact on cortisol reactivity.

In addition to cortisol, DHEA/S may be involved in the externalizing behavior of adolescent boys. For instance, Dmitrieva et al. (2001) reported higher levels of DHEA/S among a group of 10- to 18-year old boys with conduct disorder compared to normal controls. In addition, Van Goozen et al (1998) report that prepubertal boys with conduct disorder have higher levels of DHEA/S but not testosterone compared to normal controls. I speculate that among boys who experience poor attachment and early physical abuse, prepubertal increases in DHEA/S, a weak androgen, combined with a lack of inhibition associated with low cortisol levels, may be sufficient to lead to sexual behavior in social settings without strong social controls on adolescent males.

SUMMARY

This chapter began by arguing that an evolutionary perspective directs us to consider the fertility behavior of men because selective forces on males, as the sex with less direct energetic parental investment, may be particularly strong. Yet at the same time human males clearly do invest in offspring postnatally, adding an additional level of complexity to the way in which selection has shaped the reproductive biology and behavior of human males from that of our primate ancestors.

My description of reproductive maturation in humans as stretching from adrenarche to young adulthood suggests a distinct human version of male reproductive maturation. Changes in behavior needed for successful reproduction span this entire period, beginning with changes in cognition and social relationships during the prepubertal period, continuing with reproductive maturation during adolescence and the onset of sexual behavior, and ending in the onset of reproduction and parenting during the young adult phase.

This extended definition of reproductive maturation in human males highlights the role of both the testicular and adrenal axis in male reproductive behavior. Sufficient evidence exists to argue that pubertal maturation in males is part of individual variation in the reproductive axis that persists into adulthood and underlies individual continuity in sexual behavior. In the same way, cortisol is a marker of the adrenal axis, which underlies individual continuity in social behavior. However, the role of adrenal hormones in the onset of sexual behavior is only beginning to receive attention. While the association of cortisol and risk taking suggests a role for cortisol in the expression of sexual behavior, at this point only the slimmest of data substantiate the link.

There is even less empirical evidence demonstrating that DHEA/S is related to variation in adolescent sexual behavior, yet DHEA/S potentially is involved in a variety of mechanisms that may affect sexual behavior. On the one hand, conversion of DHEA/S to testosterone means that it may augment the essential role of gonadally produced testosterone in the maturation of the reproductive system, including promoting libido and somatic growth, both of which have been related to adolescent sexual behavior. In addition, DHEA/S and testosterone have been shown to have similar effects on gene expression in immune cells (Maurer et al., 2001). On the other hand, conversion of DHEA/S to estrogen means that it may play a suppressive effect in reproductive maturation but promote aspects of cognitive function related to the forebrain (Keenan et al., 2001).

In addition to its potential role as an androgen or estrogen, DHEA/S may play a role in adolescent behavior through more direct mechanisms. These include its role in stimulating GABA(A) neurons, with effects on precortical control of behavior. In addition, DHEA/S's antiglucocorticoid effects suggest a potentially important role for DHEA/S in memory development and the ability to produce novel behavior patterns in response to familiar stimuli, under conditions of arousal. The very fact that DHEA/S levels rise during maturation in humans represents an important evolutionary feature of the human life cycle that may shed light on the role of brain development and attachment in humans as well as fertility behavior more generally.

FUTURE RESEARCH DIRECTIONS

To more fully understand the implications of adrenarche for the development of boys, I suggest three important lines of investigation. The first of these is a better understanding of the interaction of DHEA/S and cortisol with testosterone in the disruption of normal emotional development in boys. The second is the study of cross-population differences in age-related patterns in adrenal and gonadal steroids and the insight they may provide into maturational timing. The third is a more detailed investigation of the role of adrenal and gonadal steroids on behavioral development in chimpanzees and gorillas as a background for understanding the truly human aspects of male reproductive maturation.

There is already sufficient evidence for the effects of cortisol and DHEA on major depressive disorder in adolescence to warrant further investigation (Goodyer et al., 2001). What the perspective offered here adds is a functional understanding that for adolescent boys mood dysregulation reflects not only the shifting patterns of psychosocial adjustment during this period but also the role of testosterone in producing the underlying motivations for attachment. DHEA/S, cortisol, and testosterone are only some of the many factors involved in this process, but they can help provide insight into the specific aspects of brain functioning that fail to develop normally in these conditions.

Researchers will also want to investigate the impact of variations in maturational timing across populations on the development of emotions and behavior. One very important issue in understanding the interaction of gonadal and adrenal steroids on adolescent maturation among boys is the role of DHEA/S in mediating the effects of testosterone on sexual behavior. If because of its relationship to brain growth, the timing of adrenarche is less variable than that of gonadarche (Worthman, 1993), individuals in early-maturing populations such as our own may be exposed to the maturational effects of DHEA/S for a much shorter time before being exposed to the sexually motivating effects of testosterone. Faster rates of maturation among adolescent boys may simply provide less time for the effects of

DHEA/S on the brain and hence less time to integrate attachment and emotional development with sexual behavior.

The final line of investigation involves comparison with our most closely related species, great apes, in order to more fully understand the relationship of adrenarche and gonadarche in reproductive maturation specifically in humans, given their large brains. While adrenarche has been demonstrated in both chimpanzees and gorillas (Smail et al., 1982; Collins et al., 1981), and DHEA/S has not demonstrated a relationship to reproductive behavior (Nadler et al., 1987), we have very little information on the timing and tempo of increases in DHEA/S and its relationship to the development of reproductive behavior. It is only by comparing such patterns from great apes with those from humans that we will be able to understand the contribution of adrenal steroids to a uniquely human reproductive maturation.

REFERENCES

Aiello, L.C., and J.C.K. Wells
2002 Energetics and the evolution of the genus *Homo*. *Annual Review of Anthropology* 31:323-338.

Alexander, G.M., and B.B. Sherwin
1991 The association between testosterone, sexual arousal and selective attention for erotic stimuli in men. *Hormones and Behavior* 25(3):367-381.

Anderson, M.J., and A.F. Dixon
2002 Sperm competition: Motility and the midpiece in primates. *Nature* 416(6880):496.

Anderson, R.A., J. Bancroft, and F.C. Wu
1992 The effects of exogenous testosterone on sexuality and mood of normal men. *Journal of Clinical Endocrinology and Metabolism* 75(6):1503-1507.

Argquitt, A.B., B.J. Stoecker, J.S. Hermann, and E.A. Winterfeldt
1991 Dehydroepiandrosterone sulfate, cholesterol, hemoglobin, and anthropometric measures related to growth in male adolescents. *Journal of the American Dietetic Association* 91(5):575-579.

Baker, R.R., and M.A. Bellis
1989 Number of sperm in human ejaculates varies in accordance with sperm competition theory. *Animal Behavior* 37:867-869.

Bateman, A.J.
1948 Intrasexual selection in *Drosophila*. *Heredity* 2:349-368.

Baulieu, E.E.
1998 Neurosteroids: A novel function of the brain. *Psychoneuroendocrinology* 23(8):963-987.

Bee, H.
1997 *The Developing Child, 8th ed.* New York: Addison-Wesley.

Belsky, J., L. Steinberg, and P. Draper
1991 Childhood experience, interpersonal development and reproductive strategy: An evolutionary theory of socialization. *Child Development* 62(4):647-670.

Bercovitch, F.B., and T.E. Ziegler
2002 Current topics in primate socioendocrinology. *Annual Review of Anthropology* 31:1-23.

Berg, S.J., and K.E. Wynne-Edwards
2001 Changes in testosterone, cortisol, and estradiol levels in men becoming fathers. *Mayo Clinic Proceedings* 76:582-592.
Bledsoe, C., S. Lerner, and J.I. Guyer
2000 *Fertility and the Male Life Cycle in the Era of Fertility Decline.* New York: Oxford University Press.
Bhasin, S., L. Woodhouse, R. Casaburi, A.B. Singh, D. Bhasin, N. Berman, X. Chen, K.E. Yarasheski, L. Magliano, C. Dzekov, J. Dzekov, R. Broos, J. Phillips, I. Sinha-Hikim, R. Shen, and T.W. Storer
2001 Testosterone dose-response relationships in healthy young men. *American Journal of Physiological Endocrinology and Metabolism* 281(6):E1172-E1181.
Bogaert, A.F., and W.A. Fischer
1995 Predictors of university men's number of sexual partners. *Journal of Sex Research* 32:119-130.
Bogin, B.
1994 Adolescence in evolutionary perspective. *Acta Paediatrica* 406(Suppl.):29-35.
1999 *Patterns of Human Growth, 2nd ed.* Cambridge University Press.
2001 *The Growth of Humanity.* New York: Wiley-Liss.
Booth, A., and J. Dabbs
1993 Testosterone and men's marriages. *Social Forces* 72(2):463-477.
Booth, A., and D.W. Osgood
1993 The influence of testosterone in deviance in adulthood: Assessing and explaining the relationship. *Criminology* 31:93-117.
Boudarene, M., and J.J. Legos
2002 Study of the stress response: Role of anxiety, cortisol and DHEA/S. *Encephale* 28(2):139-146.
Bourguignon, J.P.
1988 Variations in duration of pubertal growth: A mechanism compensating for differences in the timing of puberty and minimizing their effects on final height. Belgian Study Group for Paediatric Endocrinology. *Acta Paediatrica Scandavia* 347(Suppl.):16-24.
Bribiescas, R.G.
2001 Reproductive ecology and the life history of the human male. *American Journal of Physical Anthropology* 33(Suppl.):148-176.
Buena, F., R.S. Swerdloff, B.S. Steiner, P. Lutchmansigh, M.A. Peterson, M.R. Pandian, M. Galmarini, and S. Bhasin
1993 Sexual function does not change when serum testosterone levels are pharmacologically varied within the normal male range. *Fertility and Sterility* 59:1118-1123.
Campbell, B.C., and J.R. Udry
1995 Stress and age at menarche of mothers and daughters. *Journal of Biosocial Science* 27(2):127-134.
Cabrera, M.S., M.G. Vogiatzi, and M.I. New
2001 Long term outcome in adult males with classic congenital adrenal hyperplasia. *Journal of Clinical Endocrinology and Metabolism* 86(7):3070-3078.
Clark, P.M., P.C. Hindmarsh, A.W. Shiell, C.M. Law, J.W. Honour, and D.J. Barker
1996 Size at birth and adrenocortical function in childhood. *Clinical Endocrinology* 45(6):721-726.
Clegg, M., and L.C. Aiello
1999 A comparison of the nariokotome *Homo Erectus* with juveniles from a modern population. *American Journal of Physical Anthropology* 110(1):81-93.

Collins, D.C., R.D. Nadler, and J.R.K. Preedy
1981 Adrenarche in the great apes (Abstract). *American Journal of Primatology* 1:344.

Constantino, J.N., D. Grosz, P. Saenger, D.W. Chandler, R. Nandi, and F.J. Earls
1993 Testosterone and aggression in children. *Journal of the American Academy of Child and Adolescent Psychiatry* 32(6):1217-1222.

Cruess, D.G., M.H. Antoni, M. Kumar, G. Ironson, P. McCabe, J.B. Fernandez, M. Fletcher, and N. Schneiderman
1999 Cognitive-behavioral stress management buffer decreases in dehydroepiandrosterone sulfate (DHEA-S) and increases in the cortisol/DHEA-S ratio and reduces mood disturbance and perceived stress among HIV-seropositive men. *Psychoneuroendocrinology* 24(5):537-549.

Counts, D.R., O.H. Pescovitz, K.M. Barnes, K.D. Hench, G.P. Chrousos, R.J. Sherins, F. Comite, D.L. Loriaux, and G.B. Cutler, Jr.
1987 Dissociation of adrenarche and gonadarche in precocious puberty and in isolated hypogonadotropic hypogonadism. *Journal of Clinical Endocrinology and Metabolism* 64(6):1174-1178.

Damassio, A.R.
1999 *The Feeling of What Happens.* New York: Harcourt Brace.

Davis, M., and E. Emory
1995 Sex differences in neonatal stress reactivity. *Child Development* 66(1):14-27.

Dawes, M.A., L.D. Dorn, H.B. Moss, J.K. Yao, L. Kirisci, R.T. Ammerman, and R.E. Tarter
1999 Hormonal and behavioral homeostasis in boys at risk for substance abuse. *Drug and Alcohol Dependency* 55(1-2):165-176.

Dixson, A.F.
1998 *Primate Sexuality: Comparative Studies of the Prosimians, Monkeys, Apes, and Human Beings.* New York: Oxford University Press.

Dmitrieva, T.N., R.D. Oades, B.P. Hauffa, and C. Eggers
2001 Dehydroepiandrosterone sulphate and corticotropin levels are high in young male patients with conduct disorder: Comparisons for growth factors, thyroid and gonadal hormones. *Neuropsychobiology* 43:134-140.

Dorn, L.D., and G.P. Chrousos
1997 The neurobiology of stress: Understanding regulation of affect during female biological transitions. *Seminars in Reproductive Endocrinology* 15:19-35.

Dorn, L.D., S.F. Hitt, and D. Rotenstein
1999 Biopsychological and cognitive differences in children with premature vs. on-time adrenarche. *Archives of Pediatric and Adolescent Medicine* 153(2):137-146.

Draper, P., and H.C. Harpending
1982 Father absence and reproductive strategy: An evolutionary perspective. *Journal of Anthropological Research* 38:255-273.

Eberhard, W.G.
1985 *Sexual Selection and Animal Genitalia.* Cambridge, MA: Harvard University Press.

Ellison, P.T.
2001 *On Fertile Ground: A Natural History of Human Reproduction.* Cambridge, MA: Harvard University Press.

Erlandsson, R., J.F. Wilson, and S. Paabo
2000 Sex chromosomal transposable element accumulation and male-driven substitutional evolution in humans. *Molecular Biology and Evolution* 17:804-812.

Flinn, M.V., R.J. Guinlan, S.A. Decker, M.T. Turner, and B.G. England
1996 Male-female differences in effects of parental absence on glucocorticoid stress response. *Human Nature* 7(2):125-162.

Frankenhaeuser, M.
1980 Psychobiological aspects of life stress. Pp. 203-223 in *Coping and Health*. S. Levin and H. Ursin, eds. New York: Plenum Press.
Fredrickson, B.L.
2000 Cultivating positive emotions to optimize health and well-being. *Prevention and Treatment* 3(March).
Genazzani, A.R., F. Bernardi, P. Montetone, S. Luisi, and M. Laurie
2000 Neuropeptides, neurotransmitters, neurosteroids and the onset of puberty. *Annals of the New York Academy of Sciences* 900:1-9.
Gerra, G., A. Zaimovic, G. Giucastro, F. Folli, D. Maestri, A. Tessoni, P. Avznzini, R. Caccavari, S. Bernasconi, and F. Brambilla
1998 Neurotransmitter-hormonal responses to psychological stress in peripubertal subjects: Relationship to aggressive behavior. *Life Sciences* 62:617-625.
Goodyer, I.M., J. Herbert, P.M.F. Altham, J. Pearson, S.M. Secher, and H.M. Shiers
1996 Adrenal secretion during major depression in 8-to 16-year olds. I. Altered diurnal rhythms in salivary cortisol and dehydroepiandrosterone (DHEA) at presentation. *Psychological Medicine* 26:245-256.
Goodyer, I.M., R.J. Park, C.M. Netherton, and J. Herbert
2001 Possible role of cortisol and dehydroepiandrosterone in human development and psychopathology. *British Journal of Psychiatry* 179:243-249.
Granger, D.A., J.R. Weisz, and D. Kauneckis
1994 Neuroendocrine reactivity, internalizing behavior problems, and control-related cognitions in clinic-referred children and adolescents. *Journal of Abnormal Psychology* 103:267-276.
Gray, P.B., S.M. Kahlenbery, E.S. Barrett, S.F. Lipson, and P.T. Ellison
2002 Marriage and fatherhood are associated with lower testosterone in males. *Evolution and Human Behavior* 23:193-201.
Grumbach, M.M., J.C. Roth, S.L. Kaplan, and R.P. Kelch
1974 Hypothalamic-pituitary regulation of puberty in man: Evidence and concepts derived from clinical research. Pp. 115-166 in *Control of the Onset of Puberty*. M.M. Grumbach, G.D. Grave, and F.E. Fayer, eds. New York: Wiley.
Gunnar, M.R., L. Brodersen, M. Nachmias, K. Buss, and J. Rigatuso
1996 Stress reactivity and attachment security. *Developmental Psychobiology* 29(3):191-204.
Halpern, C.T., B.C. Campbell, C.R. Agnew, V. Thompson, J.R. Udry
2002 Associations between stress reactivity and sexual and non-sexual risk taking in young adult human males. *Hormones and Behavior* 42:387-398.
Halpern, C.T., J.R. Udry, B. Campbell, and C. Suchindran
1993 Testosterone and pubertal development as predictors of sexual activity: A panel analysis of adoloescent males. *Psychosomatic Medicine* 55:436-447.
Halpern, C.T., J.R. Udry, and C. Suchindran
1998 Monthly measures of salivary testosterone predict sexual activity in adolescent males. *Archives of Sexual Behavior* 27(5):445-465.
Handelsman, D.J.
1997 Estimating familial and genetic contributions to variability in human testicular function: A pilot twin study. *International Journal of Andrology* 20:215-221.
Harcourt, A.H., P.H. Harvey, S.G. Larson, and R.V. Short
1981 Testis weight, body weight and breeding system in primates. *Nature* 293(5827):55-57.

Hawkes, K.
2002 Grandmothers and the evolution of human longevity. Paper presented at the Human Biology Association Meeting, Buffalo, NY, April.

Heim, C., D.J. Newport, D. Wagner, M.M. Wilcox, A.H. Miller, and C.B. Nemeroff
2002 The role of early adverse experience and adulthood stress in the prediction of neuroendocrine stress reactivity in women: A multiple regression analysis. *Depression and Anxiety* 15(3):117-125.

Herdt, G., and M. McClintock
2000 The magical age of 10. *Archives of Sexual Behavior* 29(6):587-606.

Hertsgaard L., M. Gunnar, M.F. Erickson, and M. Nachmias
1995 Adrenocortical responses to the strange situation in infants with disorganized/disoriented attachment relationships. *Child Development* 66(4):1100-1106.

Huttley, G.A., I.B. Jakobsen, S.R. Wilson, and S. Easteal
2000 How important in DNA replication for mutagenesis? *Molecular Biology and Evolution* 17(6):929-937.

Keenan, P.A., W.H. Ezzat, K. Ginsburg, and G.J. Moore
2001 Prefrontal cortex as the site of estrogen's effect on cognition. *Psychoneuroendocrinology* 26(6):577-590.

Kimonides, V.G., M.G. Spillantini, M.W. Sofroniew, J.W. Fawcett, and J. Herbert
1999 Dehydroepiandrosterone (DHEA) antagonizes the neurotoxic effects of corticosterone and translocation of stress-activated protein kinase 3 in hippocampal primary cultures. *Neuroscience* 89(2):429-436.

Klimes-Dougan, B., P.D. Hastings, D.A. Granger, B.A. Usher, and C. Zahn-Waxler
2001 Adrenocortical activity in at-risk and normally developing adolescents: Individual differences in salivary cortisol basal levels, diurnal variation, and responses to social challenges. *Developmental Psychopathology* 13:695-719.

Kurtis, J.D., R. Mtalib, F.K. Onyango, and P.E. Duffy
2001 Human resistance to *Plasmodium falciparum* increases during puberty and is predicted by dehydroepiandrosterone sulfate levels. *Infection and Immunity* 69(1):123-128.

Labrie. F., A. Belanger, J. Simard, Van Luu-The, and C. Labrie
1995 DHEA and peripheral androgen and estrogen formation: Intracinology. *Annals of the New York Academy of Sciences* 774:16-28.

Lancaster, J., and C.S. Lancaster
1987 The watershed: Change in parental investment and family-formation strategies in the course of human evolution. Pp. 187-206 in *ParentingAacross the Lifespan: Biosocial Dimension.* J.B. Lancaster, J. Altman, A.S. Rossi, and L.R. Sherrod, eds. New York: Aldine de Gruyter.

Ledoux, J.E.
1998 *The Emotional Brain: The Mysterious Underpinnings of Emotional Life.* London: Weidenfeld and Nicolson.

Leigh, S.R.
1998 Evolution of human growth spurts. *American Journal of Physical Anthropology* 101(1):455-474.

Leigh, S.R., and B.T. Shea
1996 Ontogeny of body size variation in African apes. *American Journal of Physical Anthropology* 99(1):48-65.

Levitt, N.S., E.V. Lambert, D. Woods, C.N. Hales, R. Andrew, and J.R. Seckl
2000 Impaired glucose tolerance and elevated blood pressure in low birth weight, nonobese, young South African adults: Early programming of the cortisol axis. *Journal of Clinical Endocrinology and Metabolism* 85(12):4611-4618.

Maggioncalda, A.N., N.M. Czekala, and R.M. Sapolsky

2002 Male orangutan subadulthood: A new twist on the relationship between chronic stress and developmental arrest. *American Journal of Physical Anthropology* 118(1):25-32.

Majewska, M.D.

1995 Neuronal actions of dehydroepiandrosterone. Possible role in brain development, aging, memory and affect. *Annals of the New York Academy of Sciences* 774:111-120.

Manning, J.T., D. Scutt, J. Wilson, and D.I. Lewis-Jones

1998 The ratio of 2nd to 4th digit length: A predictor of sperm numbers and concentrations of testosterone, luteinizing hormone and oestrogen. *Human Reproduction* 13(11):3000-3004.

Maurer, M., Z. Trajanoski, G. Frey, N. Hiroi, J. Galon, H.S. Willenberg, P.W. Gold, G.R. Chrousos, W.A. Scherbaum, and S.R. Bornstein

2001 Differential gene expression profile of glucocorticoids, testosterone, and dehydroepiandrosterone in human cells. *Hormone and Metabolic Research* 33:691-695.

Mazur, A., and J. Michalek

1998 Marriage, divorce and male testosterone. *Social Forces* 77:315-330.

McBurnett, K., B.B. Lahey, P.J. Rathouz, and R. Loeber

2000 Low salivary cortisol and persistent aggression in boys referred for disruptive behavior. *Archives of General Psychiatry* 57(1):38-43.

McEwen, B.S.

1999 Stress and the aging hippocampus. *Frontiers in Neuroendocrinology* 20:49-70.

Meikle, A.W., J.D. Stringham, M.G. Woodward, and D.T. Bishop

1988 Heritability of plasma cortisol levels. *Metabolism* 37(6):514-517.

Meikle, A.W., R.A. Stephenson, C.M. Lewis, G.A. Wiebke, and R.G. Middleton

1997 Age, genetic and nongenetic factors influencing variation in serum sex steroids and zonal volume of the prostate and benign prostate hyperplasia in twins. *Prostate* 33:105-111.

Miller, G.

2000 *The Mating Mind: How Sexual Choice Shaped the Evolution of Human Nature.* New York: Anchor Books.

Miller, W.B., D.J. Pasta, J. MacMurray, C. Chiu, H. Wu, and D.E. Comings

1999 Dopamine receptor genes are associated with age at first sexual intercourse. *Journal of Biosocial Science* 31(1):43-54.

Moss, H.B., M. Vanyukov, J.K. Yao, and G.P. Kirillova

1999 Salivary cortisol responses in prepubertal boys: The effects of parental substance abuse and association with drug use during adolescence. *Biological Psychiatry* 45(10):1293-1299.

Mott, F.L., and R.J. Haurin

1988 Linkages between sexual activity and alcohol and drug use among American adolescents. *Family Planning Perspectives* 20(3):128-136.

Muhlenbein, M.P., B.C. Campbell, M.A. Murchison, and K.M. Phillipi

2002 Morphological and hormonal parameters in two species of Macaques: Impact of seasonal breeding. *American Journal of Physical Anthropology* 117:218-227.

Nadler, R.D., J. Wallis, C. Roth-Meyer, R.W. Cooper, and E.E. Baulieu

1987 Hormones and behavior of prepubertal and peripubertal chimpanzees. *Hormones and Behavior* 21(1):118-131.

Nass, R., S. Baker, A.E. Sadler, and J.J. Sidtis

1990 The effects of precocious adrenarche on cognition and hemispheric specialization. *Brain and Cognition* 14(1):59-69.

Nelson, K.
1996 Memory development from 4 to 7 years. Pp. 141-160 in *The Five to Seven Year Shift.* A.J. Sameroff and M.M. Haith, eds. Chicago: University of Chicago Press.

Niehoff, D.
1999 *The Biology of Violence: How Understanding the Brain, Behavior and Environment Can Break the Vicious Circle of Aggression.* New York: The Free Press.

Nielsen, C.T., N.E. Skakkebaek, J.A. Darling, W.M. Hunter, D.W. Richarson, M. Jorgensen, and N. Keiding
1986 Longitudinal study of testosterone and luteinizing hormone (LH) in relation to spermarche, pubic hair, height and sitting height in normal boys. *Acta Endocrinologica Supplement* (Copenhagen) 279:98-106.

Orentreich, N., J.L. Brind, J.H. Vogelman, R. Andres, and H. Baldwin
1992 Long-term longitudinal measures of plasma dehydroepiandrosterone sulfate in normal men. *Journal of Clinical Endocrinology and Metabolism* 75(4):1002-1014.

Parker, C.R., Jr.
1999 Dehydroepiandrosterone and dehydroepiandrosterone sulfate production in the human adrenal during development and aging. *Steroids* 64(9):640-647.

Pawlowski, B., R.I. Dunbar, and A. Lipowicz
2000 Tall men have more reproductive success. *Nature* 403(6766):156.

Phillips, D.I.W., D.J.P. Barker, C.H.D. Fall, J.R. Seckl, C.B. Whorwood, P.J. Wood, and B.R. Walker
1998 Elevated plasma cortisol concentrations: A link between low birthweight and the insulin resistance syndrome? *Journal of Clinical Endocrinology and Metabolism* 83:757-760.

Phillips, D.I., R.B. Walker, R.M. Reynolds, D.E. Flanagan, P.J. Wood, C. Osmond, D.J. Barker, and C.B. Whorwood
2000 Low birth weight predicts elevated plasma cortisol concentrations in adults from 3 populations. *Hypertension* 35:1301-1306.

Reynolds, R.M., B.R. Walker, H.E. Syddall, R. Andrew, P.J. Wood, C.B. Whorwood, and D.I. Phillips
2001 Altered control of cortisol secretion in adult men with low birth weight and cardiovascular risk factors. *Journal of Clinical Endocrinology and Metabolism* 86(1):245-250.

Remer, T.
2000 Adrenarche and nutritional status. *Journal of Pediatric Endocrinology and Metabolism* 13(Suppl. 5):1253-1255.

Remer, T., and F. Manz
1999 Role of nutritional status in the regulation of adrenarche. *Journal of Clinical Endocrinology and Metabolism* 84(11):3936-3944.

Robel, P., and E.E. Baulieu
1995 Dehydroepiandrosterone (DHEA) is a neuroactive steroid. *Annals of the New York Academy of Sciences* 774:82-110.

Rodgers, J.L., D.C. Rowe, and M. Buster
1999 Nature, nurture and first sexual intercourse in the USA: Fitting behavioral genetic models to NLSY kinship data. *Journal of Biosocial Science* 31(1):29-41.

Rosenblitt, J.C., H. Soler, S.E. Johnson, and D.M. Quadango
2001 Sensation-seeking and hormones in men and women: Exploring the link. *Hormones and Behavior* 40:396-402.

Rosenthal, D.A., A.M.A. Smith, and R. deVisser
1999 Personal and social factors influencing age at first sexual intercourse. *Archives of Sexual Behavior* 28:319-333.

Rosa Neto, P., H. Lou, P. Cumming, O. Pryds, and A. Gjedde
2002 Methylphenidate-evoked potentiation of extracellular dopamine in the brain of adolescents with premature birth: Correlation with attentional deficit. *Annals of the New York Academy of Sciences* 965:434-439.

Sanchez-Martin, J.R., E. Fano, L. Ahedo, J. Cardas, P.F. Brain, and A. Azpiroz
2000 Relating testosterone levels and free play social behavior in male-female preschool children. *Psychoneuroendocrinology* 25(8):773-783.

Scerbo, A.S., and D.J. Kolko
1994 Salivary testosterone and cortisol in disruptive children: Relationship to aggressive, hyperactive and internalizing behaviors. *Journal of the American Academy of Child and Adolescent Psychiatry* 33(8):1174-1184.

Smail, P.J., C. Faiman, W.C. Hobson, G.B. Fuller, and J.D. Winter
1982 Further studies on adrenarche in non-human primates. *Endocrinology* 111:844-848.

Small, M.F.
1988 Female primate behavior and conception: Are there enough sperm to spare? *Current Anthropology* 29(1):81-100.

Smith, B.H.
1993 Physiological age of KMN-WT 1500 and its significance for growth and development of early *Homo*. Pp. 195-220 in *The Nariokotome Homo Erectus Skeleton.* A.C. Walker and R.F. Leakey, eds. Cambridge MA: Belknap, Harvard University Press.

Smith, R.L.
1984 Human sperm competition. Pp. 601-659 in *Sperm Competition and the Evolution of Animal Matings Systems.* R.L. Smith, ed. New York: Academic Press.

Stansbury, K., and M.R. Gunnar
1994 Adrenocortical activity and emotion regulation. In *The Development of Emotion Regulation: Biological and Behavioral Considerations.* N.A. Fox, ed. *Monographs of the Society for Research in Child Development* 59(240):108-134.

Stikkelbroeck, N.M., B.J. Otten, A. Pasic, G.J. Jager, C.G. Sweep, K. Noordam, and A.R. Hermus
2001 High prevalence of testicular adrenal rest tumors, impaired spermatogenesis, and Leydig cell failure in adolescent and adult males with congenital adrenal hyperplasia. *Journal of Clinical Endocrinology and Metabolism* 86(12):5721-5728.

Storey, A.E., C.J. Walsh, R.L. Quinton, and K.E. Wynne-Edwards
2000 Hormonal correlates of paternal responsiveness in new and expectant fathers. *Evolution and Human Behavior* 21(2):79-95.

Tanner, J.M.
1978 *Fetus in Man: Physical Growth from Conception to Maturity.* Cambridge MA: Harvard University Press.

Tapert, S.F., G.A. Aarons, G.R. Sedlar, and S.A. Brown
2001 Adolescent substance use and sexual risk-taking. *Journal of Adolescent Health* 28(3):181-189.

Tubman, J.G., M. Windle, and R.C. Windle
1996 Cumulative sexual intercourse patterns among middle adolescents: Problem behavior precursors and concurrent health risk behaviors. *Journal of Adolescent Health* 18(3):182-191.

Udry, J.R., and J.O.G. Billy
1987 Initiation of coitus in early adolescence. *American Sociological Review* 52(6):841-855.

Udry, J.R., J.O.G. Billy, N.M. Morris, T. Groff, and M. Raj
1985 Serum androgenic hormones motivate sexual behavior in adolescent boys. *Fertility and Sterility* 43:90-94.

Van Goozen, S.H., W. Matthys, P.T. Cohen-Kettenis, J.H. Thijssen, and H. van Engeland
1998 Adrenal androgens and aggression in conduct disorder prepubertal boys and normal controls. *Biological Psychiatry* 43(2):156-158.

Van Niekerk, J.K., F.A. Huppert, and J. Herbert
2001 Salivary cortisol and DHEA: Association with measures of cognition and well-being in normal older men, and effects of three months of DHEA supplementation. *Psychoneuroendocrinology* 26(6):591-612.

Virkkunen, M., E. Kallio, R. Rawlings, R. Tokola, R.E. Poland, A. Guidotti, C. Nemeroff, G. Bissette, K. Kalogeras, S.L. Karonen, and M. Limmoila
1994 Personality profiles and state aggressiveness in Finnish alcoholic, violent offenders, fire setters, and healthy volunteers. *Archives of General Psychiatry* 51:28-33.

Vizmanos, B., and C. Marti-Henneberg
2000 Puberty begins with a characteristic body fat mass in each sex. *European Journal of Clinical Nutrition* 54:203-208.

Vizmanos, B., C. Marti-Henneberg, R. Cliville, A. Moreno, and J. Fernandez-Ballart
2001 Age of pubertal onset affects the intensity and duration of pubertal growth peak but not final height. *American Journal of Human Biology* 13(3):409-416.

Vogel, F., and R. Ratherberg
1975 Spontaneous mutations in humans. Pp. 5-223 in *Advances in Human Genetics.* H. Harris and K. Hirschhord, eds. New York: Plenum Press.

Wagner, M.K.
2001 Behavioral characteristics related to substance abuse and risk-taking, sensation-seeking, anxiety sensitivity, and self-reinforcement. *Addictive Behavior* 26(1):115-120.

Walker, E.F., D.J. Walder, and F. Reynolds
2001 Developmental changes in cortisol secretion in normal and at-risk youth. *Developmental Psychopathology* 13(3):721-732.

Wang, S., J. Mason, D. Charney, R. Yehuda, S. Riney, and S. Southwick
1997 Relationships between hormonal profile and novelty seeking in combat-related posttraumatic stress disorder. *Biological Psychiatry* 41(2):145-151.

Weisfeld, G.
1999 *Evolutionary Principles of Human Adolescence.* New York: Basic Books.

Worthman, C.M.
1993 Biocultural interactions in human development. Pp. 339-358 in *Juvenile Primates: Life History, Development and Behavior.* M.E. Pereira and L.A. Fairbanks, eds. New York: Oxford University Press.
1999 The epidemiology of human development. Pp. 47-104 in *Hormones, Health and Behavior.* C.M. Worthman and C. Panter-Brick, eds. Cambridge: Cambridge University Press.

Wyckoff, G.J., W. Wang, and C.I. Wu
2000 Rapid evolution of male reproductive genes in the descent of man. *Nature* 403(6767):304-309.

Yoo, A., J. Harris, and B. Dubrovsky
1996 Dose-response study of dehydroepiandrosterone sulfate on dentate gyrus long-term potentiation. *Experimental Neurology* 137(1):151-156.

Zemel, B.S., and S.H. Katz

1986 The contribution of adrenal and gonadal steroids to the growth in the height of adolescent males. *American Journal of Physical Anthropology* 71(4):459-466.

Zuckerman, M.

1995 Good and bad humors: Biochemical bases of personality and its disorders. *Psychological Science* 6:325-332.

10

Energetics, Sociality, and Human Reproduction: Life History Theory in Real Life

Carol M. Worthman

Understanding the determinants of human fertility remains a matter of urgent practical as well as scientific concern. Many fields, including demography, economics, health sciences, and policy and political science, offer theories at varying levels of explanation and predictive power. Only one theory, evolutionary theory, offers an account at the ultimate level of design.

Since its formulation, however, evolutionary theory has challenged the efforts of anthropologists and evolutionary biologists to apply the grand theory to variation within particular species and populations, or among individuals. Ideally, these efforts involve dialectic between epistemological and empirical work, between model building and model testing. Yet even outstanding empiricists in the field emphasize the remaining challenges, reporting, for instance, "the realization that no current models that adequately *explain* fertility variation in traditional societies have withstood empirical scrutiny" (Hill and Hurtado, 1995:396). Both theory and the models derived from it therefore require further work.

This essay attempts to develop a fresh view of human fertility behavior and family formation by considering the intersection of three approaches—life history theory, behavioral and reproductive ecology, and developmental psychobiology. On the theoretical front, life history theory aims to integrate comparative, cross-taxonomic data into a framework comprising life course attributes such as the timing, pace, and forms of reproduction and reproductive effort. On the population level, human evolutionary and reproductive ecologists have sought to probe the value of adaptationist models for understanding variations in reproductive behavior and biology.

On the individual level, developmental psychobiologists have unpacked the roles of rearing environments in temperament, sociality and parenting, and life history strategy.

The evolutionary and functional analyses presented below suggest the need to expand current demographic models of human fertility behavior to include considerations of design and human development. Each level of analysis–evolutionary, ecological, and developmental–suggests that human reproduction involves much more than fertility, and identifies critical variables for successful human reproduction that merit more attention in demographic analysis.

IMPORTANCE OF A BIOCULTURAL PERSPECTIVE

For over 25 years, adaptationist accounts of human behavior (first under the rubric of sociobiology, then behavioral ecology) have been dominated by the calculus of cost and benefits reckoned against the bottom line of limited available resources. Reproduction occupies a central place in this calculus because fitness, or differential reproductive success, is the currency of adaptation. The logic is simple: Reproductive effort will be determined by the availability of finite resources, principally energy and time, balanced against competing demands for subsistence or survival. Human evolutionary or behavioral ecology proceeds from the assumption that "humans should have evolved fertility and mortality patterns that lead to highest contribution to the future gene pool, given the constraints provided by general human morphological, physiological, and social characteristics, and the environments in which our species lives" (Hill and Hurtado, 1995:13).

This bold proposition—that human behavior has been shaped by selective pressures to optimize fitness—inspired a wave of empirical research, the best of which sought to test the validity of this claim and probe its ability to illuminate human behavior. This research builds on an older foundation of evolutionary biology to assess whether and how adaptive design may explain the inter- and intrapopulation variations in human reproductive function. The proposition that reproductive function itself reflects design constraints posed by evolutionary processes has yielded a series of novel hypotheses that have met with empirical support while also providing fresh perspectives on both adaptation and reproduction (Ellison, 1994; Wood, 1994). Yet even the best of these studies seldom cover beliefs, values, and schemas that inform behavior—that is, culture and experiential worlds (Borgerhoff Mulder, 1995). Research on impacts on fertility of workload, nutritional status, breastfeeding and supplementation, and maternal age rarely pursues the cultural dimensions woven into the biocultural dynamics (McDade and Worthman, 1998).

Inattention to culture, human experience, and cognition (in behavioral and reproductive ecology) reflects gaps in evolutionary thinking that are only slowly being addressed in evolutionary psychology (Crawford and Krebs, 1998; Henrich, 2001; Henrich et al., 2001). But the gaps also mirror the absence of powerful dual-inheritance models that incorporate contemporary advances in developmental and behavioral biology. Such advances demonstrate that the distinction between biological and cultural modes of transmission is gratuitous, since inheritance operates through biocultural mechanisms across ontogeny (Oyama, 1985). Using this insight, evolutionary models, reformulated as biocultural inheritance models, could build in developmental psychobiology to provide a more complete picture of human reproductive behavior that incorporates social viability as a goal for offspring, an absolute prerequisite for successful human reproduction.

The analysis here begins with an examination of life history design, particularly resource allocation over the life course to growth, reproduction, and maintenance, as effected through neuroendocrine-endocrine regulators (abbreviated as neuro-endocrine). In addition to the well-studied ecological effects on reproductive biology, less studied trade-offs with social effort are identified in foundational pathways for neuro-endocrine regulation. Thus, human physiology reflects the adaptive significance of social life and the demands for social competence and participation in that life. Then, pathways by which social ecology instructs ontogeny are reviewed, which leads directly to consideration of the environments of evolutionary adaptedness. Both sets of analyses—endocrine and epigenetic—delineate components of biocultural inheritance central to human reproduction. Thus, inheritance for humans is not appropriately viewed as dual, genetic and cultural. Rather, it has a dominant biocultural coevolutionary component that is not divisible into biological (genes) and cultural (memes) units of inheritance but runs through the mechanisms and components of epigenesis. (If we wish to model this space, we would do well to commence with close readings of Baldwin [1895] and his modern counterpart, Gottlieb [1991, 1998].)

Biocultural inheritance and the redefinition of fertility outcomes to include viability of offspring imply possibilities for parallel changes in demographic thinking. Such possibilities are exemplified in the classic formulation of the "theoretical maximum" of fertility for humans (see Figure 10-1). The maximum is intended as a biological starting point from which the components that expand interbirth intervals pare away fertility potential to determine actual fertility. But this formulation, though merely theoretical, is patently absurd.

Better models of proximate determinants of effective fertility may be constructed from schedules for actual populations, such as the Hutterites and Gainj, from which we could begin to derive general patterns of the kind represented in the top three boxes of the figure. This is the classic work of

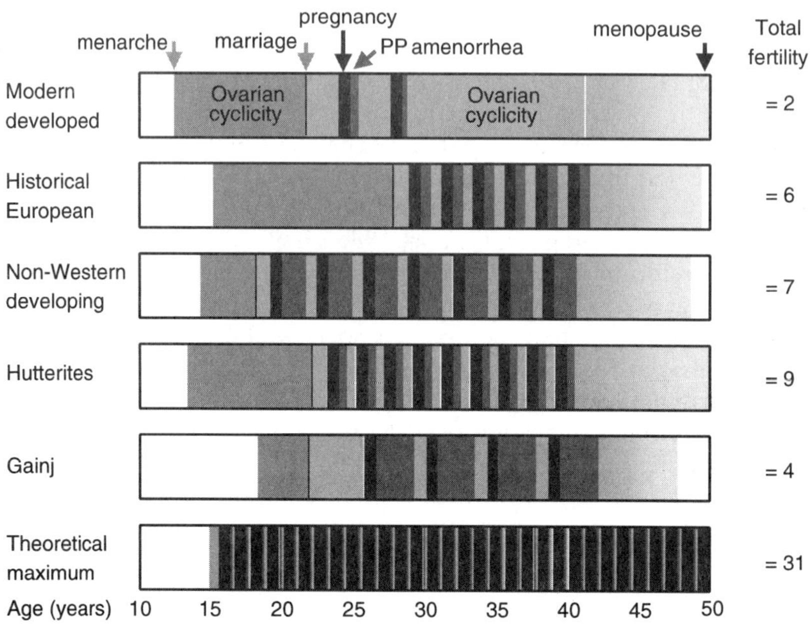

FIGURE 10-1 Scheduling in timing of reproductive events in diverse human populations (modified from Wood, 1994, which was based on Bongaarts and Potter, 1983).

demographers, which has shaped present understanding of fertility and could generate new, expanded models of determinants to help us think about fertility in creative ways. This analysis shows, however, that models of fertility behavior cannot stop with birth or lactation but must move on to identify and incorporate the key components of development that drive the production of viable offspring or the achievement of effective fertility.

LIFE HISTORY THEORY AND ENERGETICS

Life history theory concerns the evolved design constraints that shape species-specific phenotypes across the life course and that underlie the striking contrasts in life histories across the animal kingdom and even within taxa. Theorists seek design features from comparative evolutionary biology that will explain fertility and mortality schedules—classic demographic concerns. Consider the contrasts among any conceivable set of organisms, such as coelenterata, insectivora, and mammalia or sardines, whales, mice, and albatrosses (Charnov, 1993; Promislow and Harvey, 1990). Rather than focusing on differential transgenerational genetic representation (fitness) as a basis of evolutionary analysis, life history theory concentrates on resource allocation as intrinsic to adaptive strategy. The life course is viewed as the product of an integrated suite of strategies for resource allocation, of which reproduction and its translation into fitness are a central feature.

Energy and Time

Resource allocation involves deploying energy and time across the spatiotemporal place carved out of entropy that comprises a life. The calculus is simple in principle but challenging to operationalize in detail.

First, energy. This is actually better conceived as energy (e.g., calories) plus valuable, limited material resources (e.g., micronutrients). The acquisition and the disposition of resources are both components of life history strategy, but current life history theory attends little to the input or acquisition side (a focus of behavioral ecology; Smith and Winterhalder, 1992).

The total energy captured by an organism is allocated among three domains: maintenance, growth, and reproduction. Maintenance includes (1) the metabolic cost of being alive, which covers processing and distributing food, air, and other inputs, the operation of membrane potentials, biosynthesis, resource recycling, and waste treatment; (2) materials and energy required for continuous maintenance and replacement, as in the constant turnover in bone and most other organs, cells, and cellular constituents, DNA checking and repair, and barrier maintenance through dermal and mucosal production; (3) healing from injury or unusual wear and tear; and (4) defense against, removal of, and cohabitation with micropredators (pathogens and parasites), as well as detection and evasion of macropredators (non- and conspecifics). In other words, maintenance involves all the investments that allay causes of mortality, intrinsic (e.g., aging) or extrinsic (e.g., accident and predation). The extent and quality of such investments in maintenance determine mortality schedules, or age-specific probabilities and causes of death.

Growth includes increases in body size—in length, height, weight, and overall mass. Two issues with respect to growth are the distinction between determinate and indeterminate growers and the value of size. Many species confine growth to an early period of life, ceasing to grow when adult body size is attained; others grow throughout life. The contrast in resource allocation strategies is apparent. Body size within taxa increases through evolutionary time, prompting the inference that size itself may have adaptive value (Charnov, 1993).

Reproduction comprises producing viable offspring that successfully reproduce. Life history strategy for accomplishing this may vary in many dimensions, including timing of first reproduction; adult size and proportionate size of offspring at birth; number of offspring per reproductive event and spacing between events, types, amounts, and duration of postnatal care of offspring (parental effort); sex determination and the relative contributions of males and females to reproduction; and the slope of reproductive value with age. Evolutionary analysis has focused, virtually from its inception, on the necessary reproductive effort (Darwin 1871; Maynard Smith, 1978; Trivers, 1972; Williams, 1985), which has various costs (Borgerhoff Mulder, 1992), basically including (1) the biological costs of producing a new life (gametes, gestation, parturition) and (2) the costs of sustaining new life (parental care, including lactation, provisioning, defense, and solicitude for physical and emotional security). Costs may be expanded to cover (3) mating effort—finding, recruiting, and keeping a mate. Taxa show widely divergent mating strategies, which may comprise a significant portion of reproductive effort, particularly for males. A further dramatic expansion of the costs that can be counted as reproductive effort comes from defining inclusive fitness to incorporate reproduction by others, discounted by degree of relatedness to ego (Hamilton, 1964). This adds to the list (4) the costs of inclusive fitness, such as any form of altruism (to benefit others at one's own expense) as well as aspects of social behavior and environmental modification. Particularly for social species, and especially when culture is employed as a major adaptive strategy, there is a final component of reproductive effort: (5) socialization cost. Socializing the young includes nurturing them (attending to emotional-cognitive needs as well as material ones), instructing them or guiding their participation in adult activities while tolerating juvenile ineptitude; providing opportunities to obtain and practice knowledge, attitudes, behaviors, and skills required for viable sociality requisite to survival and reproduction; and even actively advancing their social prospects (Blurton Jones et al., 1989, 1992).

Second, time. Like energy, time is a finite resource that must be apportioned among the same three domains as material resources and for reproduction, particularly, among the subdomains outlined above. The time invested in any reproductive event, weighed against life expectancy, determines reproductive potential or value.

The intersection of energy and time drives rates of resource demand and use, and lies at the heart of energetics. Energetic balance can be adjusted by modulating the rate of throughput. Lower throughput, due to late and infrequent reproduction, involves lower reproductive demand per unit of time than early and frequent reproduction. Lower throughput therefore relaxes the constraint of resource availability but carries the risk of dying before completing reproduction.

Trade-Offs

Such considerations demonstrate a central principle of life history organization, namely, to establish optimal trade-offs among competing demands under consistently unpredictable circumstances. Modeling trade-offs is essential for understanding the design or the biological organization of the functions and capacities of the human organism. Life history strategies can be usefully viewed, on the level of the organismic design of a species, as a set of algorithms that negotiate the trade-offs to optimize spatiotemporal allocation of limited resources.

One cardinal rule underlies the ubiquity of trade-offs: the allocation rule. Related to thermodynamic notions of energy conservation, the allocation rule states that consumable resources used for one purpose cannot be used for another. This rule will be critically examined below.

In schematic terms, maintenance may be subtracted from resource intake to determine the net resources available for growth or reproduction, which is labeled productivity. In comparison to productivity estimated from juvenile growth rates in other determinate growers, the productivity of primates appears remarkably low, only 40 percent of that of mammals in general—and the productivity of humans is only 20 percent of that of mammals, because human children grow very slowly between the ages of 5 and 10 (Kaplan et al., 2000). Slow growth affects life history strategy in several ways. It reduces the burden of energetic demands for growth (given the species has relatively low juvenile mortality). This effect may be particularly important for easing the demands on human parents, who provision their young throughout juvenility (Bogin, 1997, 1999). Slow growth may also permit greater investments in the maintenance required to reduce juvenile mortality or to meet the high metabolic costs of large brain size. Finally, low productivity may be the product of increased developmental costs not reflected in growth (e.g., play) but required for attaining adult competence.

Human Life History Strategy

Humans are large, long lived, and obligately social primates that have altricial singleton births, spaced at 2 to 5 years, which are first breastfed and then provisioned well into the second decade. Young are carried, tended, defended, instructed, and systematically exposed to experiences or adult-driven ecologies aimed not only at teaching attitudes and techniques for survival but also developing social competence and coherence as well as adult productivity. Reproductive timing is set through distinctive physiological switches that inhibit gonadal function in childhood and activate it in puberty.

Humans are determinate growers who grow slowly over a protracted period and then exhibit a growth spurt during a relatively late puberty. In puberty, adult height is achieved and energy previously used for growth becomes available for reproduction. Shifts in energy storage through changes in body composition (girls to fat, boys to muscle) attend this transition. After a phase of subfecundity, women enter a period of reproductive activity sustained over roughly two decades. Notably, they possess the unusual feature of programmed cessation of reproductive function—menopause—whereby ovarian potency declines and ceases decades before life ends. Reproductive aging leads to a remarkably ubiquitous average age at last birth of around 40 years (Bongaarts and Potter, 1983). The reproductive careers of men are not so curtailed, although they also show signs of reproductive aging.

Challenges for Life History Theory

Life history theory has excited interest because it applies formal and game theoretical models to comparative data; provides a life span, time-integrated framework; integrates across components of phenotype rather than focusing on specific features; identifies key cost-benefit trade-offs in the design of life history strategies; and thus suggests organic design criteria and evolutionary constraints. It promises to be generalizable, predictive, and hypothesis generating. Formerly, life history analysis was primarily based on species averages for the various life history parameters; variance was not included in formal analysis. However, the range of behavioral decisions used has been expanded to include state-dependent action (condition-, context-, or density-dependent) in models that can evaluate variations within and between individuals (Brommer, 2000). Notable limitations remain. These limitations do not impugn the importance and value of life history theory but should inform its application to fertility behavior.

First, variations within taxa should be distinguished from variations across taxa. Life history theory is based on formal comparative analysis across taxa, yet the goal of the present volume is to address fertility behavior within one taxon, humans. The hierarchy of life history trade-offs derived from analysis encompassing macrotaxonomic variations (between classes or phyla—e.g. fishes versus mammals) does not necessarily generalize directly to variations within species. By definition, different taxa do not share evolutionary history and thus have different design features and life history strategies, so each taxon has a different hierarchy of allocation trade-offs, as allometric analysis confirms. Analysis involving restriction of the phyletic range (within rather than across orders or families) would narrow the sweep of organic design questions and help focus on the relevant variance to partition.

Second, like evolutionary theory itself, the formal models of life history theory are highly abstract and aphysiological and do not support direct inferences about mediating mechanisms responsible for resource allocation or constraining life history design. A given life history constraint or trade-off can be met through diverse mechanisms. An additional empirical step is required to link life history to function in specific taxa. This step is abetted by identification of design patterns and constraints that do support testable hypotheses about organic design. For instance, comparative life history analysis identified adult mortality as the prime factor explaining variations among life history strategies. But a distinction between intrinsic and extrinsic sources of mortality (Charnov, 1993) proved difficult to sustain at the level of the functioning organism, though it generated a body of work that has illuminated relationships between these two sources of mortality (Ricklefs, 1998) as well as mechanisms of aging in general (Holliday, 1995; Kirkwood, 1981; Williams, 1957). A later section will deal with endocrine architecture and attempt to link this aspect of organic design and function with life history to show how trade-offs are embodied and shape fertility in humans.

A third limitation of the life history literature concerns the allocation rule and the need for more attention to the trade-offs around sociality. Perhaps the allocation rule has not received adequate critical or empirical scrutiny. The rule may actually be "bendable," particularly with regard to the fertility behavior of highly social primates, a possibility evaluated below.

The following sections bring the strengths of life history analysis to bear on human fertility behavior while addressing limitations and expanding the scope of adaptationist thinking to substantially strengthen the analytic purchase on human reproduction.

TRANSLATION AND TRANSMISSION OF EVOLVED DESIGN

An integrated theory of reproductive ecology requires linkage of life history theory with phenotype and the mechanisms that produce life history, particularly reproductive careers. Phenotype comprises all the manifest features of an individual, including behavior. As in most species, human phenotypes adjust to environmental quality. The capacity for facultative adjustment can be gauged by the norm of reaction, or the phenotypic variation shown by a given genotype across diverse environments (Stearns and Koella, 1986). Cultural variations and the complexities associated with sociality lead to large reaction norms in human behaviors such as parenting practices or timing of marriage, but humans also exhibit substantial reaction norms in the biological bases of reproductive capacities and behavior.

Age at Menarche

One of the most thoroughly documented reaction norms for humans is age at menarche, which has been found to vary by nearly 50 percent across populations, from a low median age of just over 12 years in consistently well-nourished, healthy populations, to up to 18 years in persistently poorly nourished, less healthy ones (Eveleth and Tanner, 1990; Worthman, 1999a).

One might argue that the correlation of environmental quality with age at menarche reflects the impact of environmental insult rather than adaptive biological response, but the case of girls adopted at different ages into radically improved circumstances contradicts this interpretation. Girls from disadvantaged south Indian populations adopted at age 3 or later had an earlier age at menarche (11.1 years) than those adopted at 2 years or less (11.8 years); Proos et al., 1991). Furthermore, recent epidemiological studies of the effects of early environment on systems that drive resource allocation (Barker, 1991, 1997; Clark et al., 1996; Fall et al., 1995) have documented that fetal programming of neuro-endocrine regulation alters developmental and health outcomes across the life span (Adair, 2001; Godfrey, 1998; McDade et al., 2001; Susser and Levin, 1999; Williams and Poulton, 1999).

Secular trends and population variations in timing of reproductive maturation (indexed by menarche for girls) are related to variations in the timing of the onset of puberty in both sexes. Intensive investigation into these variations has identified maternal well-being, infant and child health, nutrition, and psychological well-being as salient ecological correlates. In teleological terms of life history theory (see Figure 10-2), maternal well-being (health, nutrition, and low stress), low juvenile mortality risk (indexed by morbidity), and sustained good nutrition reduce the resources needed for maintenance, with the net effect of increasing productivity.

Greater productivity increases the energy available for growth (in height or weight, fat or muscle) or reproduction and reduces the marginal costs of reproduction. This allows faster growth and accelerated maturation, conducive to earlier puberty. Good conditions from gestation through childhood also signal that the risk or relative cost of reproduction likely will be low (the dashed line in the figure).

At this point, limitations on the applicability of life history theory to intraspecific variations become clear, for life history predicts that adult mortality risk will be associated with earlier onset of the reproductive career (Charnov, 1993). Humans show the opposite pattern, with mortality risk associated with later puberty. As child health and survival improve in a population, child maturation accelerates, as evidenced by increased height for age and earlier age at menarche. Indeed, so close is this link that child

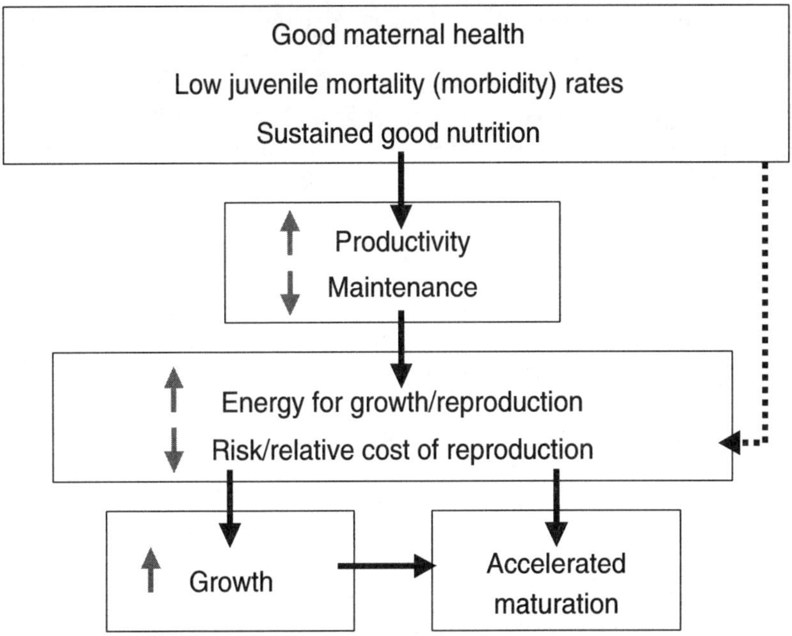

FIGURE 10-2 Secular trend in timing of puberty in terms of life history.

growth indices are used as a sensitive measure of population nutrition and health (World Health Organization, 1995).

Two Mediating Mechanisms

Phenotypic variations in reproductive behavior, such as variations in the timing of puberty, must originate somehow from evolved life history design. Two issues are involved, and lead to two distinctive but ultimately related sets of mediating mechanisms.

First is design for information use: how is life history design translated into phenotype? A case will be made here for the place of neuroendocrine-endocrine systems in the translation process. Endocrine architecture provides the concrete physiological structure for realizing the intersection of constitutional genetic endowment of the individual, fixed at conception, with environmental inputs, demands, and chance.

Second is transmission of life history design across generations. How can all the information that an organism needs to develop, survive, and succeed be communicated across generations? This is an enormous bioinformatics challenge that cannot have a purely organic solution but must be seen as a problem of biocultural inheritance.

The following sections explore these two set of reproductive mechanisms—endocrine architecture for translating life history design into phenotype and biocultural inheritance for transmitting information to instruct translation.

Endocrine Architecture of Life History

Physiological mechanisms for producing life history phenotypes remain unspecified in life history theory, but neuroendocrine-endocrine (or neuroendocrine) systems are obvious candidates (Finch and Rose, 1995). Hormones act like pacemakers for growth and developmental transitions. They are responsible for establishing the prolonged juvenile period in humans and govern the timing of puberty and the progression to reproductive maturity. Neuro-endocrine action thereafter orchestrates adult reproductive function, including the production of gametes, establishment and course of pregnancy, parturition, lactation, reproductive aging, and menopause.

The large array of neuro-endocrine regulatory systems handles resource partitioning among growth, reproduction, and maintenance. Interactions across this array determine productivity and negotiate resource allocation to short- and long-term life history projects, balancing the immediate demands of survival (e.g., metabolism, immune function) against long-term needs for growth or reproduction.

For instance, neuro-endocrine responses to psychosocial distress antagonize gonadal activity, for such distress arises from conditions likely to be less favorable for reproduction. Moreover, psychological distress and poor nutritional state each reduce sexual interest, and thereby dampen reproduction by both physiologic and behavioral routes. Hence, hormones mediate the interface between individual and environment, effecting triage to meet shifting demands and exigencies. They also present the means for facultative adjustment of life history parameters, mediating for instance the relationship of maternal workload to duration of postpartum amenorrhea.

Figure 10-3 presents the principal endocrine regulatory pathways that mediate energy allocation and trade-offs among growth, reproduction, and maintenance (reviewed in Worthman, 1999b, 2002). All these pathways traffic between brain and periphery, and four of them run from the hypothalamus at the floor of the brain, which regulates pituitary activity by releasing hormones or inhibitory factors (CRH, GnRH, etc.). Hypothalamic-releasing hormones stimulate or suppress pituitary output of trophic hormones (ACTH, LH/FSH, etc.) that act on target glands in the periphery (adrenals, gonads, etc.). In turn, target glands release hormones that mediate the stress response, reproductive function and behavior, growth, and metabolism.

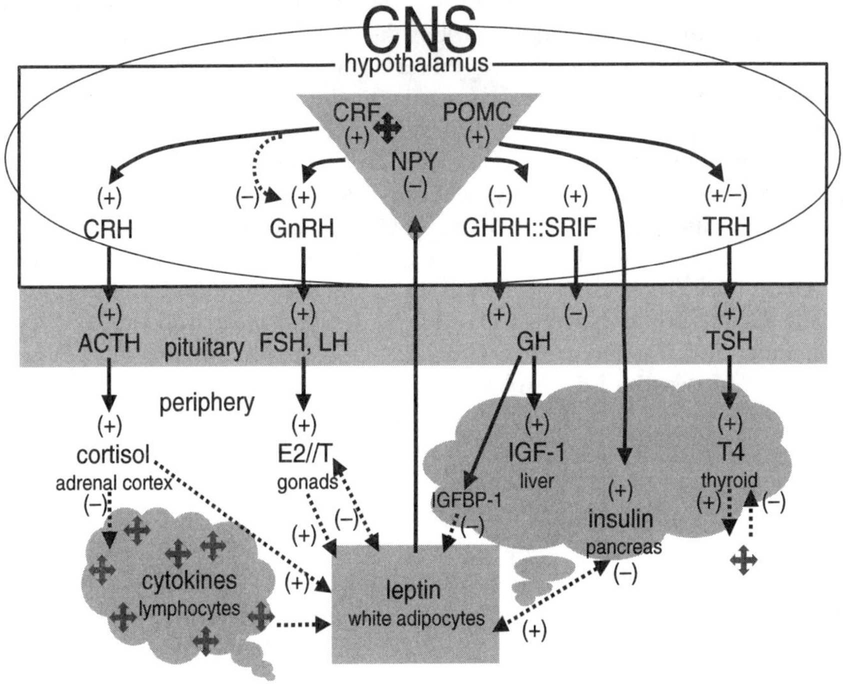

FIGURE 10-3 Representative endocrine axes, pathways, and interrelations, with particular regard to resource partitioning.
NOTE: Based on Anderson et al. (2001), Arnalich et al. (1999), Baskin et al. (1999), Bruunsgaard et al. (2000), Harris (2000), Imura et al. (1991), Mantzoros and Moschos (1998), Mantzoros et al. (2001), Owen et al. (2001, Rasmussen (2000), Straub et al. (2000), Wauters et al. (2000), and reviews in Worthman (1999a, 2002).

From the upper left to the right in Figure 10-3, the axes are (1) the hypothalamic-pituitary-adrenal (HPA) axis, which regulates arousal and stress via cortisol, a hormone that also extensively affects the other axes; (2) the hypothalamic-pituitary-gonadal (HPG) axis, which regulates gonadal function, including output of gonadal steroids (estradiol, E2; testosterone, T), which are responsible for reproductive functions and behaviors and many sex differences; (3) the somatotropic axis, which regulates growth and resource allocation via a cascade of trophic factors and binding proteins produced in the liver and locally; and (4) the thyrotropic axis, responsible for regulating metabolic rate and required for neurological development and alertness. The relationship of growth to energy availability is built into the organization of this axis.

The next two axes, at the bottom of Figure 10-3, differ from the others, involving not central coordination but distributive production and regulation, with the brain as a primary target organ. The (5) adiposal axis (bottom center) comprises white adipocytes in fat depots throughout the periphery that produce leptin, which acts in the brain and periphery with metabolic, reproductive, affective, and even hemopoeitic effects (Harris, 2000; Mantzoros, 1999; Wauters et al., 2000). This axis is significant for the present discussion because it clearly ties energetic status (not just energy stores but the balance of intake and expenditure) not only to prioritization of energy use (reproduction, metabolism) but also to mood and behavior (Baile et al., 2000; Havel, 2001; Maes, 1999; Mantzoros et al., 2001; Trayhurn and Rayner, 1996). Gonadal steroids also influence adipocyte activity and distribution (Anderson et al., 2001). Multiple neuropeptides, chiefly neuropeptide Y (NPY), proopiomelanocortin (POMC), and agouti-related peptide, mediate the actions of leptin on thermogenesis and energy metabolism and its hypothalamically mediated impact on other axes, including the gonadal. Indeed, one of the earliest observed stigmata of leptin-deficient mice was infertility (Caprio et al., 2001; Caro et al., 1996). But dense neuroendocrine pathways also tie leptin and a closely allied hormone, insulin, to motivation, affect, and behavior, which may be represented by hunger, irritability, and food intake, respectively (Mantzoros and Moschos, 1998; Schwartz et al., 1997).

The last axis, (6) the immunologic (bottom left), is stunningly complex and highly distributive. In addition to its primary place in the maintenance of physical health and integrity, the immune system strongly affects mood and behavior via cytokines released in the course of its normal pathogen-defense and repair actions (Anisman et al., 1999; Owen et al., 2001). This effect is most vividly manifested in sickness behavior—the listlessness, anorexia, social withdrawal, and cognitive blunting that accompany illness or injury (Dantzer, 2001; Hart, 1988; Yirmiya et al., 2000). Cytokine activation also suppresses sexual behavior, although animal models suggest that this effect is much more pronounced in females than males (Avitsur and Yirmiya, 1999). In addition to their potent psychobehavioral effects, cytokines trigger shunting of energy away from growth or reproduction via activation of the HPA axis and direct central effects on the HPG and somatotropic axes, suppression of thyroid activity, and peripheral actions on target organs (Rasmussen, 2000; Rivest and Rivier, 1995; von Laue and Ross, 2000).

This brief survey of endocrine architecture reveals that life history parameters have demonstrable physiological bases and furthermore raises several points about neuro-endocrine function. First, neuro-endocrine activity can be seen as clearly aimed at allocating resources among the domains of growth, reproduction, and maintenance. Neuro-endocrine pathways are organized to reflect the nature of life history demands, as in the contrast between the centrally regulated, clearly localized operation in reproduction versus the decentralized, distributive organization of the immune system. Potentially expensive and risky reproductive behaviors are under high selective pressure for appropriate timing, prolonged reallocation of resources, maintenance of biological states (cyclicity, pregnancy, parturition), and target orientation (e.g., placental [i.e., fetal] regulation of pregnancy, lactation dependence on infant stimuli).

Second, contrary to the classic silo model of endocrine organization reflected in the vertical pathways of Figure 10-3, each axis demonstrates systematic cross-talk. Cross-talk is understood rather differently when viewed from a life history perspective that throws into relief the necessity for mechanisms to allocate and reallocate energetic resources. Cross-talk provides the means to reallocate energy and modulate axis activity to meet ongoing relative demands and to do so in a physiologically integrated and synchronized manner.

Third, the neuro-endocrine architecture of life history not only supports biological functions comprising reproduction, growth, and maintenance but also integrally involves cognition and behavior. This involvement runs both ways: Hormones directly inform affect and behavior, as exemplified in the operation of the adiposal axis and the immune system, but behavior and cognition also influence hormones, as most directly exemplified by the HPA axis (McEwen, 2000; Seeman and McEwen, 1996). Such mechanisms coordinate the endocrine with the behavioral architectures of life history, as reflected in the functions of the brain as a primary site for experiential processing and memory, a center for physiological regulation and integration, and a target of peripheral modulation and signaling through endocrine action.

Fourth, the timing and course of life history events depend on ecological signals of environmental quality. Neuro-endocrine mechanisms transduce this information into physiological responses over the short term and long term. In the case of humans, favorable ecological circumstances include energetic conditions that are at least permissive, which are signaled by hormones like leptin, insulin, or cytokines, as well as positive social conditions, which are indexed through central processing (cognition and memory), emotion systems, and the HPA. These systems embody the individual's knowledge of the surrounding social ecology (a formulation analogous to Kaplan's [1995] notion of embodied capital).

Biocultural Inheritance and Fertility Behavior

The problem of intergenerational transmission for reproduction in the fullest, phenotypic, life history sense has concerned Western biologists and philosophers for several hundred years (Gould, 1977). For much of that time, progress was hampered by an unduly materialist emphasis on an organic solution, whereas an epigenetic, biocontextual (or, for the case of humans, biocultural) inheritance model now appears more appropriate. Most recently, developmental biology and genetics have documented the significance of nongenetic factors in ontogeny. In brief, postconception environments can convey most of what the individual needs to know about the inputs and demands with which it must deal effectively (Reeve and Sherman, 1993). Accordingly, ontogeny is designed to reliably capture available information to instruct development (Changeux, 1985; Gottlieb, 1991; Oyama, 1985).

Human development therefore is integral to human reproduction, perhaps more than in any other species. Human reproduction cannot be said to have succeeded until offspring development is complete. The coevolution of biocultural mechanisms for reproduction through development is distinctively elaborated among humans. Williams (1957:400) observed that: "Any individual, of whatever age, who is caring for dependent offspring is acting in a way that promotes the survival of his own genes and is properly considered a part of the breeding population. No one is post-reproductive until his youngest child is self-sufficient."

Recognizing the role of human development could help fill some of the gaps in life history models of fertility and bring them more in line with empirical observations. The substantial literatures on development and sociocultural processes would have to be integrated into the models of fitness determinants. Such integration sheds a different light on human reproduction and the selective pressures on it. If human development is coextensive with fertility in determining successful reproduction, the proximate determinants of fertility will require significant expansion to account for effective fertility, that is, for successful transmission of not only genotype but also biocultural patterns. Expansion of the concept of fertility to include postnatal processes requires incorporation not only of mortality risk but also components of developmental ecology required for biocultural transmission.

Individuals grow up in specific niches or proximal spatiotemporal envelopes. These may be labeled the effective environments of rearing. These environments can be diverse, given stratification and niche partitioning in human societies. Environments intersect with individual characteristics to create a wide range of developmental microniches (Bronfenbrenner, 1979; Super and Harkness, 1993), which produce diversity across individuals in embodied capital. This diversity is essential to complex human societies, so that variations in effective environments of rearing are critical to biocultural inheritance.

Diversity is possible partly because of human behavioral plasticity. Plasticity is rooted in a learning- and knowledge-oriented central nervous system structurally and functionally organized around a life history strategy grounded in sociality allied with high-end extractiveness (Deacon, 1997; Kaplan et al., 2000). But the basis for plasticity also resides in reproductive adaptations for biocultural inheritance.

SOCIALITY AND MULTITASKING IN LIFE HISTORY

Life history theory recognizes ecological, cognitive, and behavioral dimensions but does not adequately consider sociality. Humans must belong to social groups to survive and develop and even to reproduce. Human reproduction depends on relationships, and on sharing resources with others.

The Need for Resource Sharing

The design of the species includes an unusually pronounced pattern of asynchronous energy consumption and production (Kaplan, 1997). In foraging societies, over 25 percent of lifetime energy needs is expended by children in the first 15 years, during which time they generate only 5 percent of lifetime energy production (Kaplan et al., 2000). Furthermore, forager women do not produce as much as they consume until the end of their reproductive careers, although they do show a substantial increase in productivity in the second decade. Males, by contrast, sharply escalate production over adolescence to generate a net energy excess by age 20 and produce double their own calorie consumption over most of the next three decades. Among elders, individual production falls below consumption at age 70 in women and age 60 in men (Kaplan, 1994).

In short, among foragers, provisioning of young and subvention of reproductive-age women are necessary because of asynchrony between production and consumption. Early consumption is returned in later adult production that supports children and grandchildren. The social-cognitive fabric that sustains provisioning others and concomitant lagged reciprocity is critical to human life history strategy. Yet life history models include neither social production and consumption nor social costs and benefits.

Sociodynamics, Cognition, and Learning

Sociodynamics create or influence conditions for virtually all aspects of life history—timing of weaning, growth rates and adult body size, timing of maturation and first reproduction, pace and degree of fertility, mortality risk, and so forth. Although humans are highly diverse in their beliefs, values, practices, and resultant human ecologies, they share one important similarity: social relationships universally dominate human experience and shape the material and social worlds that individuals must navigate.

Human relationships have specific properties. They persist, through time and space. They are reciprocal. They may be ascribed (kinship, group membership) or attained (friendship). They may be displaced through time and space. They are cognition intensive, mediated largely through language, the expressiveness of face and voice, and coordinated activity.

The cognitive and social impacts of language have been extensively explored. Evolution of the human face as a communicative organ and recognition marker extends a primate trend to visual orientation, freeing of the upper lip, and snout reduction and is reflected in hairlessness (incomplete in men); high integration of muscle and skin; complexity of musculature, including muscle-muscle insertions; different central neuroregulation of voluntary versus involuntary emotional expressions; and dramatically expanded representation of the face on sensory and motor cortices. Identification, reading, and tracking of faces are supported by expanded cortical regions and specific cell subsets within them for visual and emotion processing. Individually distinctive faces also aid recognition and recall of individual-specific information (social positionality, past behaviors) to guide behavior toward, treatment by, and social interactions with others.

The importance of cognition in human social relationships is attested to by high information and processing overhead. Acquisition of social knowledge is at least as important for survival and reproduction as acquisition of productive knowledge, being crucial for successful relationships. Additionally, emotional intelligence is required to navigate relationships, and all individuals must learn how to read the emotional content of situations and behaviors, communicative and otherwise, and develop the ability to regulate their own emotions and emotional expression. In this regard, emotional-cognitive bases for deferred gratification are critical to the spatiotemporally displaced reciprocity patterns humans pursue. Experiments with chimpanzees suggest that symbolic representation of "goods," allowing abstraction and distancing, is a prerequisite (Beran et al., 1999; Boysen and Berntson, 1995). Performances of social reciprocity (e.g., conversation) are crucial to form and maintain social relationships in the short term and long term, and require integrated use of memory, signal processing, social intelligence, empathy, emotion processing, and behavior production (language, expression, gesture).

The skills necessary for such performances require extensive learning through observation, practice, and neurobehavioral honing during development. Reading emotion in others involves a formidable array of capacities: sense of self, theory of mind, cross-modality sensory mapping, integration of self and other (empathy), and expressive reciprocity to moderate ambiguity. Childhood may be extended to allow development of these emotional-cognitive skills.

Children learn to read others' emotional expression rather slowly: of the set of internationally recognized facial expressions of emotion, only happiness is reliably recognized at ages 3 to 5, anger by age 7, fear by age 10, and surprise by age 11 (Massaro, 1998). Since both language and facial expressions of emotion suffer from signal deterioration (due to, for example, darkness, distance, poor reception, and averted face) children must learn to bridge ambiguity. They must observe, mimic, and practice not only productive skills but also social ones (Tomasello, 1993, 1999). Adult tolerance for social incompetence and support for learning (via exegesis of imitative behaviors, commands and instructions, and guided performance) create the space for social learning analogous to that created for production learning. Social skills will, if anything, be more critical to successful reproduction, and it is significant that rites of passage at adolescence emphasize implicit and explicit social instruction over or in conjunction with production.

The Adaptive Value of Social Relationships

Social relationships have high adaptive value, for they regulate access to resources. On the one hand are the tangible resources emphasized in life history analysis that constitute material capital: food, shelter, safety, labor, and mates. On the other hand are immaterial resources largely overlooked in life history theory and that comprise social capital: information, social connections and memberships, social support and opportunity, assistance and cooperation, coordination and triage, and economies of scale. Deferred reciprocities allow social capital to be translated into material capital at spatially and temporally remote situations. Conversely, material capital can be converted to social capital through sharing and obligation.

Information and opportunities to acquire information through observation, association, or assisted implementation are critical resources in human life history because they facilitate access to material and social resources. Information can be of durable or ephemeral value, but given the vicissitudes of social life and ecological circumstances, ephemeral knowledge of the immediate and transient contributes just as importantly to life history as does durable knowledge of people, places, and processes. Thus, the value of social relationships inheres also in access to information, which may be regarded as the third good in limited supply, after energy and time.

In sum, human ecology and social relationships largely define the context of individual life history and determine access to resources. Virtually all aspects of reproduction–mate acquisition, mating, fertility, parenting–are framed and mediated through social behavior and social ecology. Offspring viability is also shaped through social dynamics. The very low adult mortality on which human reproductive strategy relies depends heavily on social variables. Human life history strategy includes cognitive and behavioral adaptations to acquire knowledge and skills to negotiate the social world and the material world it gates. Hence, social costs and benefits should be included in the energy calculus of life history theory.

The Costs of Sociality

Sociality requires energy and exacts costs that alter the calculus of resource allocation. First, social interaction places cognitive demands on the body's most expensive organ, the brain. Such demands include attention and emotion regulation, memory and recall, and production and processing of signals (language, face and other ethological cues, symbols) according to culture- and person-specific schemas and usages. Language use greatly increases the density of information and the elliptical and inferential content in communication, increasing the need to escalate computational speed and enhance processing modes (Beran et al., 1999; Deacon, 1997).

Second, the complexity of life in a group expands exponentially with the number of members. One must track, store, and instantaneously recall each individual's history, relationship with and interactions with oneself and with all other members of the group, inferred properties (e.g., trustworthiness), and history of social and material exchanges. The escalating computational demands imposed by group size may have contributed substantially to pressures for cortical expansion in humans. Whether or not this is true historically, humans now must meet the costly performance demands.

Third, relationships are based on spatiotemporally displaced reciprocities involving exchanges of time, material goods, and social resources. Resource sharing mitigates against acute shortfalls and helps smooth out resource availability over the life course (Kaplan, 1997). Habitual sharing comes with a cost, however. Obligations to others represent a tax on an individual, but reciprocity converts that tax into social insurance for self or offspring.

Finally, sociality brings not only support but also competition (Geary and Flinn, 2001). It is a truism of evolutionary biology and ecology that conspecifics represent the keenest competition. The costs of competition with and defense against predation by other people contribute significantly to maintenance costs. Still, the pressure of potential human competition and predation further reinforces the pressure for group membership and compliance with its costs and complex reciprocities.

Bending the Allocation Rule

Anyone who has observed and tried to code human behavior knows that multitasking is pervasive (Gosling and Petrie, 1981). Men guard goats while mending fences, gossiping with neighbors, and watching weather patterns; women clean living areas while supervising a cooking pot, tending a fire, overseeing children, and listening to the neighbors argue. Notably, children do not stay on task and show less concurrent behavioral layering, in part because cognitive skills for multitasking are acquired gradually. The allocation rule–that resources expended for one purpose cannot be used for another–requires that resources be partible. Moderating the constraints of the rule, "bending" it even while it cannot be circumvented, should provide great adaptive advantage. Such potential advantage places a premium on strategies that increase the density of purposes achieved or constraints met in a given interval with given expenditures. Parallel processing and multitasking are therefore adaptive strategies. Multitasking is facilitated by language, bipedalism with manual dexterity and tool use, cooperative foraging, a large capacity for planning, recall, and rumination; and family and group life.

Most components of reproductive effort are amenable to multitasking. Biological processes like gamete production, pregnancy, and lactation proceed concurrently with many or all other activities. Mating effort and parenting also are layered with many other activities. Everyday tasks are integrated with social relations that in turn regulate access to mates for oneself or for offspring. Men traversing the distance to a foraging site, who on the way discuss marriageable daughters for themselves or their sons, are pursuing both food acquisition and mating or parenting advantage as well as reinforcing their social bonds and refreshing their command of the social landscape. Likewise, many aspects of child care are performed in parallel with other activities. Infants and small children are carried and tended usually as a secondary or tertiary activity. Carrying and tending exact physical and cognitive costs, but their time costs are greatly diminished by integrating them with parallel activities (as with the Hiwi and Ache, in Hurtado, 1990, 1992).

Indeed, the differential reproductive burden imposed by types of labor may relate to their compatibility with multitasking (as with the Hadza, in Hawkes et al., 1997). Among Hadza foragers, for example, the value of grandmaternal care for easing a daughter's reproductive effort emerges as significant only in seasons when a mother's foraging involves tasks incompatible with concurrent child care. In a radically different postindustrial setting, the costs of parenting are greatly increased for mothers working long, inflexible hours in remote offices and lacking kin support for child care. Another form of parenting effort readily or even necessarily integrated with other tasks is child socialization. Children learn essential skills, including language, subsistence activities, social negotiation, and even child care, passively and informally through observation, imitation, and guided participation rather than direct instruction (Blurton Jones and Konner, 1976;

Rogoff, 1990; Vygotsky, 1978, 1986). Finally, high productivity, generosity, and social effort by parents generate not only social capital for themselves but also future material benefits for offspring—access to scarce social and material resources (e.g., marriage opportunities or food, respectively) that may serve as a hedge against premature parental illness or death.

Implications for Life History

How, then, should sociality and multitasking be counted in life history terms? Existing theory should be pushed to cope with these realities of human reproductive behavior. Sociality raises productivity through its impact on intake and maintenance via the pathways described above. It represents a major overlooked approach to meeting other maintenance and reproductive demands. Though sociality exacts real costs, it yields tangible benefits. Social effort accordingly represents an important arena for the allocation of trade-offs. Similarly, multitasking represents a challenging phenomenon for parsing allocation in behavior analysis and adaptationist logic. The ubiquity of multitasking relating to reproduction and involving social life indicates that its omission may limit the capacity of current behavioral ecology and life history theory to contribute to the understanding of human reproductive behavior.

The importance of social relationships, their role in fertility behavior, and their value in determining long-term offspring viability are not unique to humans. The data on baboons presented by Altmann and Alberts in this volume provide compelling nuanced evidence of this. Reproductive effort comprises complex social strategizing, not just copulating and giving birth, and the insight that such strategic capacities are both significant in humans and not unique to them should broaden our view of the determinants of fertility schedules. Efforts directed at social relationships, including relationships with group members who are neither coparents nor primary kin, yield costs and benefits over time that determine mating and parenting success. Therefore, from a life history perspective, strategies to establish, maintain, and enhance social relationships are essential components of reproductive effort.

EPIGENESIS AND REARING ENVIRONMENTS

Epigenesis in Human Reproduction

As noted above, reproduction faces an information problem: how the blueprint for a fully functional adult organism can be conveyed through the union of two parent cells. It was suggested that biocultural inheritance was an aspect of the solution. This is part of the broader process of epigenesis, the dynamic between genes and environment that informs phenotype. More formally, epigenesis comprises nonlinear developmental processes, not reducible to genes or genetic programs, that involve interactions within and among many levels of the organism and its environment (Gottlieb, 1998; Maleszka et al., 1998). Some of the most exciting work in developmental and behavioral biology over the last two decades yields insights into the nature of these interactions, and has transformed scientific views of ontogeny and adaptive design.

The problem of intergenerational transfer of information to guide ontogeny was apparently resolved by the (re)discovery of Mendelian genetics in 1900 (cited in International Human Genome Sequencing Consortium, 2001), and the blueprint analogy was reinforced by elucidation of DNA structure and function in the 1960s. But the genome simply cannot convey enough information to specify phenotype in its myriad details; indeed, initial human genome maps reported in 2001 gauge the number of protein-coding genes at 30,000 to 40,000 (International Human Genome Sequencing Consortium, 2001; Venter et al., 2001), merely double those in a fly or worm. The number of genes does not correspond to phenotypic complexity. As a crude example, the mammals mouse, whale, and human have a similar numbers of genes but possess 40, 200,000, and 85,000 million neurons, respectively (Miklos and Maleszka, 2000).

Genes provide at least the minimum information to code essential proteins and establish basic body plans. But use of the genome involves a complex metaarchitecture that is demand or context driven, and one might even say that, in ecological terms, what reproduces is the environment (Bonner, 1974). The environment is implicated in epigenesis at many levels, including replication, gene expression, splicing, posttranslational modifications, and context-dependent protein interactions (Miklos and Maleszka, 2001). Much of ontogeny–particularly that of humans, with the high premium on plasticity and longevity–is designed to capture information from the environment to "instruct" development of the organism. Environmental context can convey far more information than genes can about what the organism needs for adequate functioning.

Present knowledge of epigenesis rests on the well-studied nervous and immune systems. Epigenesis operates through (1) the proliferation of variants (e.g., neurons and neural connections, or unique cell lines) and production of transient redundancy, (2) the retention of variants that "work" best, and (3) the pruning of those that do not. Which variants work best is determined via processing of functional throughputs provided by contextual inputs or demands (e.g., visual representation or pathogen recognition; Changeux, 1985; Edelman, 1987; McDade and Worthman, 1999). The strategem of developmental Darwinism constitutes a potent means for production of phenotypic complexity honed to the circumstances in which the organism must operate, and it does so by creating ontogenetic expectancies for functional load and contextual inputs.

Expectable Environments of Rearing

The elegant epigenetic devices for environmental programming depend on the information provided by contextual inputs and therefore can evolve only when those inputs are highly reliable. These form the expectable environments of rearing (EER), the set of environments normally encountered during ontogeny. The EER encapsulates the fitness outcomes and selective pressures to which organic design is adapted.

An overview of the human EER (see Table 10-1) integrates findings from developmental biology, developmental psychobiology, anthropology, and epidemiology to translate the epigenetic landscape into everyday human ecology. The listed features are nearly or entirely universal in human groups and have all been associated with variations in phenotypic outcomes, though of varying magnitudes.

The impact of a component of the EER on phenotype depends on several factors: (1) its predictiveness of future conditions, (2) the significance of those future conditions for fitness, (3) the timeliness of the signal for mobilization of an adaptive response, (4) the feasibility of transducing the signal into ontogenetic responses, (5) the relative fitness value versus the cost of adjusting the phenotype to one cue versus another, (6) pleiotropic effects of phenotypic adjustment on other features with adaptive value, and (7) the time horizon for realizing costs versus benefits.

This set of factors determines trade-offs around maintenance of plasticity versus reliance on context to inform ontogeny. Humans are thought to maintain an unusually high degree of plasticity in domains pertaining to information processing and behavior. Ecological circumstances, group composition, and social dynamics can range widely over the life course of an individual, so many early conditions will generalize poorly to later circumstances. Reproduction is separated from early development by over a decade or more and continues for several decades. Thus, although childhood environment strongly affects biological dimensions of life history (maturation and senescence rates), its effects on reproductive behavior (on partner relationships and infant and child care) are far more subtle than immediate ecological and cumulative sociocultural effects (Chisholm, 1993, 1996; Hill and Hurtado, 1995).

IMPLICATIONS FOR RESEARCH AND POLICY

The view of human reproduction as rooted in biocultural inheritance casts new light on current human affairs. It implies that when the fabric of

TABLE 10-1 Humans' Expectable Environments of Rearing

Social ecology

- ❑ Child care
  - Gestation: maternal stress, nutrition, activity
  - Prolonged carrying (devices may be used for holding, carrying)
  - Infant/child signaling-caregiver response (contingency, state regulation)
  - Cosleeping
  - Breastfeeding (and weaning)
  - Variable caregiver competence
  - Provisioning into adolescence with transition to productive in(ter)dependence
- ❑ Family
  - Parents
  - Coresident dependent siblings
  - Privileged emotion communication and intersubjective regulation
  - Resident in family into adolescence
- ❑ Social group
  - Multiage, mixed-sex with changeable composition (mobility, mortality)
  - Presence of kin and nonkin
- ❑ Pervasive language use, multiple registers (e.g., information exchange, narrative)
- ❑ Collaboration
- ❑ Sharing and exchange (socially and spatiotemporally displaced reciprocities)
- ❑ Contexts for play, practice, and exploration (risk taking)
  - Multiage, mixed-sex play groups
  - Tolerance of low productivity, incompetence
  - Surveillance, safe spaces
- ❑ Participant observation in adult activities and competent performances
  - Feedback on imitation, provision of instruction, guided participation
- ❑ Use of analogs and symbols (visual, acoustic)
- ❑ Tool use
- ❑ Fire and thermal buffering (possibly with clothing, coverings)
- ❑ Sanctions (physical, verbal, social)

Bioecology

- ❑ Food constituents and gut activity
- ❑ Energetics (resource reliability and quality, maintenance costs) and metabolic regulation
- ❑ Exposures to pathogens, parasites, and dirt and immune development
- ❑ Sensory inputs, activity patterns, and brain development
- ❑ Perceived safety or security and vigilance (attention and arousal regulation)

human social life and culture is repatterned or rent, fertility outcomes (in terms of effective fertility) are changed.

We can expect a large measure of robustness in biocultural transmission for critical features such as language and for those under previous selection for retention of plasticity. Other areas of human developmental ecology may be more vulnerable, particularly (1) emotion and arousal regulation, particularly in affiliation, anxiety, violence and aggression, and tolerance of novelty and threat; (2) modes of learning; (3) capacities for behavior change; (4) risk for psychopathology, particularly depression, suicide, and substance use; and (5) health and mortality risk associated with metabolic and eating dysregulation (diabetes, obesity), bioreproductive morbidities (polycystic ovarian disease, breast cancer), and hyperarousal and vigilance.

Demographic and epidemiologic data worldwide suggest that human development, and hence human reproduction, currently face enormous pressures (not all unfavorable). These are well documented in recent surveys of world mental health (Desjarlais et al., 1995), the global burden of disease (Murray and Lopez, 1996), inequity and health (Chen and Berlinguer 2001; Dasgupta, 1993; Deaton, 2001; Gwatkin, 2000; Wilkinson, 1996), and globalization in virtually all domains (World Bank, 2001; Dollar and Collier, 2001). These pressures require attention because some may strain even the large evolved human capacities for plasticity, accommodation, and successful adaptation (Nesse and Williams, 1994; Trevathan et al., 1999). Such pressures may need to be met with thoughtful planning and action.

The issues are biocultural. To get a sense of this, consider the well-documented worldwide shift in growth and maturation rates (Eveleth and Tanner, 1990; Worthman, 1999a) and concurrent dramatic transformations in the ecology of child rearing: changing family composition and maternal employment; widespread schooling of children; urbanization and increased densities; demographic effects of emerging diseases, specifically AIDS; and escalating rates of population dislocation. These formidable challenges raise the bar for effective theory that will support new hypotheses about human behavior, stimulate research, and inform policy. Pushing past dual thinking about the human condition and operationalizing biocultural inheritance models may provide the start to understanding the human implications of these challenges.

ACKNOWLEDGMENTS

Thanks are owed to Kristen Hawkes, Daniel Lende, and Ryan Brown for close reading, critique, and significant additions to this work, and to Randy Bulatao for heroic editorial input.

REFERENCES

Adair, L.S.
2001 Size at birth predicts age at menarche. *Pediatrics* 107:E59.

Anderson, L.A., P.G. McTernan, A.H. Barnett, and S. Kumar
2001 The effects of androgens and estrogens on preadipocyte proliferation in human adipose tissue: Influence of gender and site. *Journal of Clinical Endocrinology and Metabolism* 86:4951-5956.

Anisman, H., A.V. Ravindran, J. Griffiths, and Z. Merali
1999 Endocrine and cytokine correlates of major depression and dysthymia with typical or atypical features. *Molecular Psychiatry* 4:182-188.

Avitsur, R., and R. Yirmiya
1999 The immunobiology of sexual behavior: Gender differences in the suppression of sexual activity during illness. *Pharmacology, Biochemistry and Behavior* 64:787-796.

Baile, C.A., T.M. Della-Fera, and R.J. Martin
2000 Regulation of metabolism and body fat mass by leptin. *Annual Review of Nutrition* 20:105-127.

Baldwin, J.M.
1895 A new factor in evolution. *American Naturalist* 30:441-451, 536-553.

Barker, D.J.P.
1991 *Fetal and Infant Origins of Adult Disease*. London: British Medical Journal Publishing.
1997 Intra-uterine programming of the adult cardiovascular system. *Current Opinion in Nephrology and Hypertension* 6:106-110.

Baskin, D.G., T.M. Hahn, and M.W. Schwartz
1999 Leptin sensitive neurons in the hypothalamus. *Hormone and Metabolic Research* 31:345-350.

Beran, M.J., E.S. Savage-Rumbaugh, J.L. Pate, and D.M. Rumbaugh
1999 Delay of gratification in chimpanzees (Pan troglodytes). *Developmental Psychobiology* 34:119-127.

Blurton Jones, N., and M.J. Konner
1976 !Kung knowledge of animal behavior. In *Kalahari Hunter-Gatherers*. R.B. Lee and I. DeVore, eds. Cambridge, MA: Harvard University Press.

Blurton Jones, N.G., K. Hawkes, and J.F. O'Connell
1989 Studying costs of children in two foraging societies: Implications for schedules of reproduction. Pp. 365-390 in *Comparative Socioecology of Mammals and Man*. V. Standon and R. Foley, eds. London: Blackwell.

Blurton Jones, N., L.C. Smith, J. O'Connell, K. Hawkes, and C. Kamazura
1992 Demography of the Hadza, an increasing and high-density population of savanna foragers. *American Journal of Physical Anthropology* 89:159-181.

Bogin, B.
1997 Evolutionary hypotheses for human childhood. *Yearbook of Physical Anthropology* 40:63-89.
1999 Evolutionary perspectives on human growth. *Annual Review of Anthropology* 28:109-153.

Bongaarts, J., and R.G. Potter
1983 *Fertility, Biology, and Behavior: An Analysis of the Proximate Determinants*. New York: Academic Press.

Bonner, J.T.
1974 *On Development. The Biology of Form*. Cambridge, MA: Harvard University Press.

Borgerhoff Mulder, M.
1992 Reproductive decisions. Pp. 339-374 in *Evolutionary Ecology and Human Behavior*. E.A. Smith and B. Winterhalder, eds. New York: Aldine de Gruyter.
1995 Bridewealth and its correlates—quantifying changes over time. *Current Anthropology* 36:573-603.

Boysen, S.T., and G.G. Berntson
1995 Responses to quantity: Perceptual versus cognitive mechanisms in chimpanzees (Pan troglodytes). *Journal of Experimental Psychology: Animal Behavior Processes* 109:47-51.

Brommer, J.E.
2000 The evolution of fitness in life-history theory. *Biological Reviews of the Cambridge Philosophical Society* 75:377-404.
Bronfenbrenner, U.
1979 *The Ecology of Human Development: Experiments by Nature and Design*. Cambridge, MA: Harvard University Press.
Bruunsgaard, H., A.N. Pedersen, M. Schroll, P. Skinhøj, and B.K. Pedersen
2000 TNF-a, leptin, and lymphocyte function in human aging. *Life Sciences* 67:2721-2731.
Caprio, M., E. Fabbrini, A.M. Isidori, A. Aversa, and A. Fabbri
2001 Leptin in reproduction. *Trends in Endocrinology and Metabolism* 12:65-72.
Caro, J.F., M.K. Sinha, J.W. Kolaczynski, P.L. Zhang, and R.V. Considine
1996 Leptin: The tale of an obesity gene. *Diabetes* 45:1455-1462.
Changeux, J.-P.
1985 *Neuronal Man*. New York: Pantheon.
Charnov, E.L.
1993 *Life History Invariants: Some Explorations of Symmetry in Evolutionary Ecology*. Oxford: Oxford University Press.
Chen, L.C., and G. Berlinguer
2001 Health equity in a globalizing world. In *Challenging Inequities in Health: From Ethics to Action*. T. Evans, M. Whitehead, F. Diderichsen, A. Bhuiya, and M. Wirth, eds. Oxford: Oxford University Press.
Chisholm, J.S.
1993 Death, hope, and sex—Life history theory and the development of reproductive strategies. *Current Anthropology* 34:1-24.
1996 The evolutionary ecology of attachment organization. *Human Nature* 7:1-37.
Clark, P.M., P.C. Hindmarsh, A.W. Shiell, C.M. Law, J.W. Honour, and D.J. Barker
1996 Size at birth and adrenocortical function in childhood. *Clinical Endocrinology* 45(6):721-726.
Crawford, C., and D.L. Krebs, eds.
1998 *Handbook of Evolutionary Psychology: Ideas, Issues, and Applications*. Mahwah, NJ: Lawrence Erlbaum Associates.
Dantzer, R.
2001 Cytokine-induced sickness behavior: Where do we stand? *Brain, Behavior, and Immunity* 15:7-24.
Darwin, C.
1871 *Descent of Man, and Selection in Relation to Sex*. London: John Murray.
Dasgupta, P.
1993 *An Inquiry into Well-Being and Destitution*. Oxford: Clarendon Press.
Deacon, T.W.
1997 *The Symbolic Species: The Co-evolution of Language and the Brain*. New York: W. W. Norton.
Deaton, A.
2001 *Health, Inequality, and Economic Development*. Princeton, NJ: Princeton University.
Desjarlais, R., L. Eisenberg, B. Good, and A. Kleinman
1995 *World Mental Health: Problems and Priorities in Low-Income Countries*. New York: Oxford University Press.
Dollar, D., and P. Collier
2001 *Globalization, Growth, and Poverty: Building an Inclusive World Economy*. New York: Oxford University Press.

Edelman, G.M.
1987 *Neural Darwinism: The Theory of Neuronal Group Selection*. New York: Basic Books.

Ellison, P.T.
1994 Advances in human reproductive ecology. *Annual Review of Anthropology* 23:255-275.

Eveleth, P.B., and J.M. Tanner
1990 *Worldwide Variation in Human Growth*. New York: Cambridge University Press.

Fall, C.H., A.N. Pandit, C.M. Law, C.S. Yajnik, P.M. Clark, B. Breier, C. Osmond, A.W. Shiell, P.D. Gluckman, and D.J. Barker
1995 Size at birth and plasma insulin-like growth factor-1 concentrations. *Archives of Disease in Childhood* 73(4):287-293.

Finch, C.E., and M.R. Rose
1995 Hormones and the physiological architecture of life history evolution. *The Quarterly Review of Biology* 70(1):1-52.

Geary, D.C., and M.V. Flinn
2001 Evolution of human parental behavior and the human family. *Parenting Science and Practice* 1:5-61.

Godfrey, K.M.
1998 Maternal regulation of fetal development and health in adult life. *European Journal of Obstetrics, Gynecology, and Reproductive Biology* 78:141-150.

Gosling, L.M., and M. Petrie
1981 The economics of social organization. Pp. 315-345 in *Physiological Ecology: An Evolutionary Approach to Resource Use*. C.R. Townsend and P. Calow, eds. Sunderland, MA: Sinauer Associates.

Gottlieb, G.
1991 Experiential canalization of behavioral development: Theory. *Developmental Psychology* 27:4-13.
1998 Normally occurring environmental and behavioral influences on gene activity: From central dogma to probabilistic epigenesis. *Psychological Review* 105:792-902.

Gould, S.J.
1977 *Ontogeny and Phylogeny*. Cambridge, MA: Harvard University Press.

Gwatkin, D.R.
2000 Health inequalities and the health of the poor: What do we know? What can we do? *Bulletin of the World Health Organization* 78:3-18.

Hamilton, W.D.
1964 The evolution of social behavior. *Journal of Theoretical Biology* 12:12-45.

Harris, R.B.S.
2000 Leptin—much more than a satiety signal. *Annual Review of Nutrition* 20:45-75.

Hart, B.L.
1988 Biological basis of the behavior of sick animals. *Neuroscience and Biobehavioral Reviews* 12:123-137.

Havel, P.J.
2001 Peripheral signals conveying metabolic information to the brain: Short-term and long-term regulation of food intake and energy homeostasis. *Experimental Biology and Medicine* 226:963-977.

Hawkes, K., J.F. O'Connell, and N.G. Blurton Jones
1997 Hadza women's time allocation, offspring provisioning, and the evolution of long postmenopausal life spans. *Current Anthropology* 36:551-577.

Henrich, J.
2001 Cultural transmission and the diffusion of innovations: Adoption dynamics indicate that biased cultural transmission is the predominate force in behavioral change. *American Anthropologist* 103:992-1013.

Henrich, J., R. Boyd, S. Bowles, C. Camerer, E. Fehr, H. Gintis, and R. McElreath
2001 In search of Homo economicus: Behavioral experiments in 15 small-scale societies. *American Economic Review* 91:73-78.

Hill, K., and A.M. Hurtado
1995 *Ache Life History: The Ecology and Demography of a Foraging People.* New York: Aldine de Gruyter.

Holliday, R.
1995 *Understanding Aging.* New York: Cambridge University Press.

Hurtado, A.M.
1990 Seasonality in a foraging society—Variation in diet, work effort, fertility, and sexual division-of-labor among the Hiwi of Venezuela. *J Anthropol Res* 46:293-346.

Hurtado, A.M., K. Hill , H. Kaplan, and I. Hurtado
1992 Trade-offs between female food acquisition and child care among Hiwi and Ache foragers. *Human Nature* 3(3):185-216.

International Human Genome Sequencing Consortium
2001 Initial sequencing and analysis of the human genome. *Nature* 409:860-892.

Kaplan, H.
1994 Evolutionary and wealth flows theories of fertility: Empirical tests and new models. *Population Development Review* 20:753-791.
1995 Does observed fertility maximize fitness among New Mexican men? A test of an optimality model and a new theory of parental investment in the embodied capital of offspring. *Human Nature* 6:325-360.
1997 The evolution of the human life course. Pp. 175-211 in *Between Zeus and the Salmon.* K.W. Wachter and C.E. Finch, eds. Washington, DC: National Academy Press.

Kaplan, H., K.R. Hill, J. Lancaster, and A.M. Hurtado
2000 A theory of human life history evolution: Diet, intelligence, and longevity. *Evolutionary Anthropology* 9:156-185.

Kirkwood, T.B.L.
1981 Repair and its evolution: Survival versus reproduction. Pp. 165-189 in *Physiological Ecology: An Evolutionary Approach to Resource Use.* C.R. Townsend and P. Calow, eds. Sunderland, MA: Sinauer Associates.

Maes, M.
1999 Major depression and activation of the inflammatory response system. *Advances in Experimental Medicine and Biology* 461:25-46.

Maleszka, R., H.G. de Couet, and G.L.G. Miklos
1998 Data transferability from model organisms to human beings: Insights from the functional genomics of the flightless region of *Drosophila. Proceedings of the National Academy of Sciences of the United States of America* 95:3731-3736.

Mantzoros, C.S.
1999 The role of leptin in human obesity and disease: A review of current evidence. *Annals of Internal Medicine* 130:671-680.

Mantzoros, C.S., and S.J. Moschos
1998 Leptin: In search of role(s) in human physiology and pathophysiology. *Clinical Endocrinology* 49:551-567.

Mantzoros, C.S., M. Ozata, A.B. Negrao, M.A. Suchard, M. Ziotopoulou, S. Caglayan, R.M. Elashoff, R.J. Cogswell, P. Negro, V. Liberty, M.L. Wong, J. Veldhuis, I.C. Ozdemir, P.W. Gold, J.S. Flier, and J. Licinio

2001 Synchronicity of frequently sampled thyrotropin (TSH) and leptin concentrations in healthy adults and leptin-deficient subjects: Evidence for possible partial TSH regulation by leptin in humans. *Journal of Clinical Endocrinology and Metabolism* 86:3284-3291.

Massaro, D.W.

1998 *Perceiving Talking Faces: From Speech Perception to a Behavioral Principle.* Cambridge, MA: MIT Press.

Maynard Smith, J.

1978 *The Evolution of Sex.* Cambridge: Cambridge University Press.

McDade, T.W., and C.M. Worthman

1998 The weanling's dilemma revisited: A biocultural analysis of breastfeeding ecology. *Journal of Developmental Behavioral Pediatrics*, 19:286-299.

1999 Evolutionary process and the ecology of human immune function. *American Journal of Human Biology* 11:705-717.

McDade, T.W., M.A. Beck, C. Kuzawa, and L.S. Adair

2001 Prenatal undernutrition, postnatal environments, and antibody response to vaccination in adolescence. *American Journal of Clinical Nutrition* 74(4):543-548.

McEwen, B.S.

2000 Allostasis and allostatic load: Implications for neuropsychopharmacology. *Neuropsychopharmacology* 22:108-124.

Miklos, G.L.G., and R. Maleszka

2000 Deus ex genomix. *Nature Neuroscience* 3:424-425.

2001 Protein functions and biological contexts. *Proteomics* 1:169-178.

Murray, C.J.L., and A.D. Lopez

1996 *The Global Burden of Disease.* Cambridge, MA: Harvard University Press/World Health Organization.

Nesse, R.M., and G.C. Williams

1994 *Why We Get Sick: The New Science of Darwinian Medicine.* New York: Time Books.

Owen, B.M., D. Eccleston, I.N. Ferrier, and A.H. Young

2001 Raised levels of plasma interleukin-1 beta in major and postviral depression. *Acta Psychiatrica Scandinavia* 103:226-228.

Oyama, S.

1985 *The Ontogeny of Information: Developmental Systems and Evolution.* Cambridge: Cambridge University Press.

Promislow, D., and P.H. Harvey

1990 Living fast and dying young: A comparative analysis of life history variation among mammals. *Journal of the Zoological Society of London* 220:431-437.

Proos, L.A., Y. Hofvander, and T. Tuverno

1991 Menarcheal age and growth pattern of Indian girls adopted in Sweden. *Acta Paediatrica Scandinavica* 80:852-858.

Rasmussen, A.K.

2000 Cytokine actions on the thyroid gland. *Danish Medical Bulletin* 47:94-114.

Reeve, H.K., and P.W. Sherman

1993 Adaptation and the goals of evolutionary research. *Quarterly Review of Biology* 68:1-32.

Ricklefs, R.E.
1998 Evolutionary theories of aging: Confirmation of a fundamental prediction, with implications for the genetic basis and evolution of life span. *American Naturalist* 152:24-44.
Rivest, S., and C. Rivier
1995 The role of corticotropin-releasing factor and interleukin-1 in the regulation of neurons controlling reproductive functions. *Endocrine Reviews* 16:177-199.
Rogoff, B.
1990 *Apprenticeship in Thinking: Cognitive Development in Social Context.* New York: Oxford University Press.
Schwartz, M.W., R.L. Prigeon, S.E. Kahn, M. Nicolson, J. Moore, A. Morawiecki, E.J. Boyko, and D.Porte
1997 Evidence that plasma leptin and insulin levels are associated with body adiposity via different mechanisms. *Diabetes Care* 20:1476-1481.
Seeman, T.E., and B.S. McEwen
1996 Impact of social environment characteristics on neuroendocrine regulation. *Psychosomatic Medicine* 58:459-471.
Smith, E.A., and B. Winterhalder, eds.
1992 *Evolutionary Ecology and Human Behavior*. New York: Aldine de Gruyter.
Stearns, S.C., and J. Koella
1986 The evolution of phenotypic plasticity in life-history traits: Predictions for norms of reaction for age- and size-at-maturity. *Evolution* 40:893-913.
Straub, R.H., L.E. Miller, J. Scholmerich, and B. Zietz
2000 Cytokines and hormones: Possible links between endocrinosenescence and immunosenescence. *Journal of Neuroimmunology* 109:10-15.
Super, C.M., and S. Harkness
1993 The developmental niche: A conceptualization at the interface of child and culture. *International Journal of Behavioral Development* 9:545-569.
Susser, M., and B. Levin
1999 Ordeals for the fetal programming hypothesis: The hypothesis largely survives one ordeal but not another. *British Medical Journal* 318:885-886.
Tomasello, M.
1993 Cultural learning. *Behavioral and Brain Sciences* 16:495-511.
1999 The human adaptation for culture. *Annual Review of Anthropology* 28:509-529.
Trayhurn, P., and D.V. Rayner
1996 Hormones and the *ob* gene product (leptin) in the control of energy balance. *Biochemical Society Transactions* 24(2):565-570.
Trevathan, W.R., E.O. Smith, and J.J. McKenna
1999 *Evolutionary Medicine*. New York: Oxford University Press.
Trivers, R.L.
1972 Parental investment and sexual selection. Pp. 136-179 in *Sexual Selection and the Descent of Man 1871-1971*. B. Campbell, ed. Chicago: Aldine.
Venter, J.C., M.D. Adams, E.W. Myers, P.W. Li, R.J. Mural, G.G. Sutton, and H.O. Smith, et al.
2001 The sequence of the human genome. *Science* 291:1304-1351.
von Laue, S., and R.J. Ross
2000 Inflammatory cytokines and acquired growth hormone resistance. *Growth Hormone and IGF Research* 10 (Suppl. B):S9-S14.
Vygotsky, L.S.
1978 *Mind in Society*. Cambridge, MA: Harvard University Press.
1986 *Thought and Language*. Cambridge, MA: MIT Press.

Wauters, M., R.V. Considine, and L.F. Van Gaal
2000 Human leptin: From an adipocyte hormone to an endocrine mediator. *European Journal of Endocinology* 143:293-311.
Wilkinson, R.G.
1996 *Unhealthy Societies: The Afflictions of Inequality*. London: Routledge.
Williams, G.C.
1957 Pleiotropy, natural selection, and the evolution of senescence. *Evolution* 11:398-411.
1985 *Sex and Evolution*. Princeton, NJ: Princeton University Press.
Williams, S., and R. Poulton
1999 Twins and maternal smoking: Ordeals for the fetal origins hypothesis? A cohort study. *British Medical Journal* 318:897-900.
Wood, J.W.
1994 *Dynamics of Human Reproduction*. New York: Aldine de Gruter.
Worthman, C.M.
1999a Evolutionary perspectives on the onset of puberty. Pp. 135-163 in *Evolutionary Medicine*. W. Trevathan, J. McKenna, and E. Smith, eds. New York: Oxford University Press.
1999b The epidemiology of human development. Pp. 47-104 in *Hormones, Health and Behavior*. C. Panter-Brick and C.M. Worthman, eds. Cambridge: Cambridge University Press.
2002 Endocrine pathways to differential well-being across the life course. In *A Life Course Approach to Women's Health*, D. Kuh and R. Hardy, eds. Oxford: Oxford University Press.
Yirmiya, R., Y. Pollak, M. Morag, S.A. Reichenberg, O. Barak, R. Avitsur, H. Ovadia, J. Weidenfeld, A. Morag, M.E. Newman, and T. Pollmacher
2000 Illness, cytokines, and depression. *New York Academy of Sciences* 917:478-487.
World Bank
2001 *Facets of Globalization*. New York: Oxford University Press.
World Health Organization
1995 *Physical Status: The Use and Interpretation of Anthropometry*. Geneva: WHO.

11

Evolutionary Biology and Rational Choice in Models of Fertility

David Lam

There is perhaps no bigger challenge for any theoretical model of human fertility behavior than the model's ability to explain the large fertility declines that have accompanied the enormous increases in human living standards in high-income countries since the 19th century and in low-income countries in more recent decades. Today, the great majority of couples in the high-income countries of the world are spectacularly rich by any historical standards, but most of them choose to have no more than one or two children. Similarly, fertility has fallen dramatically in virtually every developing country that has had significant increases in living standards in the past 20 years, with high-income couples generally leading the way to low fertility. Analyzed in the cross section, it is almost universally observed that higher-income, better-educated couples have lower fertility than poorer and less educated couples across a wide variety of cultural and institutional settings.

These stylized facts have been the focus of extensive theorizing from a wide variety of disciplinary and theoretical perspectives. The negative relationship between income and fertility has posed a particular challenge to economic and evolutionary models of fertility. Both economic and evolutionary models—at least in their most naive form—might have been expected to predict a positive relationship between income and fertility. Considerable effort has been put into fitting the observed empirical patterns into economic and evolutionary theoretical perspectives, with some important successes. One of the most important features of these analyses in both economic and evolutionary approaches has been the recognition that decreased fertility is almost universally associated with increased investments in children. It is somewhat less surprising that humans would have chosen to have fewer children as their incomes increased when one recognizes that the decrease in numbers of children was offset by enormous increases in the amount of resources invested in each child. Quality-quantity trade-offs have been central to both economic and evolutionary models of fertility and arguably offer the most plausible way for reconciling both types of models with the observed empirical patterns.

This chapter discusses the intersection between rational choice models of fertility—especially models developed by economists—and evolutionary biology models of human fertility. The focus is primarily on the issue of quantity-quality trade-offs, an area in which there is considerable theoretical overlap in the two approaches. A central motivating question is whether evolutionary perspectives on the biodemography of fertility can help us understand the negative relationship between income and fertility and how these evolutionary approaches compare to economic models of fertility behavior. The chapter begins with the presentation of a generic economic model of fertility that includes both quality-quantity trade-offs and the time cost of children. Particular emphasis is placed on the effect that increased productivity of parental time may have on choices about the quantity and quality of children and on time allocation. Then empirical evidence is presented from Brazil and South Africa that supports the view that quality-quantity trade-offs are fundamentally important in understanding fertility decline. The relationship between economic models and models drawn from evolutionary biology is then discussed. The paper points out the potential contributions that an evolutionary approach can make to economic models and considers potential differences in predictions coming from evolutionary and economic models.

THE RELATIONSHIP BETWEEN INCOME AND FERTILITY

The relationship between fertility and income has always been a fundamental issue for economists interested in fertility and the family. Becker's seminal first paper on the economics of fertility (1960) heavily focused on the question of why we do not observe a stronger positive relationship between income and fertility. Becker found the observed lack of a positive relationship curious enough that he partially attempted to explain it as a statistical anomaly, suggesting that more complete data would in fact reveal a stronger positive association. But he also introduced the notion that quantity-quality trade-offs might be at the heart of the issue, noting that in the case of many goods that have an important quality dimension, higher incomes lead to much larger increases in quality than quantity. As will be discussed below, Becker would later appeal to evolutionary biology as part of the motivation for quality-quantity trade-offs in human fertility. In his later work on time allocation, Becker (1965) added another important piece of the story, noting that high-income couples are usually high-wage couples, making time-intensive commodities like children relatively more expensive than they are for low-wage couples. These two issues—quantity-quality trade-offs and the opportunity cost of time—continue to be the most important components of economic models of fertility, especially as they relate to explaining historical patterns in fertility and cross-section differentials as a function of income, wages, and schooling.

An Economic Model of Quality-Quantity Trade-Offs

It is useful to organize the discussion around a simple economic model of child quantity and quality of the type developed by Willis (1973), Becker and Lewis (1973), and Becker (1991). Assume that parents maximize a utility function $U(N, Q, Z)$, where N is the number of children, Q is the children's average quality (where quality refers to outcomes such as children's health and schooling), and Z represents all nonchild uses of time and goods. The nature and origins of the preferences embedded in this utility function are taken as outside the model and are one area in which evolutionary models are potentially informative. One of the useful features of these types of models is that they can also incorporate issues of time allocation and the opportunity cost of children by assuming that child quality is produced using inputs of time and goods according to some production function:

$$Q = F_q(T_{qw}, T_{qh}, X_q)$$

where T_{qw} and T_{qh} are the amount of the wife's time and the husband's time used to produce child quality (summed across all children), and X_q is the amount of purchased goods used to produce child quality. Nonchild consumption, Z, is produced by an analogous production function. A standard simplifying assumption that keeps the analysis tractable is that the production functions for both child quality and nonchild consumption are constant returns to scale, implying that doubling all inputs causes a doubling of child quality, and that producing N children who are each of quality q requires exactly N times as much of all inputs as producing one child of quality q. This assumes that there is a unit production function $q = f_q(t_{qw}, t_{qh}, x_q)$, where t_{qw} and t_{qh} are the amount of the wife's time and the husband's time used for each unit of child quality per child, and x_q is the amount of purchased goods used for each unit of quality.

The wife's total time, T_w, is allocated between market work, T_{mw}, children, and nonchild consumption, subject to the time constraint $T_w = T_{mw} + NQT_{qw} + ZT_{zw}$. An analogous time constraint describes the allocation of the husband's time, T_h. The simplest case is to assume that both the wife and the husband are at an interior solution at which some time is allocated to all activities, implying that each partner's market wage is an appropriate marginal valuation of his or her time. Labor market earnings of the husband and wife plus unearned income A are used to purchase the market inputs for children and nonchild consumption, $A + w_w T_{mw} + w_h T_{mh} = NQx_q p_x + Zx_z p_x$. One of the important implications of the constant returns to scale assumption is that it means the choices of optimal inputs of time and goods into home production are a function only of the production technology and the input prices and can be separated from household consumption and fertility decisions. This separability implies that we can define the shadow price $p_q = w_w t_{qw} + w_h t_{qh} + p_x x_q$, the cost of producing one unit of child quality for a single child, a cost that is independent of the amount of quality produced.

The shadow price of Q, the average quality of all children, is $\pi_q = Np_q$. This shadow price depends on N, child quantity, and thus cannot be separated from the household's consumption decisions. Similarly, the shadow price of N is $\pi_n = Qp_q$ and is directly dependent on the choice of child quality. The endogeneity of these shadow prices with respect to the chosen levels of quantity and quality is at the heart of the complex price and income responses implied by quality-quantity models, as discussed by Willis (1973), Becker and Lewis (1973), and Becker (1991).

Several important points come out of analyzing a model such as this. The intrinsic interaction between quantity and quality means that a simple change like increasing unearned income can have complicated effects on quantity and quality. In contrast with simple models of consumer expenditures, for example, doubling income cannot lead to a doubling of both quantity and quality, since that would require four times—not two times—as much income.[1] Becker argues that in the case of other goods that have both quantity and quality dimensions, there is strong empirical evidence that increases in income lead to much larger increases in quality than quantity. The same might plausibly be expected for children. Given the nonlinearities of the model, it is possible to generate a negative effect of income on child quantity even in the case where both child quantity and child quality are "normal" goods in the usual economic sense.

Lam and Duryea (1999) and Lam and Anderson (2002) adapt this type of model to consider the impact of parental schooling on quantity-quality

[1]Although this may seem to be making too much of the simple multiplicative model of quantity and quality, the basic point will be true for more general representations of the problem. As long as couples care about both the number of children and the amount invested in them, complex nonlinearities will be introduced into the usual consumer demand analysis.

trade-offs, looking at empirical evidence from Brazil and South Africa. The case of schooling is interesting in the context of evolutionary approaches, since it might be thought of as representing the general class of increases in parental productivity in producing healthy and productive children. In the case of the model outlined here, an increase in the schooling of either parent may lower the amount of time or goods required to produce a unit of quality, thus reducing the shadow price of a unit of quality, p_q. Market wages may increase at the same time, with the partial effect of raising p_q. Whatever the resulting change in p_q, the effects of this price change on Q and N are complicated by the nonlinearity of the budget constraint. A reduction in p_q will reduce the shadow price of both quality and quantity, which are intrinsically connected, and any adjustments in N or Q in response to the change can be thought of as causing further changes in these endogenous shadow prices. A large increase in Q, for example, implies a large increase in the shadow price of N.

As shown in Lam and Anderson (2002), it is theoretically possible that an increase in parents' ability to produce higher-quality children may lead to a decrease in either fertility or child quality but not both. An additional implication of this type of quality-quantity model is that responses can be greatly exaggerated beyond those of a standard linear budget constraint. This effect, as noted by Becker (1991), may help explain the rapid declines in fertility and corresponding rapid increases in children's human capital in response to relatively modest changes in the shadow price of children. It is entirely reasonable in the context of an economic model of quantity-quality trade-offs that we could observe substantial decreases in child quantity offset by large increases in child quality in response to increased productivity of parents in producing child quality.

Labor Market Productivity and the Price of Children

It is often remarked that children are much more expensive today than they were 100 years ago, an observation that in turn is often used to help explain why fertility is so low in today's high-income countries. The quantity-quality model outlined above provides some useful insights into the issue of the cost of children. One of the most important points is that the "price" of children is an endogenous outcome of the parents' trade-off between quantity and quality. While it is fair to say that people who choose high-quality children have "expensive" children, it is quite misleading in the context of the model presented above to say that it is the high price of children that explains the low quantity. They might have chosen a combination of low quality and high quantity, in which case it would be similarly misleading to say that they had many children because they were so cheap.

It should also be noted that even the high-quality children being chosen by the rich today probably consume a substantially smaller proportion of parents' lifetime income than did the children of 100 or 1,000 years ago.

The model also helps us think about other components of the price of children that are more exogenous, and some important points are worth noting. In addition to trading off child quality for child quantity, the second dimension in which couples are making trade-offs is in the allocation of time between the labor market and care for children. The mother's schooling may have important effects here, as emphasized in many economic theories of fertility decline. As noted above, increases in a mother's schooling can be expected to simultaneously increase her productivity in home production (including child care) and in the labor market. It is often assumed that increases in market wages associated with higher schooling represent an increase in the relative price of labor market time versus home production time. This clearly does not have to be the case, however, since it is possible that an increase in schooling raises home productivity by as much as it raises wages. This could occur because wages do not adjust to the actual increase in productivity or simply because the increase in home productivity is as large as the increase in labor market productivity.[2]

A woman will work in the labor market if and only if her labor earnings are worth more to the couple than the foregone productivity of her time at home. Increased schooling will increase the probability that a woman works in the labor market if that schooling causes a larger increase in her market wage than in her home productivity. While the experience of high-income countries suggests that labor market productivity increases faster than home productivity, it may well be the case that for women with low levels of schooling (and large numbers of children) the increase in home productivity from an additional year of schooling is large. It may also be the case that, while all levels of schooling raise labor market productivity, the effects of schooling on home productivity face diminishing returns. It may thus be the case that increased schooling causes home productivity to rise as fast as market productivity at low levels of schooling, but market productivity eventually rises faster at higher levels of schooling. In this case increases in schooling would not increase labor force participation at low levels of schooling but would increase participation at higher levels of schooling.

[2]Although it is simplest to think of the labor market as the alternative use of a mother's time, a very similar story could be told about a mother's decision of how much time to spend in agricultural cultivation or even food gathering, if these activities compete with time invested in children.

The important point of this case is that children do not necessarily become relatively more expensive as market wages increase. If the mother's home productivity (including her productivity in producing high quality-children) is rising as fast as the market wage, the decline in the time inputs to produce child quality can offset the higher wage. For women who are not in the labor market initially, the increased home productivity will lower the effective price of child quality. This can plausibly lead to an increase in child quality, a decrease in child quantity, and no change in the amount of time spent in the labor market.

In this economic model, then, the effect of schooling on fertility, child quality, and women's labor supply can be viewed theoretically as being driven by trade-offs along two margins. On the one hand is the race between home productivity and labor market productivity, driving the extent to which better-educated women are pulled into the labor force by higher wages. On the other hand is the adjustment in child quality and child quantity that results from the effects of schooling on home productivity. It is important to note that the economic model offers no strong unambiguous predictions regarding the effect of income or schooling on either child quantity or quality.

If the total fertility rate in Italy today were 6.0, we could easily explain it in this model as resulting from a positive income elasticity of demand for children, whether child quality were higher or lower than is observed under the current low-fertility regime. While the model does not make sharp a priori predictions, it does suggest that decisions about child quality, child quantity, and time allocation are best analyzed jointly, with a great deal potentially learned from looking at the combined set of outcomes. One prediction the model does make is that we should never see both the numbers of children and the quality of children fall in response to increases in income or schooling. The joint responses in fertility, investments in children, and women's employment can potentially be informative about the mechanisms that drive fertility decline.

EMPIRICAL EVIDENCE FROM BRAZIL AND SOUTH AFRICA

The observed cross-sectional relationship between schooling and fertility is potentially informative about the kinds of changes that may take place during the demographic transition and therefore provides a useful reference point for thinking about the relationship between economic and evolutionary models of fertility. Figures 11-1 to 11-4 present empirical patterns from Brazil and South Africa. These are particularly interesting cases to consider because their extremely high levels of inequality generate a distribution of education that has significant percentages of adults spread across the schooling distribution from zero years to university. Both countries also have

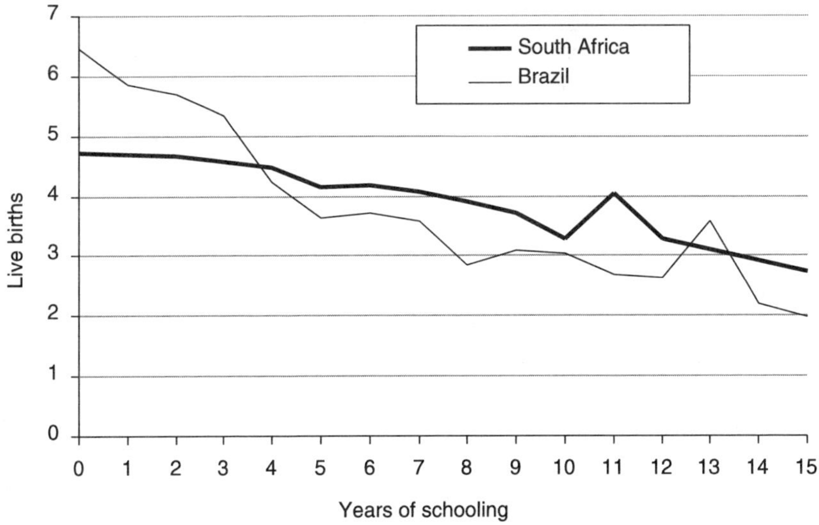

FIGURE 11-1 Number of live births by years of schooling for married women, ages 45 to 54, in Brazil 1984, and for black South Africans, 1995-1998.
SOURCE: 1984 Brazil PNAD and 1995-1998 South Africa October Household Survey.

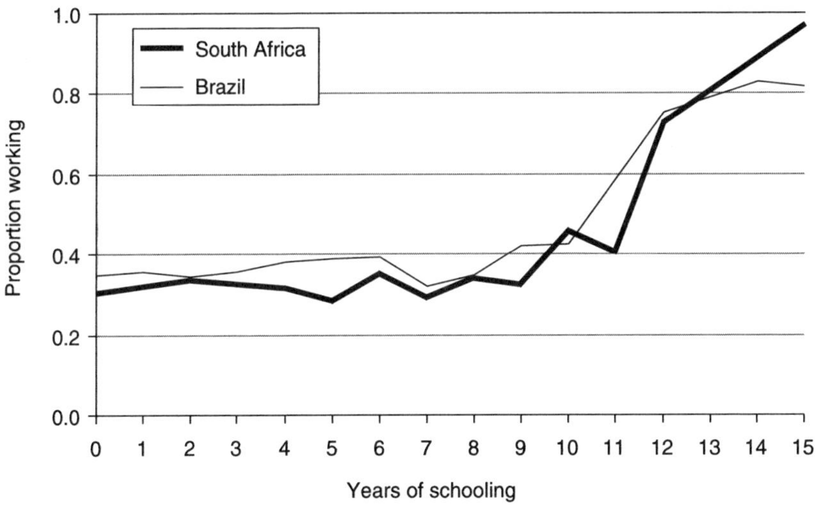

FIGURE 11-2 Employment rates by years of schooling for married women, ages 35 to 44, in Brazil, 1984, and for black South Africans, 1995-1998.
SOURCE: 1984 Brazil PNAD and 1995-1998 South Africa October Household Survey.

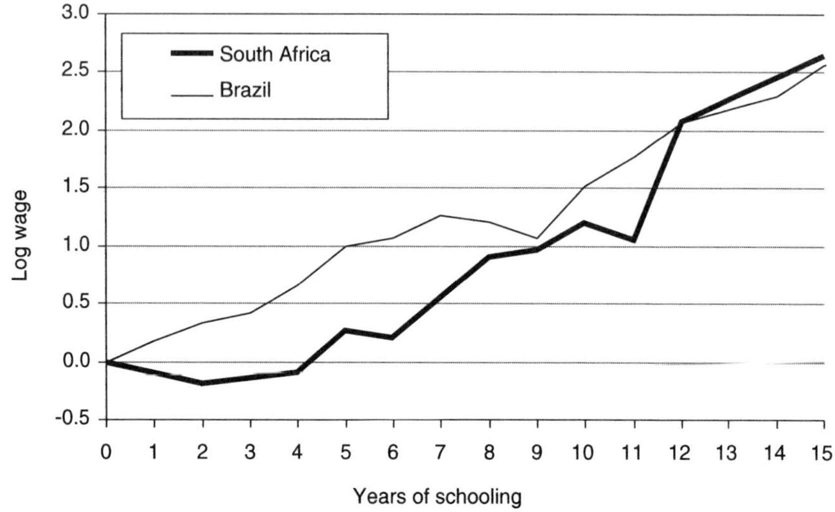

FIGURE 11-3 Natural logarithm of monthly wages by years of schooling (relative to women with zero schooling) for married women, ages 35 to 44, with positive wages, in Brazil, 1984, and for black South Africans, 1995-1998.
SOURCE: 1984 Brazil PNAD and 1995-1998 South Africa October Household Survey.

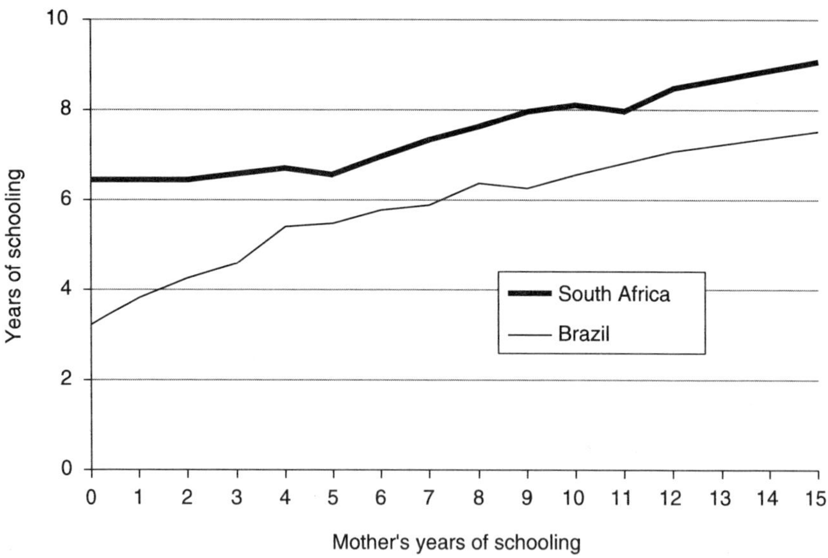

FIGURE 11-4 Mean years of schooling of 15-year-olds by mother's education, in Brazil, 1984, and for black South Africans, 1995-1998.
SOURCE: 1984 Brazil PNAD and 1995-1998 South Africa October Household Survey.

large nationally representative household surveys that make it possible to look at detailed relationships between schooling and fertility.[3]

Figure 11-1 shows the number of children ever born by years of completed schooling for women ages 45 to 54 in Brazil in 1984 and for black women in South Africa using pooled data from the October household surveys for 1995, 1997, and 1998. The results for Brazil are similar to those of Lam and Duryea (1999). The results for South Africa are similar to those of Lam and Anderson (2002). The figure demonstrates the large differences in fertility across years of women's schooling in both countries. For Brazilian women in 1984 there was a decline of over three births between women with zero years of schooling and women with 8 years of schooling. The schooling gradient in contemporary black South Africa is more modest, but there is still a decline of about 0.75 births over the first 8 years of schooling. The difference between black women who have completed grade 12 and black women with no schooling is about 1.5 births. Regression analysis using additional control variables indicates that these simple bivariate relationships between schooling and fertility are somewhat attenuated but remain substantial when controls for region, husband's schooling, and husband's income are included (Lam and Duryea, 1999; Lam and Anderson, 2002).

Although fertility falls relatively steeply with schooling in both Brazil and South Africa, there is surprisingly little effect of the first 8 years of schooling on the probability that women are employed in the labor market. Figure 11-2 plots the proportion of all women ages 35 to 44 that reported being employed in the previous 7 days by years of schooling. Very similar patterns are observed at both younger and older ages in both countries. The patterns for Brazil and South Africa are surprisingly similar, with the proportion of women employed being between 30 and 40 percent until about 8 years of education. Employment rates increase dramatically at higher levels of schooling in both countries, reaching levels typical of high-income countries. Employment rates among university-educated women are two to three times as high as employment rates among women with primary schooling or less.

Comparing Figures 11-1 and 11-2, there is surprisingly little relationship between fertility and employment as schooling increases. This pattern is even more surprising when the effect of schooling on wages is taken into account. Figure 11-3 plots the mean log wage for employed women reporting nonzero wages relative to women with no schooling. In both countries there is a strong positive relationship between schooling and wages. In Brazil this positive relationship is observed beginning at grade 1, with

[3]The Brazil results are based on the 1984 Pesquisa Nacional por Amostra de Domicilios (PNAD), a nationally representative survey of over 100,000 households. The South African results are based on the pooled October household surveys from 1995, 1997, and 1998, a pooled dataset of about 80,000 households.

increases on the order of 15 to 20 percent per year of schooling over the first seven grades. In South Africa the implied rate of return to schooling is in the range of 15 to 25 percent per completed grade after grade 4.

Comparing Figures 11-2 and 11-3, it is striking that employment rates for women remain low and relatively constant over ranges of schooling in which wages are rising substantially. In both Brazil and South Africa, among 35- to 44-year-old women who work, those with 8 years of schooling report wages about 1.0 log points higher than those with zero years of schooling, implying about three times higher wages. The percentage of women working at these two schooling levels is almost identical, however, only slightly above 30 percent. Women with 8 years of schooling have considerably fewer births in both countries, but this lower fertility does not translate into higher involvement in the labor force.

In both Brazil and South Africa we observe a situation in which schooling appears to have a negative effect on fertility over ranges in which there is very little relationship between employment and fertility. This suggests that the effect of education on fertility is not working primarily through price-of-time effects. Wages increase substantially over this range, without any corresponding increase in women's employment, additional evidence that there is some aspect of women's time allocation other than labor market activity to explain the link between education and fertility. As suggested in the theoretical discussion above, investments in child quality may be the margin in which education and time allocation interact with fertility.

Figure 11-4 plots the schooling attainment of 15-year-old children as a function of their mother's schooling. The gradient of children's schooling by mother's schooling is substantial in both countries, with stronger effects in Brazil. In Brazil in 1984, 15-year-old children whose mothers had 12 years of schooling were about four grades ahead of children whose mothers had no schooling. The gap in South Africa between these extremes is about two grades. One of the important features of Figure 11-4 is that the gradient is quite steep over the range of schooling in which fertility falls without any corresponding change in women's employment, the range up to 8 or 9 years of schooling.

These empirical patterns suggest that an increase in the opportunity cost of children due to rising wages is unlikely to be the major reason that increases in women's schooling are associated with declines in fertility in Brazil and South Africa. Despite increases in market wages, women do not substantially increase their market labor supply as their schooling increases. The evidence suggests that quality-quantity trade-offs are a more plausible explanation for the link between maternal schooling and fertility.

These results suggest there is a strong link between fertility and investments in children. Increases in schooling at low levels lead to increases in the productivity of both mothers and fathers in producing better-educated children. Parents respond to this increased productivity in a way consistent with the theoretical model outlined above—they choose higher levels of child quality and reduce the number of children. As argued by Becker (1991), one of the interesting implications of a model of quality-quantity interactions is that an increase in income or a reduction in the unit price of quality can lead to large responses, with large increases in quality and large decreases in quantity. Increases in women's schooling also lead to increased labor market productivity, as evidenced by the large rise in wages. In making labor supply decisions, however, women are faced with simultaneous increases in home productivity and labor market productivity. Over a large range of schooling it appears that increases in home productivity are large enough to offset even large increases in wages. Until about 8 years of schooling we do not see women responding to rising wages with significant increases in labor supply. The driving mechanism through which schooling reduces fertility, then, does not appear to be rising opportunity cost of time due to rising wages. Rather, couples respond to their increased productivity in producing child quality by reducing the number of children and investing more resources in each child.

QUALITY-QUANTITY TRADE-OFFS AND FERTILITY DECLINE

While the cross-sectional relationships between education and the quality and quantity of children shown in Figures 11-1 to 11-4 do not necessarily have implications for the time series changes observed across populations, there would seem to be at least a rough correspondence between the cross-sectional and time series patterns over the broad sweep of historical fertility declines. Declining fertility has almost universally gone hand in hand with increased investments in children, as indicated by improvements in child health, survival, and education. While the specific causal mechanisms are difficult to identify, it is virtually impossible to separate declining numbers of children from the increased investments in those children in any population in which fertility has declined. Indeed, it is the almost universal increase in the "cost" of children that has caused many observers to see this higher cost as a mechanism inducing parents to have fewer children. In the context of the economic model of quality-quantity trade-offs, however, this higher cost is itself a matter of choice, with the simultaneous decisions about quantity and quality impossible to separate from each other.

Evolutionary Approaches to Quality-Quantity Trade-Offs

The trade-off between the quality and quantity of offspring plays an important role in evolutionary biology, including applications of evolutionary biology to human fertility. As argued by Kaplan and Lancaster elsewhere in this volume, evolutionary forces may well have produced a tendency to trade off child quality and quantity in hunting and gathering populations, with parents responding to the perceived payoff to investments in quality given environmental conditions. For example, humans may have adapted to postpone subsequent births in favor of increased investment in existing children when perceived payoffs to such investments were high. Such trade-offs may well have been fitness maximizing in a hunting and gathering setting.

From an evolutionary perspective, the link between the quantity and quality of offspring may offer one of the most plausible mechanisms for explaining the reductions in fertility that have accompanied the large increase in standards of living in both high-income and low-income countries. In developing his economic model of fertility, Becker (1991) suggests that the quantity-quality trade-off can help provide a link between Darwinian theory and the decline in family size associated with rising family incomes in the past hundred years. In *A Treatise on the Family*, Becker (1991:137) argues, "a reduction in the number of children born to a couple can increase the representation in the next generation if this enables the couple to invest sufficiently more in the education, training, and 'attractiveness' of each child to increase markedly their probability of survival to reproductive ages and the reproduction of each survivor." The quantity-quality calculus may be affected by the environment in which parents make such decisions, including factors that affect their ability to produce child quality and the returns to those investments. Writing from an evolutionary perspective, Low (2000:144-145) writes that "complexities in either the ecological or social environment that result in increased effectiveness of parental investment should result in more investment, even at the expense of fertility itself."

Low's discussion suggests that high eventual reproductive payoffs to trading off child quantity for child quality in the current generation might hold the promise of reconciling evolutionary models of fertility with the awkward empirical evidence of declining fertility in the face of rapidly rising incomes over time. Parents might find it optimal to reduce child quantity in favor of quality in their own offspring, with the payoff coming in the form of increased numbers of grandchildren born to their well-endowed children. As noted by Kaplan and Lancaster (this volume), however, the weight of empirical evidence suggests that the payoff to increased investments in child quality in terms of increased numbers of grandchildren or other descendants is very unlikely to make up for the direct effect of reduced numbers of children in the next generation, at least in contemporary high-income settings. The study by Kaplan et al. (1995) of Albuquerque men indicates that the men who had the greatest number of grandchildren were those who had the greatest number of children.

The argument that investments in child quality may increase the number of offspring in the long run raises theoretical complications as well. A model in which numbers of children are reduced as a strategy to maximize numbers of grandchildren (or great grandchildren) has the unappealing feature that it requires children to make the opposite calculation from their parents, producing large quantities of children at the expense of child quality. This implies a kind of dynastic time inconsistency that seems unlikely to generate a stable equilibrium path within a lineage and is unlikely to be consistent with adaptive evolutionary processes. If it were rational for high-income couples in the current generation to reduce quantity in favor of quality, given the observed trade-offs in the environment, why wouldn't their highly endowed children come to the same conclusion? The payoff must come in some generation eventually having very high fertility, with an ever-increasing baby boom required to generate a sufficient return on the initial investment as more generations choose low fertility.

It seems unlikely, then, that reductions in fertility in favor of child quality are ever likely to be fitness maximizing in a modern setting, at least not to a degree that can fit the large fertility reductions of the past 100 years into a simple evolutionary framework. In this sense it might be concluded that the issue of quantity-quality trade-offs cannot rescue an evolutionary model from a fundamental inconsistency with the observed declines in fertility that have accompanied large increases in income. It might further be argued that the rational choice economic model is therefore better able to explain modern low fertility than is the evolutionary model, since the observed fertility behavior is consistent with standard economic models. The apparent superiority of the economic model should not be overstated, however. Low fertility is consistent with an economic model simply because almost any level of fertility is consistent with the economic model, as long as both quantity and quality are not simultaneously reduced in response to increases in income.

Evolutionary Origins of Indifference Curves

Although economic and evolutionary models might be viewed as offering competing approaches to understanding the trade-off between quality and quantity of children, they may in fact be highly complementary. As noted above, Becker (1991) appealed to evolutionary interpretations in discussing his own economic model of quality-quantity trade-offs. Economists have generally been much more attracted to evolutionary models of demographic behavior than most noneconomist demographers. As Bergstrom (1996:1903) writes in his survey of evolutionary and biological approaches to the family, "Because of the intimate connection between reproduction and the family, it should not be surprising that the theory of evolutionary biology has fundamental implications for the economics of the family." One of the important contributions of evolutionary models is that they potentially help explain the origins of the utility functions that economists traditionally take as given. This could be especially valuable in developing models of fertility and the family, since evolutionary approaches may provide guidance in thinking about issues such as intrafamily altruism, preferences about having children, and the trade-off between child quantity and child quality.

In the case of quantity-quality trade-offs, the focus of this paper, it is worth considering whether evolutionary biology can help inform the economic model laid out above. While one does not necessarily need an evolutionary approach to explain why there might be a utility trade-off between the quantity and quality of children—any more than one needs an evolutionary approach to explain a utility trade-off between the quantity and quality of televisions—it is nonetheless useful to realize that a quality-quantity trade-off in offspring is a highly plausible evolutionary adaptation. Even if observed quality-quantity trade-offs in the modern environment do not appear to be fitness maximizing, this does not imply that these behaviors do not have an evolutionary origin. We may be observing an evolutionary adaptation operating in a very different environment than the environment in which it evolved.

As argued by Kaplan and Lancaster, it may well have been fitness maximizing in a hunting and gathering setting to shift from quantity of offspring to quality of offspring when the rate of return to investments in quality was high. In economic terms the "indifference curves" describing the trade-off between quantity and quality may have been developed in this early human environment. The returns to investments in child quality today, as measured for example by returns to giving a child a college education, may be many times higher than the returns ever experienced in early human populations. The response to these high returns, given the indifference curves developed in a very different setting, is to reduce fertility to very low levels and make very large investments in each child. This behavior is not in fact fitness maximizing, but it may reflect trade-offs that have an evolutionary origin. A strong quantity-quality fertility trade-off that responds to high returns to investments in children may be one of the most fundamental elements in the biodemography of fertility, helping us understand both the time series and the cross-section relationships between income and fertility.

While this argument has considerable appeal, a criticism of this sort of explanation is that it allows the evolutionary model to potentially fit almost any kind of observed relationship between income and fertility. We may have a story of where the utility function came from, but we have no sharp predictions about what that utility function might imply in any particular setting. This is a criticism of both the economic and the evolutionary models, since both models can potentially be reconciled with any relationship between income and fertility. The trade-off between quality and quantity appears to be a compelling piece of the puzzle, but we are left with models from both economic and evolutionary approaches that in principle are consistent with either a positive or a negative relationship between income and fertility.

CONCLUSIONS

This paper has explored how economic rational choice models and evolutionary biology models can be used to explain the widely observed negative relationship between income and fertility within populations and over time. The focus has been on quality-quantity trade-offs, an issue that has been fundamental in both economic and evolutionary models. Standard economic models of fertility are theoretically consistent with a negative relationship between income and fertility, especially if there is a positive relationship between income and investments in children. This prediction can also be applied to the effects of increased productivity of parents, resulting for example from increased schooling.

Empirical evidence from Brazil and South Africa suggests that the strong negative effect of mother's schooling on fertility is the result of a strong quality-quantity trade-off over the first 8 years of schooling. Although women's labor market productivity, as measured by the market wage, rises rapidly over the first 8 years of schooling in both countries, only about 30 percent of women are employed over the entire range. Child quality, as measured by the schooling of 15-year-olds, rises rapidly with mother's schooling, however. If these cross-sectional patterns apply to historical changes over time, they suggest that increasing parental productivity leads to a large increase in child quality and an offsetting decrease in fertility. This quantity-quality trade-off appears to be far more important in explaining fertility decline than an increase in the price of children resulting from higher women's wages.

Evolutionary biology models have also emphasized quality-quantity trade-offs, which offer at least the potential to reconcile evolutionary predictions with an observed negative relationship between income and fertility over time. Some authors suggest that such trade-offs may in fact maximize reproductive fitness because of the eventual increase in the numbers of grandchildren or great-grandchildren resulting from increased endowments in current children. Empirical evidence suggests that payoffs in offspring from later generations are unlikely to be large enough to offset the reduction in current children in contemporary settings, however. A simple quantity-quality model is therefore unlikely to explain current low fertility as being adaptive in an evolutionary sense. This does not mean that quality-quantity trade-offs may not have been highly adaptive in hunting and gathering settings, however, and may therefore have had an important effect in shaping the preferences that guide the behavior of modern humans. We observe almost universal patterns of declining fertility and increased investments in children in response to rising incomes and rising productivity in a wide variety of cultural, environmental, and institutional settings. It does not seem unreasonable to believe that rational economic choices about quality-quantity trade-offs in our modern setting are being driven at least in part by preferences that were influenced by the process of evolution in a much different early human environment.

REFERENCES

Becker, G.S.

1960 An economic analysis of fertility. Pp. 209-231 in *Demographic and Economic Change in Developed Countries.* Princeton, NJ: National Bureau of Economic Research.

1965 A theory of the allocation of time. *Economic Journal* 75:493-517.

1991 *A Treatise on the Family.* Cambridge, MA: Harvard University Press.

Becker, G.S., and H.G. Lewis

1973 On the interaction between the quantity and quality of children. *Journal of Political Economy* 81:S279-S288.

Bergstrom, T.C.

1996 Economics in a family way. *Journal of Economic Literature* 34:1903-1934.

Kaplan, H., J. Lancaster, J. Bock, and J. Johnson

1995 Does observed fertility maximize fitness among New Mexico men? A test of an optimality model and a new theory of parental investment in the embodied capital of offspring. *Human Nature* 6:325-360.

Lam, D., and S. Duryea

1999 Effects of schooling on fertility, labor supply, and investments in children, with evidence from Brazil. *Journal of Human Resources* 34:160-192.

Lam, D., and K. Anderson

2002 Women's schooling, fertility, and investments in children in South Africa. Paper presented at the annual meeting of the Population Association of America, Atlanta, GA.

Low, B.

2000 *Why Sex Matters: A Darwinian Look at Human Behavior.* Princeton, NJ: Princeton University Press.

Willis, R.J.

1973 A new approach to the economic theory of fertility behavior. *Journal of Political Economy* (March-April):S14-S64.

12

Reflections on Demographic, Evolutionary, and Genetic Approaches to the Study of Human Reproductive Behavior

John N. Hobcraft

Demographers have long specialized in documenting, measuring, and trying to explain levels, trends, and differentials in human fertility. Traditional demographic approaches are nevertheless lacking in several respects. First, much of the explanatory literature neglects potential biological pathways, except in the very narrow reproductive biology area. The papers in this volume amply demonstrate the need to consider the roles of genetic, cognitive, and neuroendocrine pathways in shaping reproductive behavior. Second, far too little attention is paid to the fact that births initiate the process of parenthood, rather than being an end in themselves, and that reproductive choice and evolution have been shaped by the need to ensure survival and nurture of children. Exceptions to this omission have included some of the economics literature, which fairly unsuccessfully evaluates the benefits of children as a source of family production in traditional societies and as old age insurance (see Das Gupta, 1993, for a good overview). In a contemporary low-fertility context, Hobcraft and Kiernan (1995) proposed a framework for examining the decision processes and constraint involved in becoming a parent in Europe (see also Hobcraft, 1993, for an emphasis on child welfare above and beyond child survival). This issue of parenthood rather than fertility per se is also well illustrated by Worthman's chapter in this volume.

The long-standing recognition of the critical importance of both reproductive biology and behavior and their interplays in determining human fertility has been especially clear in the various treatments of the proximate determinants of fertility (Bongaarts and Potter, 1983; Davis and Blake, 1956; Wood, 1994). In theoretical essence these studies examine variations through the life course and among populations in fecundability (the monthly capacity to reproduce) and in sexual activity, combined with behavior to limit conception and the study of the biology and behavior of the determination of whether conceptions result in a live birth. Practical measurement often falls far short of the ideal.

This approach of working outward from the proximate determinants through to broader determinants of fertility (and related behavior and biology) has been prevalent and perhaps explains the rarity of attempts to include genetic or evolutionary components explicitly. This view can be illustrated by posing the question of whether it is more useful to know that 40 percent of the variance in fertility in some population at some time is attributable to contraceptive behavior in a proximate determinants framework or whether the same fraction can be attributed to genetic variation in an ACE (Additive, Common, and Environment) model (a model that attempts to partition the variance in behavior into three components: an additive genetic component, a common or shared-environment component, and a nonshared environment element). There may be doubts about the pathways that determine contraceptive behavior, but we can be sure that the links with fertility are fairly direct; on the other hand, the genetic association reveals very little about pathways at all.

Yet the more interesting questions for the future involve exploring the pathways forward from an observed genetic association or backward from an observed pattern of contraceptive behavior. Of course, the interconnecting pathways are much closer to being established for the biological components of fertility through endocrinological and neural links to genetic markers than for the behavioral components. In view of the huge range of potential pathways it makes considerable sense for exploratory work to ensure the identification of and discrimination among elements in the paths that are proximal forwards from genetic variability (or markers), emphasizing brain and endocrine links to fertility, and among those that are proximal backward from fertility and the proximate determinants. These two threads should ultimately interplay and meet. Nevertheless, some conceptual and measurement progress is occurring concerning pathways from genetic or evolutionary origins through to human bonding (Miller and Rodgers, 2001) or childbearing motivation (Miller et al., 2000).

A fairly separate strand of theorizing about fertility and related behavior goes under a variety of labels, including the almost defunct sociobiology, evolutionary psychology, evolutionary anthropology, human behavioral ecology, and gene-environment coevolution; these fields often disagree substantially, but they all grapple with evolutionary aspects of human fertility and related behavior. A central challenge facing these approaches, as far as a contemporary demographer is concerned, is the extent to which they are relevant to our understanding of the demographic transition and changes in fertility behavior, especially to very low levels of fertility. For some proponents of an evolutionary perspective it seems that Darwinism (sometimes very broadly interpreted) has become a new form of quasi-religious belief (the frequent use of the term "ultimate cause" is indicative—e.g., Clark and Low, 2001), so that any regularity in human behavior is deemed by definition of evolutionary origin and any variation simply reflects different adaptive strategies. Well-written and lively accounts of plausible mechanisms, which either cannot be tested or regard testing as irrelevant, often involve writing history backward rather than providing useful insights into modern behavior. However, some serious attempts to make hypotheses more precise and testable do occur, although many pitfalls and areas of dispute often remain. A recent illustration of the difficulties is provided by the exchange regarding the Trivers-Willard hypothesis (see Freese and Powell, 1999, 2001; Kanazawa, 2001).

To express such caution and skepticism does not mean that I dismiss these approaches out of hand or that I take the blinkered social science approach that reproduction is "all in the jeans." The problem is rather to get a clearer and better-defined set of mechanisms and then to explore the extent to which they are relevant to modern reproductive behavior. For example, in a framework for understanding "becoming a parent in Europe," Hobcraft and Kiernan (1995) posed the question of whether evolution predisposed us to have sex or to reproduce, since either mechanism would suffice to ensure regular conception in a traditional society. However, they have different consequences for understanding current fertility behavior, since the separation of sex and reproduction is achievable. How could we distinguish between these two plausible "determinants" of past reproductive behavior? If we are predisposed to reproduce in some direct pronatalist sense, achieving very low fertility would require stronger behavioral desires and controls to offset this innate tendency than if the pathway was through recreational sex (Diamond, 1997; Foster, 2000; Hobcraft and Kiernan, 1995; Morgan and King, 2001).

An interesting issue to explore is the extent to which evolutionary and genetic approaches to understanding human fertility, which diverge considerably in their approaches at the moment, will come back together as we refine our understanding of the pathways involved in the complexities of human reproduction.

We will almost surely find that the genetic associations with modern fertility behavior are mediated through other forms of behavior. For example, there is some evidence that risk taking is partly genetically mediated and risk taking is also associated with many aspects of reproductive behavior, such as early sex and pregnancy, lower and less effective use of contraception, early partnership and partnership breakdown; risk taking could also be associated with the biology of reproduction, for example, with a higher incidence of sexually transmitted infections and consequent fecundity impairment. Part of the genetic variability in fertility might thus arise from variation in risk taking that affected many outcomes, all of which are related to reproduction.

BEHAVIORAL GENETICS MODELS OF REPRODUCTION

One of the key features of behavioral genetics approaches to the analysis of human behavior is the increasing attention to the design of their studies (Plomin, 1994; Rutter et al., 2001). Moreover, there is increasing attention to interplays of nature and nurture, or gene-environment correlations and interactions. Teasing out these elements requires strong identifying and theoretical assumptions for the models used and is likely to demand longitudinal information too. By comparison with Reiss et al. (2000), for example, most behavioral genetics studies of fertility-related behavior seem fairly primitive, though it is of course early days.

Most of the studies on fertility-related behavior to date have relied on standard ACE or DCE models (Additive and Dominant; the latter include a dominant instead of an additive genetic component). Since many fertility-related studies rely on samples of twins (and occasionally siblings or other close relatives), we begin here. Essentially siblings and especially twins are *defined* as having a common environment, and monozygotic (MZ) twins are 100 percent genetically related, whereas dizygotic (DZ) twins and siblings share half their genes. The nature of the models and their fitting means that any gene-environment correlations are swept into the additive genetic component and that all unexplained residual variance is swept into the nonshared environment term (see, for example, Rutter's chapter in this volume; Rutter and Silberg, 2002; Turkheimer and Waldron, 2000; Rutter et al., 2001; and for an accessible account of the basic models and ideas, Plomin et al., 1997 and Plomin, 1994). For a lively discussion of the use of such models in a demographic context, see the comments on Morgan and King (2001) by Capron and Vetta (2001) and Kohler (2001).

Since the majority of studies that have attempted partitions of variance in fertility using behavioral genetics models have been based on the information from the Danish Twin Registry (for an overview see Rodgers et al., 2001b), we shall begin by looking at these in some detail. These studies have all examined a variety of birth cohorts, including those of 1900-1923 (Kohler and Christensen, 2000), 1870-1910 and 1953-1964 (Kohler et al., 1999), 1953-59 (Rodgers et al., 2001a), 1953-1970 (this volume), and 1945-1968 (Kohler et al., 2001). No compelling rationale has been provided for these very different selections of birth cohorts, although data availability and selection issues undoubtedly play a part. The fertility-related outcomes considered have also varied, partly as result of censoring of experience for the later cohorts, but have included children ever born (completed or partial cohort fertility), childlessness or its converse of having had a least one birth, ever marriage, measures of early childbearing, and a retrospectively reported age at first attempt to get pregnant (collected in 1994).

The twin registry was first established in 1954, when those born in 1870 were already 84 years old, and information was sometimes only obtained from proxy reports from the cotwin or even other relatives (see Kohler et al., 1999). Strong selection for survival is reflected in the small sample sizes for the earliest cohorts (around 600 twin pairs of each sex for the birth cohorts of 1870 to 1889, compared with about 1,400 for those of 1890-1910). Moreover, the reported fertility for these earliest birth cohorts seems very low and apparently quite out of line with the general population, suggesting either severe misreporting or strong selection of survivors for low fertility. No indication is provided concerning conditions about survival to any age for inclusion in the analysis—it is not clear that including twins or co-twins who died early in their reproductive careers is wise (it might be defensible for studying reproductivity but not fertility behavior). No comment is made concerning the lower correlation of children ever born for MZ twin pairs than for DZ twin pairs among men born between 1870 and 1889. Moreover, smoothed estimates for the ACE and DCE models are obtained using a sophisticated weighting procedure with a "bandwidth" that concentrates 76 percent of the weights in the 7 years centered on the birth cohort in question; no indication is provided of how the end cohorts were weighted, and all results for the 1953-1964 cohorts may well be susceptible to such "end" effects. I also have unanswered concerns about the possible interactions of taking weighted averages in circumstances where both the numbers of cases included in the analysis and the levels of fertility are changing rapidly over time.

For the earlier birth cohorts the most striking finding, discussed at length by Kohler et al. (1999), is an apparent sharp increase in the genetic component of variation in completed fertility for women born during the 1880s, with a rapid return to lower levels for those born after that decade. Given that estimates were weighted over several years, it is possible that this decadal effect is an artefact of a single spike or singularity getting spread across most of the decade. In contrast, there is, if anything, a reduction in the genetic component for men born in this decade to zero or even negative estimates. One striking feature of the results that can only be examined impressionistically from Kohler et al. is the apparent almost exactly opposite movements in the genetic and shared-environment components over time. This seeming constancy of broad-range heritability (or of the nonshared-environmental component) over time is intriguing and could possibly suggest that the just-identified nature of ACE or DCE models when all pairs share a common environment (no twins reared apart) may lead to instability of the partition of the two components of the variance.

A similar observation might be made with respect to the other paper that examines time trends in these components (Kohler et al., 2001), where there is a seeming shift from 50 percent of the variation in early fertility being accounted for by shared environment, with no genetic component, for the 1945-1952 birth cohorts to exactly the reverse for the 1962-1968 birth cohorts. Again, this raises questions as to whether such shifts are real or, at least in part, artefacts of near collinearity in the components. The very large standard errors for the variance components estimates (significance is often indicated at the 10 percent level) are possibly suggestive in this respect. There are a series of other difficult assumptions that have to be made: for example, the assumption that MZ and DZ twins do not alter their environments differentially (an example of the potentially large implications of such a difference is provided in a different context by Feldman et al., 2000). Since I am no expert on models of this type, these are raised as concerns rather than explicit criticisms.

The results and their interpretation are nevertheless both intriguing and challenging enough to warrant further replication with other data sources. Kohler and his collaborators are quite comfortable with a very low genetic component of variation for the earliest cohorts considered, seeing this as being compatible with Fisher's fundamental theorem of natural selection for a society with pretransitional fertility levels, since very little genetic variation would be expected for fitness components. Hughes and Burleson (2000) give the plausible candidates for such life history traits: juvenile survival, development rates, age-specific fecundity, mating success, and longevity. Implicit in the interpretation of Kohler and colleagues is that fertility of the cohorts born during the 1870s in Denmark was almost entirely determined by fitness components. The significant early shared-environment component is thus interpreted as reflecting differentials in childbearing success (which would also probably be reinforced by survival differentials to achieve reproductive success) associated with variations in fitness that are usually interpreted as being likely to be status related in most evolutionary discussions.

The very rapid and short-term emergence of a substantial genetic component of variation in fertility of women (but not men) born during the 1880s is seen as being associated with the (first) demographic transition. Such a shift, of course, does nothing to challenge Fisher's theorem. In most fertility transitions the fertility decline is achieved through fertility limitation within marriage, although it is often also accompanied by delayed marriage. More importantly (and in many ways problematic for evolutionary interpretations—see, e.g., Foster, 2002), the differentials in fertility that emerge during the early fertility transition are usually negatively associated with status, and this situation usually continues through the first demographic transition and often during the second one too. Since new and status-related behavior is coming into play, there is a real possibility that some of the new behavioral constraints on fertility will be related to genetic origins, although of course inevitably constituting gene-environment interplays. But there is also no obvious reason why shared environment should disappear as a source of variation at the same time. And why should these features be different for men than for women?

To begin to answer such questions, we need some clarity about what pathways are likely to be involved in originating new genetic sources of variation that are associated with innovative behavior such as trying to prevent conception. Is the rise in genetic variability simply due to new behavior being adopted by the advantaged (including the better educated)? Presumably, both in light of Fisher's theorem and the lack of a genetic component for preceding cohorts, we would be justified in concluding that the genetic traits now being expressed had little to do with the fertility-related fitness components but reflected new sources of variation in changing circumstances. In this respect the conclusion that "fertility motivation rather than fecundity is subject to genetic variation" (Kohler et al., 1999:281) is hardly surprising, although the particular example of the analysis of age at first try to have a child (with potentially serious recall problems) does not show unequivocally stronger genetic variation than either censored completed fertility or ever having had a birth for the 1953-1964 birth cohorts. Moreover, there are clearly interplays between behavior and motivation on the one hand and fecundity on the other: delaying childbearing until ages of reduced fecundity can have unintended consequences.

The finding that genetic influences seem to be stronger for the transition from zero to one child than for "completed" fertility is puzzling, especially for the earlier cohorts, and the fact that such correlations could not arise across the generations (i.e., from parent to child, since parents cannot be infertile) is never addressed. Why is the increase in the genetic component of variation in fertility for women so short lived during the demographic transition (lasting less than a decade, even when spread out by the smoothing procedures)? The (over)interpretation of Kohler et al. (1999:281) is:

> Since fertility is generally a household decision reflecting the preferences of husband and wife, correlated fertility motivations among twins reveal themselves in the number of children a couple has, provided that the household decision includes the preference of the twin. The strong genetic influence on the number of children at the onset of the fertility decline and in contemporary cohorts therefore emphasizes the instrumental role of females in adopting conscious fertility control and in household bargain-

> ing about fertility: only if females have a strong influence on household decisions about fertility do genetic influences on fertility motivations reveal themselves in fertility outcomes. While it is probably undisputed that females in contemporary cohorts exercise a strong influence on household decisions the strong influence of females in cohorts born around 1885 (i.e. in cohorts facilitating the early fertility decline) may be more surprising.

Implicit in such an argument would be the notion that women were genetically more effective at bargaining over remaining childless than over family size. There is no justification for why women born in the 1880s stood out in terms of genetically mediated bargaining power over fertility control, compared with those born in immediately subsequent decades. Nor is it readily apparent why women's liberation on fertility decision making should not have shared-environment components and sources.

An important feature of this extended citation is that it acknowledges that childbearing (and marriage) involves both partners. This carries several implications for future research on fertility, marriage, and divorce. First, twin studies will never permit us to address and disentangle genetic components of variation for the dyad involved. The only way to get leverage on this aspect will be through molecular genetics (or linking back through neuroendocrine protein pathways to genetic markers), and that will require much sharper elaboration of likely pathways and identification of markers for these pathways. Second, shared environment predominantly relates to shared family of origin effects and is a concept largely introduced as a means for separating out narrow-sense heritability (that nevertheless incorporates all gene-environment interplays). In particular, it always seems odd to pay exclusive attention to shared family-of-origin environment components for adult behavior, although nevertheless a source of important and interesting pathways to adult development. A full analysis in the context of fertility would surely involve separating out shared-environment components from the family of origin of both partners and for the couple themselves, in addition to examining assortative mating by genes and by childhood shared and nonshared environments, and the roles of genotype-genotype interplays. The study of such complex differentiation would both necessitate molecular genetic indicators and new tools of analysis, although again endocrine and neural pathways may also hold some promise.

We have examined the studies of sources of variation in fertility over time in considerable detail because these are potentially extremely interesting and could lead to insights that go beyond the "black box" partitioning of variance that is usually the only result from such studies. The studies using the Danish twins are the most sophisticated yet in this context. The innovative attempt to use linkages for kinship in the National Longitudinal

Survey of Youth (Doughty and Rodgers, 2000; Rodgers et al., 1999; Rodgers and Doughty; 2000) seem beset by considerable uncertainty in the linkage process and the inability to determine the zygosity of twin pairs fully.

Some other twin-based studies of fertility-related behavior raise more puzzles than they answer. For example, McGue and Lykken (1992) used a postal sample of twins from the Minnesota Twin Registry, with an unreported response rate. For their samples of both men and women, MZ twins show a lower overall correlation in risk of divorce than do DZ twins; this inconvenient and challenging feature of their data was not discussed, nor did it preclude strong claims of results for genetic sources of variation in divorce, generally based on looking at conditional probabilities of one twin divorcing given that the other had, where MZ twins did have higher conditional probability. A more careful genetically informed study on divorce is based on the Colorado Adoption Study, which enables the authors to tease out some interesting results (O'Connor et al., 2000).

PATHWAYS TO FERTILITY BEHAVIOR

The availability of simple and cheap assays for biological markers, such as neuropeptides and endocrine proteins has led to a wide range of studies that look at links to fertility behavior. Many of these studies have looked at pathways that are involved in the biology of fertility, including puberty, menarche, ovulation, pregnancy, and lactational infecundability. Such work is very valuable in aiding our understanding of variations in some of the key proximate determinants of fertility. These findings with respect to hormonal mediation of family formation outcomes are ably reviewed in Cameron's chapter in this volume. It is striking that a large body of evidence can be reviewed concerning sexual behavior and the biology of fertility, but there seems to be a paucity of evidence on endocrine or neuroendocrine pathways related to the other behavioral aspects of fertility, such as reproductive intentions or motivations, with the exception of nurturance or parental behavior. See Panksepp (1998) for a review of neuroscience findings, especially on sexual feelings and behavior and on nurturance and maternal behavior.

There are, however, many other interesting and unanswered questions on the underpinnings of the biology of fertility that are relevant to fertility outcomes and possible sources of genetic variation. Why are there significant levels of involuntary infertility? What are the sources of the variation in the ending of the reproductive life span? Why do quite high fractions of couples experience early natural onset of secondary sterility and what are the sources of variability among couples? Are they genetic, gene-environment interactions, or environmentally induced? In a similar vein, why does heterogeneity in fecundity need to be incorporated into biometric models of fertility? Is this simply to account for differences in behavior, especially coital frequency? Or are there genuine variations among fecund couples in their biological chance of conception? All of these are questions about fitness-related aspects of fertility.

At least for the reproductive biology of fertility we do know quite a lot about which biological markers are involved and often how they operate. But fertility-related behavior, including pair bonding, coital frequency, contraceptive use, and abortion among others and fertility motivations are much less well understood. This is why serious attempts to outline the pathways involved or the ontogenies are badly required (see Miller and Rogers, 2001, on human bonding; and Foster, 2000, or Miller et al., 2000, on childbearing motivation). It is probably here that the greatest opportunities for geneticists, brain scientists, and endocrinologists to come together with demographers and those engaged in evolutionary anthropology or psychology and in behavioral ecology. It is clear that the latter group has much to learn from the harder sciences, which are already having a profound effect on their understanding of the determinants of fertility and fertility-related behavior. It is also likely that the greater knowledge of empirical patterns, differences, and regularities in such behavior among human populations will provide interesting insights and challenges for those engaged in the biology.

Improving the extent of understanding and intellectual interchange among the disciplines involved in the study of (human) reproduction does seem an important way forward. Clarity of understanding of pathways through genes, brain, endocrine system, and environment and more especially the mutual interplays and feedbacks involved and the elucidation of conditional responses is vital. Assumptions of determinism or of ultimate causality for one domain should always be challenged, whether genetic, evolutionary, or social scientific/environmental determinism.

Thus, for example, it is not enough to assume that evolution must be the source of all behavior because it is by definition the ultimate cause (see, e.g., Clarke and Low, 2001). Clarke and Low (2001:636) provide the interesting example that evolutionary scholars would never ask "why Americans want children, since genetic and lineage success are basic currencies." Yet Foster (2000) clearly addresses such an issue from an evolutionary perspective. If we cannot address questions about decisions concerning childlessness or the lowest low fertility in an evolutionary perspective, does this make such concerns irrelevant for modern reproduction? Foster (2002) argues persuasively that an evolutionary explanation for the (first) demographic transition is not needed.

PATHWAYS TO WHAT?

As already indicated above, there is a considerable body of evidence to suggest that genetic, neural, and endocrinological pathways are involved in both sexual maturation and sexual behavior and that these pathways interplay with and can be reinforced by behavior. Several authors have drawn attention to the sufficiency of an evolved sex drive among humans, one of the relatively few species to enjoy recreational sex (Diamond, 1997), to have ensured fertility in traditional societies (Foster, 2000; Hobcraft and Kiernan, 1995; Morgan and King, 2001; Potts, 1997). Foster (2000) also argued persuasively that this sufficiency would make it highly unlikely that a separate set of evolved responses to ensure fertility per se would have been necessary. The modern separation of sexuality and fertility through contraception and abortion has perhaps thus demonstrated the "blind watchmaker" aspect of evolution in this context: a purposive evolution might have ensured a mechanism tied to a need to bear children.

In this context, Hobcraft and Kiernan (1995) also posed questions as to why, if there was a strong innate disposition to be fertile, so many societies and religions found it necessary to develop strong pronatalist norms. In many cultures it is parents and other elders who maintain social controls over early access to sexual partners and who arrange marriages. Such control is linked to status, lineage, and inheritance patterns but is external to the individual involved and thus neither phenotypic nor genotypic. Equally, there is much evidence from human societies that considerable pressure for an early first birth within marriage is exerted by parents or parents-in-law or others in the older generations.

Were humans, perhaps especially women, who disproportionately bore the physical and emotional costs of childbearing and child rearing, always wont to limit reproduction once their brains evolved enough to enable free choice? And is modern family limitation simply a reflection of the increased ability (and societal tolerance) to control fertility?

There is also evidence related to human bonding and especially nurturance that is seen as relevant to fertility motivation (see Foster, 2000; Miller and Rodgers, 2001; and Morgan and King, 2001). Once again, the evidence extends, however incompletely, to genetic, neural, and endocrinological pathways and to their interplay with each other and reinforcement from environmental experiences. Demographers who have picked up on this literature differ in their interpretations as to how far the environmental mediation is lifelong and how far it is directly mediated through pregnancy, birth, and nurturance of one's own child; there is also dispute about the extent to which early gender differentiation goes beyond a learned response. An "Occam's razor" approach to evolution might see a direct response through pregnancy-mediated changes in the mother as sufficient in this respect. But there is a case to be made that such nurturance is part of a wider set of attributes required for successful long-term pair bonding to help keep mother and father together during the dependent development period for their offspring (see Panksepp, 1998; Miller and Rodgers, 2001; and Young, this volume).

An unresolved puzzle concerning nurturance arises in the context of very low fertility, as discussed by Foster (2000). She makes a persuasive case that it is the phenotypic need to nurture that means most women wish to have at least one birth and this means that fertility is unlikely to go much lower than the extremes already seen in parts of Europe. Yet if nurturance is strongly reinforced by brain changes during pregnancy and by feedback to neural receptors after a child is born, how is it that this mechanism does not then serve to make it even more likely that a woman will want further births? Presumably there have to be series of negative feedbacks to offset the nurturance drive?

On the whole, evolutionary anthropologists and evolutionary behavioral ecologists (see Symons, 1979; Wood, 1994; Campbell and Wood, 1994; Low, 2000; Ellison, 2001; and both Kaplan and Lancaster and Worthman, this volume) have been much more enthusiastic about incorporating (and sometimes co-opting) the ideas and work of demographers and related social scientists on fertility behavior into their perspectives than demographers have been to grasp evolutionary perspectives or new biological research[1] (with a few notable exceptions, e.g., Udry, 1996). This fusion is challenging, necessary, and not yet fully successful, and demographers, with their rich understanding of empirical research on contemporary and historical populations, need to play their part in any new synthesis.

HOW CAN WE EXPLAIN MODERN VERY LOW FERTILITY?

One of the truisms of many evolutionary accounts of behavior, including fertility and mating, is a clear gender differentiation of roles: in hunter-gatherer societies men were the hunters and women the gatherers, enabling the latter to nurture the children. Mate selection and infidelity are also seen as driven by quite different concerns, with men often seen as having to be "trapped" into long-term bonding and nurturance, and the more facile projections to modern society retain a breadwinner/homemaker distinction (e.g., for a variety of perspectives, Baker, 1996; Batten, 1994; Birkhead, 2000; Buss, 1994, 1999; Etcoff, 1999; Miller, 2000;

[1]Of course, this does not apply to the integration of biology and behavior in the analysis of the proximate determinants of fertility, where demographers have led the way (e.g., Davis and Blake, 1956; Bongaarts and Potter, 1983; Gray et al., 1993).

Potts and Short, 1999; Ridley, 1993). A similar role differentiation by gender is a basic postulate of much modern microeconomics theory of the family (Becker, 1981). Yet, hardly surprisingly, many modern feminists regard such postulates as provocative.

What is clear, however, is that there has been a major change in roles and independence of women and that this has had implications for partnership stability, childbearing and more especially child rearing, and the broader domestic division of labor. Adaptation of men and institutions to these changes is quite variable, and these changes and tensions have been seen by several commentators to be implicated in the so-called baby bust since the late 1960s (for a broad European perspective, see Hobcraft and Kiernan, 1995; on England and Wales, see Hobcraft, 1996; see also Folbre, 1994, 2001, and McDonald, 2000).

But there is a much broader range of factors to be looked at in the context of very low fertility. One fundamental shift of emphasis has to be to examine the factors related to becoming a parent with its long-term ramifications, rather than births (see Worthman, this volume). The framework proposed and applied for European fertility by Hobcraft and Kiernan (1995) and further to England and Wales by Hobcraft (1996) picked out several key elements involved in the decision-making process about becoming a parent, most of which have seen profound changes in the past 40 years. The separation of sex and fertility, which was made highly reliable for the first time by modern contraception and greater access to safe, legal abortion, played a key part as a proximate determinant. Our framework allowed for pronatalist phenotypic and societal pressures, although not explicitly identifying nurture needs. The main discussion was about the series of individual, partnership, and societal constraints on becoming a parent: including the biology of reproduction; time and money constraints involved in nurture and development and their competition with other activities, including work, leisure, and domestic tasks; changing ideas, tastes, and preferences on gender, reproduction, and individual rights; and security prospects over the rearing of a child.

We saw the following requirements and an assessment of their future stability as being explicitly relevant to decisions about whether to have a child at a particular point in time: having a partner, completing education or training, employment, housing, and security. In addition, we paid particular attention to gender differences in the employment domain and the domestic division of labor. The broad interpretation of historical trends and regional variations was embedded in this framework. Hobcraft (2002) provided a more detailed elaboration of measurement and conceptual issues that has influenced the proposed content of the Gender and Generation Programme under the aegis of United Nations Economic Commission for Europe (UNECE).

In many ways such an interpretive framework and analysis could be seen as having close parallels to a behavioral ecology approach represented and extended by Kaplan and Lancaster (this volume) and to the life history approach provided by Worthman (this volume), though much less constrained by the need to place all short-term behavioral changes in an evolutionary perspective. But the wide range of human behaviors and developmental, life course, and contextual factors included in this framework point up the challenges in unpicking biological (in the broad sense, including endocrinological, neural, and genetic pathways and feedbacks) roles in determining fertility behavior. In most low-fertility societies, attempts to become pregnant are largely under individual or couple control and assisted reproduction is often possible. This conscious (and possibly rational) choice manifestly involves brain-environment interactions. But will we find very few genetic or neuroendocrine protein markers each linked to the wide range of factors considered by the actors involved in such choices, or perhaps more likely discover a plethora of differing links for different elements of behavior and choice? Or is such a route the wrong path to search, since all of these behavioral elements are just constraints that the human mind imposes, which are set against an overarching innate and socially reinforced urge to reproduce or nurture? These conceptual issues clearly matter in determining where to look, and we need to pay much closer attention to designing studies that might enable us to clarify these issues.

Although human behavior is deeply affected by our genes and their interplay with environment, there is no reason to suppose that all behavior has to be adaptive or that the only genetically mediated pathways to modern fertility behavior have their origins with genes that evolved in relation to fertility behavior itself. The example of genetically mediated risk-taking behavior was given in the introduction, and several possible pathways linked to fertility were indicated. Of course, as stressed earlier, it is helpful to know the relevant pathways, both biological (in the broad sense) and behavioral, and the interactions and feedbacks within and between these domains.

CONCLUSION

Over the next few years we see a highly productive domain of research that links both fertility and fertility-related behavior backward through identifiable pathways and genetically mediated neural and endocrinological pathways forward to fertility-related behavior. As argued above, there is a huge and challenging research agenda, not the least of which will be analysis of (changing) partner-partner interplays and interactions. Moreover, we see the future of such research as being necessarily linked to molecular genetics, brain science, and endocrine systems, rather than being possible to tease out from twin or adoption studies. Nevertheless, we have discussed the insights that are being gleaned from twin and adoption studies and expect that they will provide further stimulus and insights. The novel analysis of time trends in the partitioning of components of genetic and shared-environment variance components is replicable with long-term demographic registers given modern computer linkage algorithms. But the longer-term horizon demands molecular linkages, especially if the partners are both to be considered.

Demographers concerned with such issues (and we all should be) will have to think carefully about the design of studies in order to tease out the complexities involved and most of the advances will involve learning from or engaging with molecular geneticists, brain scientists, and endocrinologists. Demographers also need to understand and work more closely with the broader interpretative disciplines rooted in evolutionary perspectives. The research agenda is an exciting one in which rapid scientific progress needs a strong social scientific perspective and vice versa. Exemplified by the National Research Council and Institute of Medicine (2000) and National Research Council (2001) and by the present volume, this recognition of the need to collaborate across disciplinary boundaries is gradually occurring in a range of fields.

REFERENCES

Baker, R.
1996 *Sperm Wars: Infidelity, Sexual Conflict and Other Bedroom Battles.* London: Fourth Estate.

Batten, M.
1994 *Sexual Strategies: How Females Choose Their Mates.* New York: G.P. Putnam.

Becker, G.S.
1981 *A Treatise on the Family.* Cambridge, MA: Harvard University Press.

Birkhead, T.
2000 *Promiscuity: An Evolutionary History of Sperm Competition and Sexual Conflict.* London: Faber and Faber.

Bongaarts, J., and R.G. Potter
1983 *Fertility, Biology, and Behavior: An Analysis of the Proximate Determinants.* New York: Academic Press.

Buss, D.M.
1994 *The Evolution of Desire: Strategies of Human Mating.* New York: Basic Books.
1999 *Evolutionary Psychology: The New Science of the Mind.* Needham Heights, MA: Allyn & Bacon.

Campbell, K.L., and J.W. Wood, eds.
1994 Human reproductive ecology: Interactions of environment, fertility, and behavior. *Annals of the New York Academy of Sciences* 709.

Capron, C., and A. Vetta
2001 Comments on "Why have children in the 21st century?" *European Journal of Population* 17:23-30.

Clarke, A.L., and B. Low
2001 Testing evolutionary hypotheses with demographic data. *Population and Development Review* 27(4):633-660.

Das Gupta, P.
1993 *An Inquiry into Well-Being and Destitution.* Oxford: Clarendon.

Davis, K., and J. Blake
1956 Social structure and fertility: An analytic framework. *Economic Development and Cultural Change* 4:211-235.

Diamond, J.
1997 *Why Is Sex Fun? The Evolution of Human Sexuality.* London: Weidenfeld and Nicolson.

Doughty, D., and J.L. Rodgers
2000 Behavior genetic modelling of menarche in U.S. females. In *Genetic Influences on Human Fertility and Sexuality: Theoretical and Empirical Contributions from the Biological and Behavioral Sciences.* J.L. Rodgers, D.C. Rowe, and W.B. Miller, eds. Dordrecht: Kluwer.

Ellison, P.T.
2001 *On Fertile Ground: A Natural History of Human Reproduction.* Cambridge, MA: Harvard University Press.

Etcoff, N.
1999 *Survival of the Prettiest: The Science of Beauty.* New York: Doubleday.

Feldman, M.W., S.P. Otto, and F.B. Christiansen
2000 Genes, culture, and inequality. In *Meritocracy and Economic Inequality.* K. Arrow, S. Bowles, and S. Durlauf, eds. Princeton, NJ: Princeton University Press.

Folbre, N.
1994 *Who Pays for the Kids? Gender and the Structures of Constraint.* London: Routledge.
2001 *The Invisible Heart: Economics and Family Values.* New York: The New Press.

Foster, C.
2000 The limits to low fertility: A biosocial approach. *Population and Development Review* 26(2):209-234.
2002 Why we don't need an evolutionary explanation for the demographic transition. *European Journal of Population.*

Freese, J., and B. Powell
1999 Sociobiology, status, and parental investment in sons and daughters: Testing the Trivers-Willard hypothesis. *American Journal of Sociology* 104:1704-1743.
2001 Comment: Making love out of nothing at all? Null findings and the Trivers-Willard hypothesis. *American Journal of Sociology* 106:1776-1789.

Gray, R., with H. Leridon and A. Spira, eds.
1993 *Biomedical and Demographic Determinants of Reproduction.* Oxford: Clarendon Press for IUSSP.

Hobcraft, J.N.
1993 Women's education, child welfare and child survival: A review of the evidence. *Health Transition Review* 3(2):159-175.
1996 Fertility in England and Wales: A fifty-year perspective. *Population Studies* 50:485-524.
2002 Moving beyond elaborate description: Towards understanding choices about parenthood. In *The Dynamics of Fertility and Partnership in Europe: Insights and Lessons from Comparative Research.* M. Macura and G. Beets, eds. New York: United Nations.

Hobcraft, J.N., and K.E. Kiernan

1995 Becoming a parent in Europe. In *Evolution or Revolution in European Population Vol I, Plenary Sessions, European Population Conference, Milan*, European Association for Population Studies/ International Union for the Scientific Study of Population. Milan: FrancoAngeli.

Hughes, K.A., and M.H. Burleson

2000 Evolutionary causes of genetic variation in fertility and other fitness components. In *Genetic Influences on Human Fertility and Sexuality: Theoretical and Empirical Contributions from the Biological and Behavioral Sciences.* J.L. Rodgers, D.C. Rowe, and W.B. Miller, eds. Dordrecht: Kluwer.

Kanazawa, S.

2001 Comment: Why we love our children. *American Journal of Sociology* 106:1761-1776.

Kohler, H.-P.

2001 Comments on Morgan and King (2001): Three reasons why demographers should pay attention to evolutionary theories and behavior genetics in the analysis of contemporary fertility. *European Journal of Population* 17:31-35.

Kohler, H.-P., and K. Christensen

2000 Genetic influences on fertility behavior: Findings from a Danish twin study, 1900-23. In *Genetic Influences on Human Fertility and Sexuality: Theoretical and Empirical Contributions from the Biological and Behavioral Sciences.* J.L. Rodgers, D.C. Rowe, and W.B. Miller, eds. Dordrecht: Kluwer.

Kohler, H.-P., J.L. Rodgers, and K. Christensen

1999 Is fertility behavior in our genes? Findings from a Danish twin study. *Population and Development Review* 25(2):253-288.

2001 From nurture to nature: The shifting determinants of early female fertility in Danish twin cohorts 1945-68. Unpublished manuscript prepared for European Research Conferences (EURESCO) Conference on the Second Demographic Transition, Bad Herrenalb.

Low, B.S.

2000 *Why Sex Matters: A Darwinian Look at Human Behavior.* Princeton, NJ: Princeton University Press.

McDonald, P.

2000 Gender equity in theories of demographic transition. *Population and Development Review* 26(3):427-439

McGue, M., and D.T. Lykken

1992 Genetic influences on risk of divorce. *Psychological Science* 3(6):368-373.

Miller, G.

2000 *The Mating Mind: How Sexual Choice Shaped the Evolution of Human Nature.* New York: Doubleday, Random House.

Miller, W.B., D.J. Pasta, J. MacMurray, D. Muhleman, and D.E. Comings

2000 Genetic influences on childbearing motivation: Further testing of a theoretical framework. In *Genetic Influences on Human Fertility and Sexuality: Theoretical and Empirical Contributions from the Biological and Behavioral Sciences.* J.L. Rodgers, D.C. Rowe, and W.B. Miller, eds. Dordrecht: Kluwer.

Miller, W.B., and J.L. Rodgers

2001 *The Ontogeny of Human Bonding Systems: Evolutionary Origins, Neural Bases, and Psychological Manifestations.* Dordrecht: Kluwer.

Morgan, S.P., and R. Berkowitz King

2001 Why have children in the 21st century? Biological predisposition, social coercion, rational choice. *European Journal of Population* 17:3-20.

National Research Council
2001 *New Horizons in Health: An Integrative Approach.* Committee on Future Directions for Behavioral and Social Sciences Research at the National Institutes of Health, B.H. Singer and C.D. Ryff, eds., Board on Behavioral, Cognitive, and Sensory Sciences. Division of Behavioral and Social Sciences and Education. Washington, DC: National Academy Press.

National Research Council and Institute of Medicine
2000 *From Neurons to Neighborhoods: The Science of Early Childhood Development.* Committee on Integrating the Science of Early Childhood Development, J. P. Shonkoff and D.A. Phillips, eds., Board on Children, Youth, and Family. Commission on Behavioral and Social Sciences and Education. Washington, DC: National Academy Press.

O'Connor, T.G., A. Caspi, J.C. DeFries, and R. Plomin
2000 Are associations between parental divorce and children's adjustment genetically mediated? An adoption study. *Developmental Psychology* 34:429-437.

Panksepp, J.
1998 *Affective Neuroscience: The Foundations of Human and Animal Emotions.* Oxford: Oxford University Press.

Plomin, R.
1994 *Genetics and Experience: The Interplay Between Nature and Nurture.* Thousand Oaks, CA: Sage.

Plomin, R., J.C. DeFries, G.E. McClearn, and M. Rutter
1997 *Behavioral Genetics, 3rd ed.* New York: W.H. Freeman.

Potts, M.
1997 Sex and the birth rate: Human biology, demographic change, and access to fertility-regulation methods. *Population and Development Review* 23(1):1-39.

Potts, M., and R. Short
1999 *Ever Since Adam and Eve: The Evolution of Human Sexuality.* Cambridge: Cambridge University Press.

Reiss, D., J.M. Neiderhiser, E.M. Hetherington, and R. Plomin
2000 *The Relationship Code: Deciphering Genetic and Social Influences on Adolescent Development.* Cambridge, MA: Harvard University Press.

Ridley, M.
1993 *The Red Queen: Sex and the Evolution of Human Nature.* London: Penguin.

Rodgers, J.L., and D. Doughty
2000 Genetic and environmental influences on fertility expectations and outcomes using NLSY kinship data. In *Genetic Influences on Human Fertility and Sexuality: Theoretical and Empirical Contributions from the Biological and Behavioral Sciences.* J.L. Rodgers, D.C. Rowe, and W.B. Miller, eds. Dordrecht: Kluwer.

Rodgers, J.L., K. Hughes, H.-P. Kohler, K. Christensen, D. Doughty, D.C. Rowe, and W.B. Miller
2001a Genetic influence helps explain variation in human fertility: Evidence from recent behavioral and molecular genetic studies. *Current Directions in Psychological Science* 10(5):184-188.

Rodgers, J.L., H.-P. Kohler, K.O. Kyvik, and K. Christensen
2001b Behavior genetic modelling of human fertility: Findings from a contemporary Danish study. *Demography* 38:29-42.

Rodgers, J.L., D.C. Rowe, and M. Buster
1999 Nature, nurture and first sexual intercourse in the USA: Fitting behavioral genetic models to NLSY kinship data. *Journal of Biosocial Science* 31:29-41.

Rutter, M., A. Pickles, R. Murray, and L. Eaves
2001 Testing hypotheses of specific environmental risk mechanisms for psychopathology. *Psychological Bulletin* 127:291-324.

Rutter, M., and J. Silberg
2002 Gene-environment interplay in relation to emotional and behavioral disturbance. *Annual Review of Psychology* 53:463-490.

Symons, D.
1979 *The Evolution of Human Sexuality*. Oxford: Oxford University Press.

Turkheimer, E., and M. Waldron
2000 Nonshared environment: A theoretical, methodological, and quantitative review. *Psychological Bulletin* 126:78-108.

Udry, R.
1996 Biosocial models of low fertility societies. Pp. 325-336 in *Fertility in the United States: New Patterns, New Theories*. J.B. Casterline, R.D. Lee, and K.A. Foote, eds. *Population and Development Review* 22 (Supplement).

Wood, J.W.
1994 *Dynamics of Human Reproduction: Biology, Biometry, Demography*. New York: Aldine De Gruyter.

Contributors and Other Workshop Participants

Susan C. Alberts is an assistant professor in the Department of Biology at Duke University. She works primarily in two lines of research. The first involves understanding how behavior impacts individual fitness in natural populations of large mammals. This research is based on detailed information about individual behavior and life histories and is focused primarily on the savannah baboon population in Amboseli National Park in southern Kenya. The second involves the relationship between genes and behavior: How does behavior affect a population's genetic structure, and how do genetic relationships influence behavior? This work includes projects on both the Amboseli baboon population and the well-studied Amboseli wild elephant population. Dr. Alberts holds a B.A. in biology from Reed College, an M.A. in biology from the University of California, Los Angeles, and a Ph.D. in ecology and evolution from the University of Chicago.

Jeanne Altmann is professor of ecology and evolutionary biology at Princeton University. She holds a Ph.D. from the University of Chicago and was previously chair of the Committee on Evolutionary Biology there. Dr. Altmann's interests focus on nonexperimental research design and analysis, ecology and evolution of family relationships and behavioral development, primate demography and life histories, conservation education, and behavioral aspects of conservation. Since 1971 she and her colleagues have conducted an intensive longitudinal study of demography, ecology, and behavior of the baboons of Amboseli National Park in Kenya, a program that has recently been extended to include noninvasive investigations of genetic structure and physiology. Dr. Altmann is a member of the American Academy of

Arts and Sciences. Her professional activities have included service as editor of *Animal Behaviour*, president of the Animal Behavior Society, vice president for conservation for the International Primatological Society, advisory board member for the National Science Foundation/Social, Behavioral and Economic Sciences, and, currently, chair of the Scientific Advisory Committee for the Integrated Nonhuman Primate Biomaterials and Information Resource.

Rodolfo A. Bulatao was staff director for the panel organizing the workshop. His research has covered psychosocial issues in population, fertility determinants, family planning program effectiveness, and program and reproductive health service costs. He previously directed the World Bank's annual population projections and has worked on projections in various areas, including causes of death. He has also helped develop and evaluate population projects in developing countries. Dr. Bulatao was previously affiliated with the East-West Center and the University of the Philippines. He served on the National Research Council's Committee on Population in 1983-1985 and on its Working Group on Population Growth and Economic Development. He has an M.A. in sociology from the University of the Philippines and a Ph.D. in sociology from the University of Chicago.

Judy L. Cameron is associate professor of psychiatry, neuroscience, and cell biology at the Oregon Primate Center. She studies the effects of exposure to mild everyday stresses on long-term health. Her laboratory work focuses on identifying the neural systems that respond to stress and understanding how changes in the functional activity of these systems modulate stress-responsive physiological systems, including behavior, neuroendocrine function, cardiovascular function, and glucose tolerance. The stresses studied include metabolic stresses (such as dieting, missing meals, and exercise) and psychosocial stress (such as being separated from familiar individuals and introduced to unfamiliar individuals). Her studies utilize nonhuman primates, and many combine experimental work with clinical work to understand the mechanisms underlying responses to chronic exposure to stress and the clinical implications. Dr. Cameron holds a Ph.D. from the University of Arizona.

Benjamin Campbell is assistant professor of anthropology at Boston University. He received his Ph.D. in anthropology from Harvard University in 1990, with additional postdoctoral training in demography at the Carolina Population Center. His intellectual interests are in the area of human evolutionary biology, namely, the implications of human evolution for the biology and behavior of living populations. His recent research focuses on human reproductive biology, including physiology and behavior, and its relationship to health. He has done research among Turkana and Ariaal pastoralists in Kenya and adolescent boys in the United States, Zimbabwe, and Zambia as well as with macaques and baboons. He is currently pursuing questions surrounding the impact of environmental fluctuations on the evolution of life history, particularly the stage of adolescence, in humans.

Steven W. Gangestad is a professor in the Department of Psychology, University of New Mexico. His interests revolve around evolutionary psychology, particularly the ways in which humans' current psychological design is a product of evolutionary selection. His recent research has focused on the evolution of adaptations involved in romantic relationships, most particularly the determinants of mate attraction. Dr. Gangestad holds a Ph.D. from the University of Minnesota.

John Hobcraft is professor of population studies in the Department of Social Policy at the London School of Economics. He is also a research associate with the Centre for Analysis of Social Exclusion and chairs the Population Investigation Committee. He is currently a member of the National Research Council's Committee on Population and of Academia Europaea. His research covers many facets of demography, including methodology and substance on the topics of child health and mortality, fertility, partnership, family, and gender. He has worked extensively on demographic behavior and its underpinnings for both the developing world and for Great Britain and Europe. He has recently been researching the life course factors involved in the emergence of multiple disadvantage or social exclusion in the United Kingdom. Prof. Hobcraft is active in population policy, among other things having been a lead negotiator for the United Kingdom at the Cairo International Conference on Population and Development in 1994. He has a B.Sc. in economics from the London School of Economics.

Hillard S. Kaplan is professor of anthropology at the University of New Mexico. A researcher in the field of human behavioral ecology, he has worked on fertility patterns and family formation in New Mexico and Botswana. He has also done fieldwork among foraging peoples and hunter-horticulturalists, such as the Ache in Paraguay; the Machiguenga, Piro, and Yora in Peru; the Tsimane in Bolivia; and the HamBukushu in Botswana. With his colleagues he has been responsible for producing some of the most detailed quantitative datasets on human foraging, sharing, parental care, and demography. Dr. Kaplan has masters' degrees from the University of Pennsylvania and Columbia University and a Ph.D. from the University of Utah.

Hans-Peter Kohler received an M.A. in demography (1994) and a Ph.D. in economics (1997) from the University of California, Berkeley, and currently is associate professor of sociology at the University of Pennsylvania. Previously, he was head of the research group on social dynamics and fertility at the Max Planck Institute for Demographic Research (1997-2002) and a visiting professor at the Department of Demography at the University of California, Berkeley (fall 2002). His research focuses on fertility and related behaviors in both developing and developed countries. A key characteristic of his research is the attempt to integrate demographic, economic, sociological, and biological approaches in empirical and theoretical models of demographic behavior. Within this broader goal, Dr. Kohler's research interests are centered around three themes: (1) the biodemography of fertility in low fertility contexts, including a particular focus on the relevance of genetic influences on fertility and related behaviors and the interaction of these influences with socioeconomic change; (2) the theoretical and empirical implications of social interactions for fertility change, behavioral responses to AIDS, and population dynamics in developing and developed countries; and (3) patterns of extremely low fertility in Southern and Eastern Europe, including also the development of new methods for measuring and forecasting below-replacement fertility.

David Lam is professor of economics and director of the Population Studies Center and the Michigan Center on the Demography of Aging at the University of Michigan. He is also a member of the National Research Council's Committee on Population. His work focuses on the interaction of economics and demography in developing countries, including research on human capital, inequality, fertility, marriage, and aging. His current research focuses on intergenerational dynamics of inequality in Brazil and South Africa. He has a master's degree in demography and a Ph.D. in economics from the University of California, Berkeley.

Jane B. Lancaster has been a professor of anthropology at the University of New Mexico since 1985. Her scholarship focuses on the evolutionary biology and behavior of humans using cross-cultural and human evolutionary ecology perspectives. Since 1990 she has collaborated with Hillard Kaplan on a multiyear project funded by the National Science Foundation on fertility and investment in children among men in Albuquerque. The project has surveyed more than 7,000 men and has done long life history interviews of 1,300. The goal was to look at trade-offs in male fertility and child quality. A second initiative has been to develop the field of human evolutionary ecology in anthropology. Dr. Lancaster established the human evolutionary ecology graduate training program at the University of New Mexico. She has also edited a series of volumes under the auspices of the Social Science Research Council: *Child Abuse and Neglect* (1987), *Parenting Across the Life Span* (1987), and *School-Age Pregnancy and Parenthood* (1986). In

1990 she established *Human Nature: An Interdisciplinary Biosocial Perspective*, a journal rated fifth among anthropology journals based on citations.

Joseph L. Rodgers is a Robert Glenn Rapp Foundation presidential professor at the University of Oklahoma. He has a B.S. in mathematics from the University of Oklahoma and an M.A. and a Ph.D. in psychology (with a minor in biostatistics) from the University of North Carolina at Chapel Hill. He has been in the quantitative psychology program at the University of Oklahoma since 1981, with visiting research and teaching positions in psychology and statistics at the University of Hawaii, Ohio State, the University of North Carolina, Duke University, and the University of Southern Denmark. Dr. Rodgers's methodological areas of interest include nonlinear dynamic modeling, scaling and measurement, behavior genetic models, and quasi-experimental design. His substantive interests include intellectual development, adolescent sexual development, adolescent deviance, and human fertility.

Michael L. Rutter is professor of developmental psychopathology at the Institute of Psychiatry, Kings College, University of London. He is also an honorary consultant psychiatrist at the South London and Maudsley National Health Service Trust in London. He was honorary director of the Medical Research Council's Unit in Child Psychiatry from 1984 to 1998 and honorary director of the Social, Genetic, and Developmental Psychiatry Research Centre from 1994 to 1998. Dr. Rutter holds a medical degree from the University of Birmingham Medical School and received postgraduate training in internal medicine, pediatrics, psychiatry, and psychology. His research interests particularly involve the interplay between nature and nurture as applied to life-span development. He is a fellow of both the Royal Society and the British Academy, a foreign associate member of the Institute of Medicine, a foreign honorary member of the American Academy of Arts and Sciences (1989) and a foreign associate member of the U.S. National Academy of Education (1990).

Kenneth W. Wachter is professor of demography and statistics and chair of the Department of Demography at the University of California, Berkeley. His research deals with the demography of aging, mathematical demography, biodemography, computer simulation of demographic and social processes, and census adjustment. He is a member of the National Academy of Sciences and a fellow of the American Academy of Arts and Sciences and the American Association for the Advancement of Science. He received the Mindel Sheps award in mathematical demography and served, until recently, on the board of directors of the Social Science Research Council. He is the chair of the National Research Council's Committee on Population. Dr. Wachter holds a Ph.D. in statistics from Cambridge University.

Carol M. Worthman currently holds the Samuel Candler Dobbs chair in the Department of Anthropology, Emory University (Atlanta), where she also directs the Laboratory for Comparative Human Biology. Her work is at the cutting edge of interdisciplinary biosocial research on human development, particularly reproductive endocrinology. She has conducted cross-cultural ethnographic and biosocial research among the Kikuyu of Kenya and the Hagahai of Papua New Guinea, as well as in rural and semiurban areas of the United States. Dr. Worthman is internationally recognized through her contributions in developing evolutionarily sophisticated models of human development and in the emerging field of evolutionary medicine generally. Since 1987 she has been principal investigator or coprincipal investigator on projects supported by such major funding agencies as the National Science Foundation, the National Geographic Society, the Ford Foundation, and the Spencer Foundation. In 1988-1993 she received a W.T. Grant faculty scholar career development award. She is currently principal investigator at the National Institutes of Health Research Center for Developmental Epidemiology. Dr. Worthman obtained her Ph.D. from Harvard University in 1978.

Larry J. Young is an associate professor at the Department of Psychiatry and Behavioral Sciences and the Center for Behavioral Neuroscience at Emory University in Atlanta. He holds a B.S. in biochemistry from the University of Georgia and a Ph.D. in zoology from the University of Texas at Austin. He has also received postdoctoral training from the Department of Psychiatry and Behavioral Sciences at Emory University. Dr. Young's research focuses primarily on the molecular and neuroendocrine bases of social behavior. Much of the work concerns the role of the neuropeptides, oxytocin and vasopressin, and their receptors on social behavior. Dr. Young is also interested in understanding how behavioral systems evolve at the level of the genome.

OTHER WORKSHOP PARTICIPANTS

Christine Bachrach
National Institute of Child Health and Human Development
Bethesda, MD

Barney Cohen
Committee on Population
National Research Council

Peter T. Ellison
Department of Anthropology
Harvard University

John Haaga
Population Reference Bureau
Washington, DC

Jennifer Harris
National Institute on Aging
Bethesda, MD

Kristin Hawkes
Department of Anthropology
University of Utah

Kim Wallen
Department of Psychology
Emory University

Maxine Weinstein
Center for Population and Health
Georgetown University

Index

B

C

D

E

F

G

H

I

L

M

N

O

P